LEADING TOPICS IN CANCER RESEARCH

HORIZONS IN CANCER RESEARCH, VOLUME 39

HORIZONS IN CANCER RESEARCH

Volume 1: Prostate Cancer
John N. Lucas (Editor)
ISBN 1-59454-100-0

Volume 2: Trends in Ovarian Cancer Research
A. P. Bardos (Editor)
ISBN 1-59454-023-3

Volume 3: Percutaneous Cryotherapy of Renal Cell Carcinoma under an Open MRI System
Junta Harada, Kazuo Miyasaka and Sajio Sumida (Editors)
ISBN 1-59454-169-8

Volume 4: Focus on Colorectal Cancer Research
Julia D. Martinez (Editor)
ISBN 1-59454-101-9

Volume 5: Focus on Leukemia Research
Rafael M. Romero (Editor)
ISBN 1-59454-093-4

Volume 6: Progress in Bladder Cancer Research
A. M. Mallory (Editor)
ISBN 1-59454-129-9

Volume 7: Trends in Prostate Cancer Research
John N. Lucas (Editor)
ISBN 1-59454-265-1

Volume 8: Tumor Budding in Colorectal Cancer Recent Progress in Colorectal Cancer Research
Tadahiko Masaki (Editor)
ISBN 1-59454-189-2

Volume 9: Trends in Breast Cancer Research
Andrew P. Yao (Editor)
ISBN 1-59454-134-5

Volume 10: Trends in Leukemia Research
Rafael M. Romero (Editor)
ISBN 1-59454-311-9

Volume 11: Liver Cancer: New Research
Felix Lee (Editor)
ISBN 1-59454-182-5

Volume 12: Focus on Lung Cancer
Robert L. Carafaro (Editor)
ISBN 1-59454-082-9

Volume 13: Treatment of Ovarian Cancer
A. P. Bardos (Editor)
ISBN 1-59454-022-5

Volume 14: Focus on Kidney Cancer Research
Kelvin R. Nunez (Editor)
ISBN 1-59454-110-8

Volume 15: Focus on Pacreatic Cancer Research
Maxwell A. Loft (Editor)
ISBN 1-59454-270-8

Volume 16: Peritoneal Carinomatosis from Ovarian Cancer
Kostantinos N. Chatzigeorgiou and John N. Bontis (Editors)
ISBN 1-59454-398-4

Volume 17: Trends in Pacreatic Cancer Research
Maxwell A. Loft (Editor)
ISBN 1-59454-524-3

Volume 18: Trends in Kidney Cancer Research
Kelvin R. Nunez (Editor)
ISBN 1-59454-141-8

Volume 19: Ovarian Cancer: New Research
A. P. Bardos (Editor)
ISBN 1-59454-241-4

Volume 20: Gene Therapy in Cancer
Grace W. Redberry (Editor)
ISBN 1-59454-288-0

Volume 21: Lung Cancer New Research
Robert L. Carafaro (Editor)
ISBN 1-59454-

Volume 22: New Developments in Bone Cancer Research
Catherine E. O'Neil (Editor)
ISBN 1-59454-337-2

Volume 23: New Developments in Breast Cancer Research
Andrew P. Yao (Editor)
ISBN 1-59454-809-9

Volume 24: Trends in Bone Cancer Research
E. V. Birch (Editor)
ISBN 1-59454-346-1

Volume 25: Focus on Brain Cancer Research
Andrew V. Yang (Editor)
ISBN 1-59454-973-7

LEADING TOPICS IN
CANCER RESEARCH
HORIZONS IN CANCER RESEARCH, VOLUME 39

LEE P. JEFFRIES
EDITOR

Nova Science Publishers, Inc.
New York

LIBRARY OF CONGRESS CATALOGING-IN-PUBLICATION DATA

Leading topics in cancer research / Lee P. Jeffries (editor).
       p. ; cm.
Includes index.
ISBN 13: 978-1-60021-332-8
ISBN 10: 1-60021-332-4
1. Cancer--Research. I. Jeffries, Lee P.
[DNLM: 1. Neoplasms. 2. Research. QZ 206 L4345 2006]
RC267.L432   2006
616.99'40072--dc22   2006020821

Published by Nova Science Publishers, Inc. ✦ *New York*

CONTENTS

PREFACE

Cancer is a group of different diseases (more than 100) characterized by uncontrolled growth and spread of abnormal cells. Cancer can arise in many sites and behave differently depending on its organ of origin. Significant progress has been made in recent years in the battle against cancer and in understanding its underlying biological mechanisms. This research progress has resulted in many experimental treatments and cures. This new book brings together important research from around the world in this frontal field.

Neoplastic transformation evolves over a period of time involving the progression of cellular immunophenotype (IP) from normal to hyperplastic to dysplastic, and finally, to fully malignant. Superimposed on these changes is the interaction of the initiated cell with its microenvironment, whereby the neoplastically transformed cells, through the regulation or dysregulation of cytoskeletal, integrin, protease and adhesion molecules among others, develop a novel manner of relation with their surrounding microenvironment. Studies of the neuroendocrine-immune network reveal that the hormonal and cytokine milieu plays an important role impacting the growth and dedifferentiation capabilities of cancer cells. This is further affected by the tumor cells themselves inasmuch as they determine and regulate the constitution of their hormonal microenvironment, allowing the most aggressive and invasive of neoplastically transformed cell clones to promote their own growth and dissemination. Chapter 1 details the clinical significance of immunohistochemistry that has developed over the last quarter century. The advancement of monoclonal antibody (MoAB) technology has been of great significance in ensuring the place of immunohistochemistry in the increasingly accurate microscopic diagnosis of human neoplasms, becoming a method of choice in neuropathology. Selected groups of target molecules of great significance in general cancer biology and of particular importance in brain tumors are discussed. The discovery of neoplasm associated antigens (NAAs) has not only made the more accurate diagnosis of human cancer feasible, but has also shed light on the extensive IP heterogeneity of even the most closely linked human malignancies. The identification of disseminated neoplastically transformed cells by immunohistochemistry has allowed for a clearer picture of cancer invasion and metastasis, as well as the malignant evolution of the tumor cell-associated IP. The sensitivity and significance of immunohistochemistry lies not only in the detection of various tumor-associated markers, but also in the use of information gleaned from extensive evaluations of a particular tumor in establishing a functional molecular biological, biochemical and humoral profile of the particular tumor. The elucidation of the steps of the progression of cancer from pre-malignant to invasive and metastatic forms is of utmost importance in the differential diagnosis of neoplasms and in the establishment of appropriate therapeutic regimens. These regimens will certainly begin to take on a more individualized form, targeting combinations of molecular markers in the increasingly more specific and efficacious management of brain tumors.

Epigenetic silencing of tumor suppressor genes plays an important role in the pathogenesis of human cancer. Especially, hypermethylation of the promoter regions of cancer-related genes is often observed in tumors. Recently, a novel tumor suppressor gene, which was termed Ras association domain family 1 (RASSF1A) gene was characterized by its frequent epigenetic silencing in human tumors. RASSF1 consists of two main variants (RASSF1A and RASSF1C), which are transcribed from distinct CpG island promoters. Aberrant methylation of the RASSF1A promoter region is one of the most frequent epigenetic inactivation events detected in human cancer and leads to silencing of RASSF1A. Silencing of RASSF1A was commonly observed in primary tumors including lung, breast, pancreas, kidney, liver, cervix, nasopharyngeal, prostate, thyroid and other cancers. Moreover, RASSF1A methylation was frequently detected in body fluids including blood, urine, nipple aspirates, sputum and bronchial alveolar lavages. Inactivation of RASSF1A was associated with an advanced tumor stage (e.g. bladder, brain, prostate, gastric tumors) and poor prognosis (e.g. lung, sarcoma and breast cancer). Detection of aberrant RASSF1A methylation may serve as a diagnostic and prognostic marker. The functional analyses of RASSF1A reveal an involvement in apoptotic signaling, microtubule stabilization and mitotic progression. As discussed in chapter 2, the tumor suppressor RASSF1A may act as a negative Ras effector inhibiting cell growth and inducing cell death. Thus, RASSF1A represents a tumor suppressor gene, which is frequently epigenetically silenced in the pathogenesis of human cancers.

Breast cancer is the most common malignancy among women. Whereas most breast cancers are sporadic that is, not inherited, some are the result of inherited predisposition. Approximately 5% to 10% of breast cancers develop in individuals who were born with mutations in highly penetrant genes. Women who carry mutations in such genes have increased lifetime risks of developing breast and ovarian cancer. These risks are modified by alterations in other genes and environmental factors, an interaction that is poorly understood at present. The purpose of this review article in chapter 3, is to provide an overview of current knowledge with regard to breast cancer susceptibility. It highlights first the genetic basis of hereditary breast cancer syndromes, in particular the role of the two major breast cancer susceptibility genes *BRCA1* and *BRCA2,* secondly the genetic testing with its benefits and limitations, and finally the management options for women with an inherited predisposition with regard to surveillance for the early detection of disease and with regard to prevention.

Ovarian cancer is the sixth most common malignancy in women and the leading cause of death from gynecologic malignancies. Seventy percent of ovarian cancers present as advanced disease, which is associated with an overall five-year survival of 30%. The earlier the stage of disease, the better the survival (Stage 1 - 85% 5-year). Risk factors associated with ovarian cancer include: advancing age and family history of breast and/or ovarian cancer or Hereditary Non-Polyposis Colon Cancer or known BRCA 1 or 2 mutation. As discussed in chapter 4, there is no known precursor status for ovarian cancer; however, if earlier stage disease could be identified then survival could be enhanced. Much work has been done addressing the role of various imaging modalities (ie., ultrasound) with or without tumor markers (ie., CA125) to identify women with early stage disease.

A genetic testing service can determine which members of a population might benefit most from prevention measures. The eligibility criteria for a service will affect the number of people who use it and the portion that test positive, and this affects both the service's costs and benefits. In chapter 5, a computer simulation model is used to estimate the effects of eligibility restrictions on the performance of a genetic testing service. In particular, restrictions might apply to someone's age, gender and family history of disease. The effects are considered in terms of the eligibility criteria's sensitivity, specificity and "post-test likelihoods" for a genetic test result. All of these measures are affected differently by eligibility restrictions, and criteria should be chosen according to outcomes that are considered most important. The authors focus on a testing service for cancer susceptibility, but the extension to other diseases is straightforward.

Cancer is an insidious disease, in which virtually every aspect of cellular control can be subverted to allow the uncontrolled, invasive cellular growth that defeats multicellular cooperation and kills an organism. In testimony to the essential role for proper execution of cell death in tumor suppression, apoptosis is widely recognized as an essential tumor-suppressor system. Indeed, defects in apoptosis are considered a hallmark of cancer, and are known to render the tumor resistant to immunosurveillance and therapy. Prion infections represent a fascinating biological phenomenon which has elicited at the interface between neuroscience and immunology. Although Prion protein (PrPc) is well known for its implication in transmissible spongiform encephalopathy, recent data in chapter 6 indicated that PrPc may participate in programmed cell death regulation. PrPc would be correlated to the acquisition of a resistance phenotype by tumor cells to cytotoxic effectors or antitumor drugs. This review revisits the molecular mechanisms of tumor resistance to apoptosis and the implication of the PrPc in this phenomenon.

Polyunsaturated fatty acids (PUFAs) are necessary for normal cellular function. However PUFAs are prone to peroxidation, which can cause cell death including apoptosis. Susceptibility to peroxidation increases with the degree of unsaturation, i.e. with greater numbers of carbon-carbon double bonds per fatty acid molecule. Studies of human cancer cell lines treated with PUFAs in vitro demonstrated that apoptosis increased with degree of fatty acid unsaturation. This suggests that the induction of apoptosis is by a peroxidative mechanism. This might translate into an anti-cancer effect in vivo, consistent with epidemiological evidence that diets rich in the highly unsaturated fatty acids, eicosapentaenoic acid (EPA; 20:5, n-3) and docosahexaenoic acid (DHA; 22:6, n-3) correlate with reduced risk of colorectal cancer. Atherosclerosis is a chronic inflammatory disease. The lipid-rich foam cells of human atherosclerotic lesions are predominantly monocyte-derived macrophages (HMM), and their death contributes to the lipid cores of plaques (advanced lesions). HMM death is implicated in destabilisation of advanced atherosclerotic lesions, leading to plaque rupture with thrombogenic consequences, including cardiovascular events and strokes. In vitro, HMM treated with PUFAs showed a general trend for increasing apoptosis with increasing degree of fatty acid unsaturation, although arachidonic acid (AA; 20:4, n-6) stood out above the trend (in contrast to its behaviour in cancer cell lines) as it induced apoptosis more strongly than both the more highly unsaturated (and more peroxidisable) EPA and DHA. In HMM in vitro, AA-induced apoptosis was diminished by the cyclo-oxygenase inhibitor indomethacin and by the lipoxygenase inhibitor nordihydroguaiaretic acid, suggesting roles for these enzymes in the induction of apoptosis by AA. Moreover 15(S)-hydroperoxy-5,8,11,13-eicosatetraenoic acid was a very strong inducer of apoptosis in HMM, whereas 15(S)-hydroxy-5,8,11,13-eicosatetraenoic acid was innocuous. A major source of PUFAs in atherosclerosis is plasma low-density lipoprotein (LDL). Much evidence implicates oxidation of LDL in atherogenesis, including the apoptosis-inducing effect of oxidised LDL (oxLDL) on HMM in vitro. LDL oxidation involves peroxidation of the PUFA chains of LDL lipids, which are predominantly esters. Various LDL oxidation products can induce death in HMM in vitro, and radical scavengers such as alpha-tocopherol and BO-653 can prevent both LDL oxidation and the ensuing HMM death. Lipoprotein-associated phospholipase A_2 (Lp-PLA$_2$) is a naturally present LDL-borne enzyme that hydrolyses oxidised phospholipids (but not non-oxidised phospholipids) forming lysophosphatidylcholine and oxidised, non-esterified fatty acids. Treatment of LDL with inhibitors of Lp-PLA$_2$, especially the highly specific inhibitor SB222657, diminished the ensuing HMM death including apoptosis, when the LDL was oxidised and added to HMM in vitro, even though the Lp-PLA$_2$ inhibitors did not diminish LDL oxidation. These findings in chapter 7, may be relevant to potential mechanisms of fatty acid influences on atherosclerosis and cancer and may suggest strategies for combating these diseases.

The employment of virus therapy to treat human neoplasms has a three decade history. One such virus that has been explored is the Newcastle Disease Virus (NDV) Vaccine (MTH-68/N). MTH-68/N vaccine therapy has been employed in a number of different neoplasms with success. This success has also been demonstrated in glioblastomas and high grade gliomas. Glioblastoma multiforme (GBM) is the most common primary brain tumor and by far it is the most aggressive form of glial tumors. This neoplasm has a poor prognosis, averaging six months to a year. Nine cases of advanced GBM and high grade glioma were treated with the NDV vaccine (MTH-68/N) after the classical modalities of anti-neoplastic therapy failed. The authors' results included survival rates of ten years, nine years, eight years, six years, five years, three years, nine months, and six months post-diagnosis for the eight surviving patients. Against all odds, these surviving patients have also returned to a lifestyle that resembles their pre-morbid daily routines. They enjoy good clinical health. These patients have regularly received the MTH-68/N vaccine for a number of years without interruption as a form of monotherapy once the classical modalities failed. The MRI and CT results have revealed an objective decrease in size of the tumors, in some cases the near total disappearance of the mass. There has also been documented decrease in mass effect following administration of the MTH-68/N vaccine. Although one of our patients did succumb to complications of his malignancy, the results are nonetheless extremely promising in that there is not only a decrease in tumor burden but also a return of pre-morbid functioning. It should be stressed that the positive results may be due to the long-term employment of the vaccine. Chapter 8 seeks to shed light on the background of NDV with a focus on the possible mechanism of action. There is also a detailed description of the clinical course of each of the cases, the revealing and convincing clinical findings, as well as of the functional improvement that the patients experienced with the use of the MTH-68/N and MTH-68/H vaccine after all classical modalities failed and hope was nearly lost.

The fundamental principle of radiotherapy is to destroy malignant cells while minimizing damage to normal tissues. Almost all patients who receive radiotherapy to the head and neck area develop some grade of acute mucositis, which is not only painful, but may compromise tumor control by determining decrease in dose intensity and interruptions of the treatment. The term 'oral mucositis' describes the adverse effect of chemotherapy or radiation induced inflammation of the oral mucosa. Symptoms of mucositis vary from pain and discomfort to an inability to tolerate food or fluids. The degree and duration of mucositis in patients receiving radiotherapy are related to radiation source, cumulative dose, dose intensity, volume of irradiated mucosa, smoking/alcohol consumption and oral hygiene conditions. To the authors' knowledge in chapter 9, there is no other controlled study which has evaluated vitamin E as a single radioprotective agent in patients with head and neck tumors treated with radiation therapy alone or post-operative. For this reason, the authors conducted a double-blind, randomized trial with the objective to investigate the potential mucosal protection of vitamin E in irradiated patients with head and neck cancer, motivated by its simplicity of administration, no severe toxicity in conventional doses, low cost and easy availability. The fundamental principle of radiotherapy is to destroy malignant cells while minimizing damage to normal tissues. Almost all patients who receive radiotherapy to the head and neck area develop some grade of acute mucositis, which is not only painful, but may compromise tumor control by determining decrease in dose intensity and interruptions of the treatment. The term 'oral mucositis' describes the adverse effect of chemotherapy or radiation induced inflammation of the oral mucosa . Symptoms of mucositis vary from pain and discomfort to an inability to tolerate food or fluids. The degree and duration of mucositis in patients receiving radiotherapy are related to radiation source, cumulative dose, dose intensity, volume of irradiated mucosa, smoking/alcohol consumption and oral hygiene conditions. The pathogenesis of oral mucositis is thought to involve direct and indirect mechanisms. It is generally believed that oral mucositis is consequent to the direct inhibitory effects of therapy on DNA replication and mucosal cell proliferation. Indirect effects result from release of inflammatory mediators, loss of protective salivary constituents, therapy-induced neutropenia, and the emergence of microorganisms on damaged mucosa. Sonys et al proposed a four phase hypothesis as to the mechanisms of the development of mucositis: 1) inflammatory or vascular phase, induced by toxic cytokines released from epithelial cells after chemotherapy or radiotherapy administration; 2) epithelial phase, characterized by atrophy and ulceration due to reduced renewal of the oral basal epithelium; 3) ulcerative or bacteriological phase, during which some areas of erosion become covered with a fibrinous pseudomembrane. Bacterial colonization occurs, producing endotoxins which contribute to further cytokines release; and 4) healing phase, with epithelial renewal and reestablishment of the local flora. Histopathologically, edema and vascular changes such as thickening of the tunica intima, reduction in the size of the lumen and destruction of the elastic and muscle fibers of the vessel walls are noted. A number of agents with potentially mucosal protection capabilities and different mechanisms of action in radioinduced mucositis has been investigated in randomized trials. Most of them have reduced number of patients, and their efficacy and safety have not been clearly established. Consequently, there is no standard intervention for oral radioinduced mucositis.

Cancer vaccines are becoming a promising approach to the treatment of cancer. Chapter 10 summarizes the scientific background for the design of therapeutic cancer vaccines, as well as the challenges in their development. The current approaches to the discovery of the tumor-associated antigens as a basis for the new cancer vaccines are reviewed. The most promising methods for cancer vaccine development are also discussed. In this chapter the authors categorize the therapeutic cancer vaccines as follows: peptide vaccines, recombinant viral vaccines, DNA vaccines, and dendritic cell-based immunotherapy. They focus on their advantages and disadvantages and their current uses in the treatment of cancer. An up-to-date description of the results of cancer vaccine clinical trials is provided. They also discuss the future prospects in the design and the utilization of the cancer vaccines.

Experimental and clinical evidences strongly indicate that the immune system can naturally prevent tumour development and provide new support to the old idea of treating tumours with therapeutic vaccines. Several cancer vaccines are currently under clinical testing, using a wide diversity of tumour antigens and platforms for delivering them to the immune system. Most of them intend to elicit citotoxic-T-lymphocyte responses or antibody responses against antigens expressed by tumour cells. However, in parallel to this mainstream, a different cancer vaccine approach has been developed, focusing the activation of an immune response against some self extra cellular proteins (mainly hormones and growth factors) which participate in the control of cell proliferation. These vaccines are composed by the self hormone linked to a carrier and administered in an adjuvant. Immunization provokes specific anti-hormone antibodies that block the binding to the receptor, avoiding the "start up" of signal transduction mechanisms derived from this binding. These vaccines are not intended to mobilize the effector's branch of the immune system for a direct cytolysis but to inhibit hormonal mechanisms which in turn, influence tumour development. The field of anticancer drugs has experienced recently a paradigm shift, beyond unspecific anti-proliferative drugs, to specific targets related to growth factors and signal transduction. Cancer vaccines aiming to interfere with hormone and growth factor mediated cell proliferation represent an equivalent idea, in the field of active immunotherapy. The rationale of hormone immunosuppresion can be found in autoimmune diseases against hormones and their receptors. Nature has created mechanisms of interaction between hormone systems and immune systems, that, when deregulated, provoke autoimmune diseases. An adequate manipulation of these interactions can be used to fight diseases where hormonal mechanisms are deregulated, i.e. cancer. In chapter 11 the authors review the current development of several hormone-suppressive active immunotherapies and they provide a wider description of the approach of active immunotherapy for Epidermal Growth Factor (EGF) deprivation developed at our own laboratory. Insegia^{TM} (G17DT) is an immunogen containing gastrin which provokes an antibody response blocking gastrin-stimulated cell growth. It is actually in clinical trials for pancreatic, colorectal and gastric carcinomas. Gonadimmune^{TM} (D17DT) is a vaccine containing the gonadotrophin releasing hormone (GnRH) which is being tested in the clinical setting for prostate cancer. AVICINE^{R} is a vaccine targeting the human chorionic gonadotrophin (hCG) currently in clinical trials for colorectal and pancreatic cancer. The EGF vaccine, finally, is a composition of Epidermal Growth Factor linked to a carrier protein, which induces anti-EGF antibodies which in turn block the binding of EGF to the EGF-Receptor (EGFR). It is currently in Phase 2 clinical trials for the treatment of non-small cell lung carcinoma (NSCLC). Additionally, a similar vaccine is being developed to target Transforming Growth Factor (TGF), an alternative ligand of the EGFR. This last vaccine is currently under pre-clinical investigation. Specific antibody responses have been obtained after vaccination with all these self molecules, and for those tested in the clinical setting this antibody response is related with decrease in the targeted hormone levels and with improved survival of vaccinated patients. Once the initial proof of the concept is becoming a reality, current challenges are how to find the best therapeutic doses and vaccination schedules to expand the immune response and how to maintain it long enough to sustain a chronic treatment.

In: Leading Topics in Cancer Research
Editor: Lee P. Jeffries, pp. 1-33

ISBN 1-60021-332-4
© 2007 Nova Science Publishers, Inc.

Chapter 1

THE SIGNIFICANCE OF IMMUNOHISTOCHEMISTRY IN BRAIN TUMOR DIAGNOSTICS AND IMMUNOTHERAPY

Bela Bodey, *Bela Bodey Jr. and Stuart E. Siegel*

Department of Pathology, Keck School of Medicine, University of Southern California, Los Angeles, and Childrens Center for Cancer and Blood Diseases, Childrens Hospital Los Angeles, Los Angeles, CA

ABSTRACT

Neoplastic transformation evolves over a period of time involving the progression of cellular immunophenotype (IP) from normal to hyperplastic to dysplastic, and finally, to fully malignant. Superimposed on these changes is the interaction of the initiated cell with its microenvironment, whereby the neoplastically transformed cells, through the regulation or dysregulation of cytoskeletal, integrin, protease and adhesion molecules among others, develop a novel manner of relation with their surrounding microenvironment. Studies of the neuroendocrine-immune network reveal that the hormonal and cytokine milieu plays an important role impacting the growth and dedifferentiation capabilities of cancer cells. This is further affected by the tumor cells themselves inasmuch as they determine and regulate the constitution of their hormonal microenvironment, allowing the most aggressive and invasive of neoplastically transformed cell clones to promote their own growth and dissemination.

This chapter details the clinical significance of immunohistochemistry that has developed over the last quarter century. The advancement of monoclonal antibody (MoAB) technology has been of great significance in ensuring the place of immunohistochemistry in the increasingly accurate microscopic diagnosis of human neoplasms, becoming a method of choice in neuropathology. Selected groups of target molecules of great significance in general cancer biology and of particular importance in brain tumors are discussed. The discovery of neoplasm associated antigens (NAAs) has not only made the more accurate diagnosis of human cancer feasible, but has also shed light on the extensive IP heterogeneity of even the most closely linked human malignancies. The identification of disseminated neoplastically transformed cells by immunohistochemistry has allowed for a clearer picture of cancer invasion and metastasis, as well as the malignant evolution of the tumor cell-associated IP. The sensitivity and significance of immunohistochemistry lies not only in the detection of various tumor-associated markers, but also in the use of information gleaned from extensive evaluations of a particular tumor in establishing a functional molecular biological, biochemical and humoral profile of the particular tumor. The elucidation of the steps of the progression of cancer from pre-malignant to invasive and metastatic forms is of utmost importance in the differential diagnosis of neoplasms and in the establishment of appropriate therapeutic regimens. These regimens will certainly begin to take on a more individualized form, targeting combinations of molecular markers in the increasingly more specific and efficacious management of brain tumors.

Keywords: Immunohistochemistry;   Monoclonal   antibody   (MoAB);   Cellular immunophenotype (IP); Cancer associated marker (CAM); Neoplasm associated antigen (NAA); Cancer/testis-antigen (CTA); Melanoma antigens (MAGE, BAGE, GAGE, and LAGE-1/NY-ESO-1); CTA-directed, individualized antineoplastic immunotherapy.

INTRODUCTION

During the last three decades, immunohistochemistry has revolutionized both the research and diagnostic endeavors of pathologists, including neuropathologists [1, 2]. It is a great feeling to know that through our extensive research observations on brain tumors, which have been well documented in numerous articles, we have been able to contribute to these exciting developments. Certainly, the rapid advancement of MoAB producing technology has been of great significance in assuring the place of immunohistochemistry in the modern accurate microscopic diagnosis of human neoplasms, as a method of choice in histopathology. A conventional histopathologic diagnosis still relies on the microscopic morphological changes in the observed tissue slides. In the case of mammalian neoplasms, a number of structural changes characterize the specimen. These usually include a serious loss of normal tissue architecture, increased basophilia, variability of cellular shapes and nuclei, disproportion between cell nucleus and cytoplasm and a various degree of nuclear enlargement. Unfortunately morphologic cell and tissue changes that take place during the neoplastic transformation are highly variable allowing somewhat a subjective evaluations by different pathologists. Certainly, the tissue changes that characterize neoplastic cell transformation are generally reduced to a neoplasm grading system. The worldwide employed grading system ranges from grades 1 to 4, with the larger numbers being assigned to more aggressive neoplastic behavior. It is the variability of neoplastic transformation that has led to the rapid development of immunohistochemical diagnostic procedures. Monoclonal antibodies (MoABs) have been employed in characterization of the fine antigenic structure of biological macromolecules. The technique take advantage of the important fact that MoABs

---

* *Corresponding author:* Bela Bodey, M.D., D. Sc., 8000-1 Canby Avenue, Reseda, CA 91335, USA. Phone and Facsimile: (818) 886-1082; Electronic Mail: Bodey18@aol.com

react with a single antigenic epitope, rather than having an immunoreactivity representing an additive binding to heterogeneous antigenic determinants as is the case with polyclonal antibodies and conventional antisera. Employing certain, chosen libraries of newly developed poly- and monoclonal antibodies greatly improved the precision of microscopic diagnosis in histopathology and also the concordance between pathologists. Certainly, the most important principle of the evaluation of an immunocytochemical result in mammalian neoplasms remains that positive immunoreactivity is significant only when it occurs in neoplastic cells previously recognized by standard (usually the routine hematoxylin and eosin stain) microscopic morphology. However, it should be kept in mind that the evaluation of immunoreactivity is proper only when there is a concomitant interpretation of appropriate control slides. The importance of immunohistochemistry in cancer biology is certain, and the aim of this chapter is to describe some of the important contributions of this technique.

BRAIN TUMOR ASSOCIATED MARKERS

The main goal of molecular oncology during the 1980s and 1990s has been the discovery of a marker which would be specific for neoplastically transformed cells, as such, or for a neoplasm of specific tissue or organ differentiation line; and we have the feeling that this goal has not been fulfilled yet [3, 4]. Presently, the literature consider a neoplastic marker as an increasing level of a substance which is not unique for neoplastically transformed or tumor cells, and is indeed expressed in normal cells. The marker could be localized in the cytoplasm of neoplastically transformed cells or on their surface. The marker may also be produced by the tumor-surrounding tissue (paracrine secretion) under the influence of the tumor cells. Therefore, the immunocytochemical results of identifying a tumor marker should be interpreted with great caution and should be always confronted with the results of routine histopathology, as well as other observations. This is valid even if the immunohistochemical results greatly improve the proper diagnosis and differential diagnosis. Immunohistological procedures should also be based on strictly standardized antigen detection techniques [5, 6]. Histopathology and immunohistochemistry continue to be increasingly popular methods for predicting outcome in patients with malignant tumors. Recently traditional histopathologic studies have stressed the importance of endothelial proliferation in the diagnosis and prognosis of a wide variety of mammalian neoplasms. Immunohistochemical proliferation markers, in particular MIB-1, may be useful in assessing unregulated cellular behavior, whereas their role in establishing neoplastic cells is less clear. Similarly, numerous studies on p53 and epidermal growth factor receptor (EGFR) immunohistochemistry in mammalian neoplasm have demonstrated serious predictive values.

Advanced immunohistochemistry employs hundreds of well-characterized, highly specific antibodies recognizing only the desired, target antigens. The highly senstitive methods of immunocytochemistry have expanded our understanding of the biology and immunobiology of brain tumors (as well as a wide array of other tumor types) and have led to the development and refinement of ever more reliable ways of diagnosis and differential diagnosis of CNS tumors, among many others. WHO Histopathological Typing of Tumors by the CNS has shown progress for both the current members and possible new special types of brain tumors that may occur, especially for the meningiomas and neuro-epithelial/neuroglial type [7]. The routine technique using light microscope examination was the most useful one for daily diagnosis for many years, but immunohistochemistry techniques are needed for difficult cases, *e.g.,* GFAP, NE 14, NSE, S100, and MBP. Diagnostic problems could be caused by tissue- or cell-sampling errors, which are influenced by the tumor location itself. Thus, neurosurgeons encounter problems with biopsy intraoperatives or with the mishandling of tissues.

Grading of CNS tumors must be put according to the clinical interest for further management of the patient. CNS grading ranges from grade I (benign looking) to IV (malignant). Morphological grading is based on Kernohan and Adson [8] or Kernohan and Sayre [9].

Classification and grading of astrocytic tumors has been the subject of several controversies and no universally accepted classification system is yet available. Nevertheless, acceptance of a common system is important for assessing prognosis as well as easy comparative evaluation and interpretation of the results of multi-center therapeutic trials. Besides WHO guidelines [10], the other systems of classification are the Kernohan, Daumas-Duport (SAM-A) [11], and TESTAST-268 [12]. Karak and co-workers set out to evaluate each system in order to establish which one is the most useful [13]. They reported the results of a single center study on comparative survival evaluation along with assessment of inter-classification concordance in 102 cases of supratentorial astrocytic tumors in adults. Hematoxylin and eosin (H&E) stained slides of these 102 cases were reviewed independently by two pathologists and each case classified or graded according to the four different classification systems. The histological grading was then correlated with the survival curves as estimated by the Kaplan-Meier method. The most important observation was that similar survival curves were obtained for any one grade of tumor by all the four classification systems. Fifty three of the 102 cases (51.9%) showed absolute grading concordance using all 4 classifications with maximum concordant cases belonging to grades 2 and 4. Intra-classification grade-wise survival analysis revealed a statistically significant difference between grade 2 and grades 3 or 4, but no difference between grades 3 and 4 in any of the classification systems. It is apparent from the results of this study that if specified criteria related to any of the classification systems are rigorously adhered to, it will produce comparable results. The group thus recommended that one system be adhered to because it would allow for objectivity and reproducibility. Their final recommendation was for the Daumas-Duport (SAM-A) system since it appears to be the simplest, most objectivized for practical application and highly reproducible with relative ease.

Molecular aspects underlying the differences of the subtypes of astrocytic glioma can also be used to classify these tumors. Godard and co-workers demonstrated that human gliomas can be differentiated according to their gene expression [14]. The researchers found that low-grade astrocytoma have the most specific and similar expression profiles while primary glioblastoma exhibit much larger variation between tumors. Secondary glioblastoma display features of both other groups. We identified several sets of genes with relatively highly correlated expression within groups that: (a). can be associated with specific biological functions; and (b). effectively differentiate tumor class. Such classification techniques allow for the development of targeted treatment strategies adapted to individual patients and allow for patient stratification [15]. Moreover, using a genetic classification approach, classification success rates of up to 89% accuracy have been obtained [16].

Immunohistochemical markers are also proving to be a useful tool for characterizing medulloblastomas (MEDs). Medulloblastomas occurring in children represent a histological spectrum of varying anaplasia and nodularity. In order to determine whether immunohistochemical markers might be useful parameters in subclassifying these neuroectodermal tumors, Son and co-workers studied 17 childhood MEDs, including nine diffuse/non-anaplastic, four diffuse/anaplastic, three nodular/non-anaplastic and one nodular/anaplastic subtypes [17]. The expression of neural cell adhesion molecule (NCAM), nerve growth factor receptor (NGFR), neurofilament (NF), synaptophysin (SYN), glial fibrillary acidic protein (GFAP), S100, Bcl-2, and Ki-67 was investigated by employing the immunohistochemistry against specific antibodies. The study showed that NGFR, NF, GFAP and S100 were not detected in anaplastic subtypes of MEDs (0/5), while non-anaplastic subtypes were mainly expressed within the nodules. All 17 tumors were reactive for NCAM, SYN and Bcl-2. In addition, Ki-67 labeling indices for anaplastic subtypes (39.0 +/- 7.42%) were significantly higher than that of non-anaplastic MEDs (11.4 +/- 8.04%; $p < 0.0001$). These results suggest, according to the authors, that immunohistochemical markers are a useful adjunct in characterizing subtypes of pediatric MEDs. In fact, scrutiny of the cytological variation found among MEDs has recently led to the concept of the anaplastic MED, which overlaps the large-cell variant and appears to share its poor prognosis. In contrast, the MEDs with extensive nodularity, a distinctive nodular/desmoplastic variant occurring in infants, has a better outcome than most MEDs in these young patients, proving that cytological and immunocytochemical data are indeed very relevant [18]. Perry conducted a similar study as Son and co-workers and found that MED grading based on anaplasia demonstrated a statistically stronger association with patient outcome than clinical staging. Therefore, histologic grading of MEDs seems warranted as a routine diagnostic aid [19]. Classification of the MEDs histopathologically and according to profiles of molecular abnormalities will help both to rationalize approaches to therapy, increasing the cure rate and reducing long-term side-effects, and to suggest novel, more individualized immunotherapeutical treatments [20].

Assessment of angiogenic potential by measuring the blood capillary density in histological sections assumes that a 4 mm thick section is representative of whole human solid neoplasm's vascularity. The number of blood capillaries was nonetheless counted at 1.0 mm^2 microscopic field (brain tumor tissue at 200x magnification), choosing microvessel hot spots on immunocytochemical slides stained by MoABs against endothelial cell markers [21].

FOURTH-MODALITY, MOLECULAR MARKER-DIRECTED TREATMENT

Cancer associated markers (CAMs) are the biochemical and immunological counterparts of the morphology of mammalian neoplasms. The expression of an immunocytochemically defined CAM is also related to the tissue of origin and is not a random event. At the same time the expression of a CAM can also be related to the particular developmental stage of tissues and organs [22, 23]. Rapid advances in immunohistochemistry have resulted in the characterization of hundreds upon hundreds of highly specific poly- and monoclonal antibodies, recognizing only desired target antigens, which are useful in the IP assessment of normal and neoplastic cells. During the past two decades, the use of MoABs against oncofetal, neoplasm associated, cell lineage specific, endothelial, and cell proliferation related antigens in the diagnosis and biological assessment of prognosis in neoplastic disease gained increased importance. A sensitive direct correlation exists between the expression of certain molecules and the development of an invasive, highly malignant IP of neoplastic cells, allowing for the occurrence of angiogenesis and metastasis [24-30]. Metastatic spread is a major factor in the prognosis of cancer patients. Early detection and eradication of circulating neoplastically transformed cells prior to the tissue development of distant metastases could help to improve the prognosis of tumor patients after therapeutical primary tumor resection. Disseminated neoplastic cells have been detected in different body compartments employing cytological and immunocytochemical methods and, more recently, employing different molecular biological techniques. The most frequently studied body compartments are the bone marrow, peritoneal cavity, blood and lymph nodes, but other body fluids such as urine, bile, pancreatic juice and sputum have also been analysed [31]. At all of these sites, neoplastic cells have been detected [32, 33]. In embracing a multidisciplinary approach to the management of breast cancer (BC) patients with sentinel node biopsy, the surgical pathologist task is to screen sentinel nodes for possible metastasis [34]. The consequences of missing sentinel node micrometastasis can directly influence treatment strategies, and this screening therefore has to be performed with more attention than usual. There is a great diversity in the histopathological work-up of sentinel nodes, with many centres employing additional observation methods such as immunohistochemistry, reverse transcription polymerase chain reaction or flow cytometry in addition to the obligatory haematoxylin and eosin staining.

The fact still remains that in order to properly assess any immunohistochemical reactivity used for differential diagnostic purposes, the target cells have to be identified as neoplastically transformed cells by routine histopathological techniques. Selected groups of target molecules of great significance in cancer biology are discussed. The discovery of neoplasm associated antigens has not only made the more accurate diagnosis of human cancer feasible, but has also shed light on the extensive cellular IP heterogeneity of even the most closely linked human malignancies. The identification of disseminated neoplastically transformed cells by immunohistochemistry has allowed for a clearer picture of cancer invasion and metastasis, as well as the evolution of the tumor cell-associated IP towards increased malignancy. Immunoassaying (immunoreactivity) is also capable of detecting specific infectious agents, from ordinary bacteria to spirochetes, fungi, parasites and especially viruses, as well as identifying possible causative agents of CNS diseases.

During our immunocytochemical observations of brain tumor cellular IP, we employed the immunohistochemical method of "antigen liberation" or "antigen retrieval" [35-40]. In the first step, antigen retrieval was sometimes achieved by single or combined enzymatic digestion (ficin, pepsin, and trypsin from Zymed Labs., South San Francisco, CA, USA) prior to the primary antigen-antibody reaction. Heat induced epitope retrieval (HIER) [41, 42], as modified by us, was also employed. Antigen retrieval required immersion of tissue sections, in a Target Retrieval Solution (DAKO Corp., Carpinteria, CA, USA) and heating in a water bath (95°C to 99°C). No single antigen retrieval solution works best with all antigenic epitopes. Our method with citrate-based (neutral pH) solution worked well with most antibodies applied in this study that required such pretreatment. Heat (microwave) targeted antigen retrieval resulted in an increase of antigen detection for a number of MoABs, and we also noticed a serious increase of immunoreactivity (*i.e.* staining intensity).

IMPLICATIONS OF BRAIN TUMOR IMMUNOHISTOCHEMISTRY

Histopathology and immunohistochemistry continue to be popular methods for predicting outcome in patients with malignant gliomas. Over the past two decades, we have employed an extensive panel of over 90 antibodies in cellular IP characterization of medulloblastomas (MEDs)/primitive neuroectodermal tumors (PNETs) and astrocytomas (ASTRs), using a sensitive, four-step, alkaline phosphatase conjugated immunohistochemical antigen detection technique. The following is the most characteristic IP in MEDs/PNETs: Synaptophysin, Chromogranin A, HLA-A,B,C, HLA-DR, Vimentin, TE4, TE7, TE8, TE15, AE1, AE3, TE3, CLA, UJ 308, Leu 2/a, Leu 3a/3b, NF-H, MAP-1, MAP-2, MAP-5, GFAP, EGFR, p53, HOX-B3, -B4, -C6, c-erb-2 (HER-2), c-erb-3 (HER-3), c-erb-4 (HER-4), Caspase-3, FasR, Survivin, CD105 (Endoglin), COX-2, IGF-R, MMP-2, -3, -9, -10, -13, and in ASTRs: GFAP, Vimentin, Tenascin, HLA-A,B,C, HLA-DR, CLA, UJ 308, UJ 167.11, A2B5, Thy-1, Chromogranin A, NF-H, TE7, Leu-2/a, Leu 3a/3b, c-erb-2, c-erb-4, p53, Caspase-3, -6, -8, -9, FasR, CD105, COX-2, IGF-R, MMP-3, -10, MAGE-1. Overall, childhood MEDs/PNET and ASTR cells display a heterogeneous IP, differentiated as well as immature neurofilament proteins are present in most of these tumors, as well as neuronal differentiation is always present in all cases. Recently, traditional histopathologic studies have stressed the importance of endothelial proliferation in the diagnosis of GBM. Immunohistochemical proliferation markers, in particular MIB-1, may be useful in assessing oligodendroglioma behavior, whereas their role in malignant ASTRs is less clear. Similarly, new studies on p53 and epidermal growth factor receptor (EGFR) immunohistochemistry in gliomas have demonstrated only limited predictive values. Nonetheless, the importance of immunohistochemistry in tumor biology is certain, and the rest of this chapter is devoted in great part to the important contributions of this technique.

In the last decade, there is increasing recognition of polyphenotypic high-grade malignancies in non-CNS tumor literature. Some of these tumors have been regarded as variants of PNET or as extrarenal malignant rhabdoid tumors (MRTs). Jay *et al.* have described two posterior fossa neoplasms, both of which displayed a "polyphenotypic" expression of neural, epithelial, myogenic, and glial markers, including synaptophysin, neurofilament, vimentin, glial fibrillary acidic protein, S-100, neuron-specific enolase, desmin, S antigen, MIC2, cytokeratin, epithelial membrane antigen, and carcinoembryonic antigen (CEA) [43]. One tumor showed complex intercellular junctions, cytoplasmic intermediate filaments, well-developed rough and smooth endoplasmic reticulum and Golgi apparatus, cilia, and neurosecretory granules. The other neoplasm showed pools of glycogen, desmosomes, and tonofilaments. The histological and ultrastructural appearances were inconsistent with glioma, PNET, meningioma, ependymoma, choroid plexus carcinoma, sarcoma, germ cell tumor, and other tumors in the WHO classification. Although the polyphenotype raises the issue that these may represent variants of MRT or the atypical teratoid-rhabdoid tumor, the morphologic findings in the two cases were very dissimilar. The two cases presented by the authors underscore the problems in nosology and classification of polyphenotypic tumors of the CNS. This is particularly significant, as therapeutic protocols for PNET, MRT, and non-CNS polyphenotypic tumors are quite different.

Mixed gliomas have been difficult to define and subsequently diagnose due to the paucity of literature specifically examining this group of tumors [44, 45]. Thirty mixed gliomas in which the minor glial component comprised at least 20% of the total tumor were observed: 20 oligoastrocytomas (OA) and ten malignant oligoastrocytomas (MOA). Nineteen patients were male (mean age 36 years) and 19 patients presented with seizures. The tumor was located in the frontal lobe in 17 patients and the temporal lobe in nine patients. The duration of preoperative symptoms in 25 patients ranged from five days to 14 years (mean 2.6 years). A mean follow-up of four years was available in 29 patients. Fourteen patients, seven with OA and seven with MOA, had recurrent tumor. One patient with MOA and four patients with OA (three with tumor progression and one with extensive leptomeningeal spread) died as a result of their tumor one to five years after diagnosis. Eighteen patients received chemotherapy and/or radiation therapy. Twenty-five tumors were immunostained with antibody to p53 protein. p53 nuclear staining was seen in 5/16 OA and 3/9 MOA. Immunoreactivity was observed only in neoplastically transformed astrocytes. One of the four patients who died with OA was p53 positive. Three recurrent MOAs were p53 positive. It was concluded that mixed gliomas most frequently occur in the frontal lobe and the majority of patients present with seizures; that there is no obvious association of p53 detection in mixed gliomas with tumor grade or behavior; and that similar to pure fibrillary astrocytomas, a subset of OA and MOA may be associated with p53 alterations.

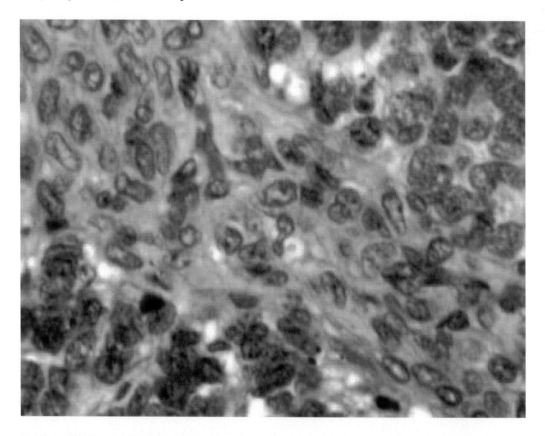

Figure 1. Childhood anaplastic ASTR. Expression of caspase-9 in the cytoplasm of neoplastically transformed cells. Routine, 10% buffered formalin fixation. Paraffin wax embedding. Alkaline phosphatase conjugated streptavidin-biotin antigen detection technique on a 4 μm thick section. Magnification: 500x.

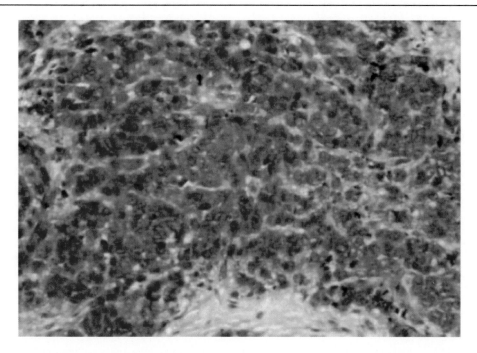

Figure 2. Childhood medulloblastoma (MED)/primitive neuroectodermal tumor (PNET). Expression of *FasR* on the surface of the neoplastically transformed cells. Routine, 10% buffered formalin fixation. Paraffin wax embedding. Alkaline phosphatase conjugated streptavidin-biotin antigen detection technique on a 4 μm thick section. Magnification: 200x.

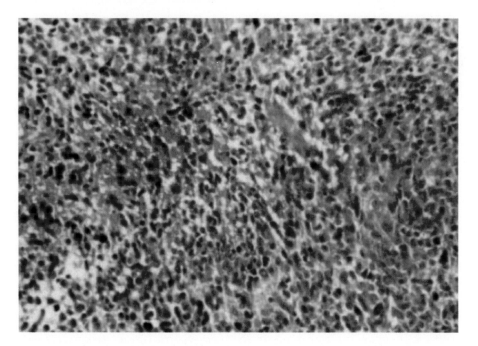

Figure 3. Childhood medulloblastoma (MED)/primitive neuroectodermal tumor (PNET). Expression of *FasR* on the surface of the neoplastically transformed cells. Routine, 10% buffered formalin fixation. Paraffin wax embedding. Alkaline phosphatase conjugated streptavidin-biotin antigen detection technique on a 4 μm thick section. Magnification: 200x.

Ganglioglioma is a rare, mixed neuronal-glial neoplasm of the central nervous system that occurs in young patients and has a benign clinical course [46]. 27 specimens were studied by routine histochemistry, 21 specimens by immunochemistry, and 14 specimens were examined at the ultrastructural level by Hirose and co-workers in an attempt to define the immunophenotypic and morphologic features of ganglioglioma. The age of the 27 patients, 14 males and 13 females, ranged from 3 to 52 years (mean 22 years). The most commonly affected site was the temporal lobe (13 patients). Three patients experienced a local recurrence. Microscopically, the tumors were comprised of well differentiated, somewhat abnormal neurons as well as glial cells, the latter including astrocytes of fibrillary (59%) and pilocytic (41%) type. Scant mitotic activity was observed in 2 tumors (7%). Glial cells of all tumors were immunoreactive for glial fibrillary acidic protein (GFAP), S-100 protein, and vimentin. Ki-67 labeling indices ranged from 0.6 to 10.5% (mean 2.7%) and p53 labeling indices between 1.1 to 42.4% (mean 15.6%). Ki-67 and p53 labeling indices in recurrent tumors were significantly higher than those of nonrecurrent ones ($p=0.036$ and $p=0.026$, respectively). No examples of anaplastic transformation were encountered. Immunohistochemically, many neuronal cells were positive for synaptophysin (100%), Class 3 β-tubulin (100%), neurofilament protein (90%), and chromogranin A (86%), in addition to S-100 protein (71%) and, occasionally, vimentin (24%). Ultrastructural characteristics of neuronal cells included the presence of numerous, 100-230 nanometer dense core granules within both perikarya and cell processes, well developed rough endoplasmic reticulum, microtubules within cell processes, and synapses associated with clear vesicles. Astrocytic cells usually contained abundant intermediate filaments; their cell membranes, when abutting the stroma, were covered by basal lamina. It is certain that gangliogliomas are comprised of well-differentiated neuronal cells and glial cells that are very often of pilocytic type. No cells with features intermediate between neurons and glia were observed. Neuronal cells are characterized by prominent neurosecretory features distinct from those of normal neurons in the central nervous system. Furthermore, higher Ki-67 and p53 labeling indices may indicate more aggressive behavior.

A recent study by Haapasalo et al. evaluated the feasibility and utility of Ultrarapid immunostaining of Ki-67 in astrocytomas [47]. It was found that the Ultrarapid technique, a method that could be carried out on frozen sections in about 10 minutes, provided reactivity comparable to that achieved with standard immunohistochemistry of paraffin embedded slides using the MIB-1 antibody. Thus, the Ultrarapid technique could certainly be utilized in the intraoperatve diagnosis of gliomas as well as other tumors.

Nerve growth factor (NGF) is important to the survival, development, and differentiation of neurons [48]. Its action is mediated by a specific cell surface transmembrane glycoprotein, nerve growth factor receptor (NGFR). NGFR expression was examined by immunohistochemistry in human fetal and adult adrenal medullary tissue, peripheral nervous system (PNS) neuroectodermal tumors (neuroblastoma, ganglioneuroblastoma, ganglioneuroma), pediatric primitive neuroectodermal tumors (PNETs) of the CNS, and CNS gliomas. Sixty-nine tumors in total were probed in this manner. Nerve growth factor receptor immunoreactivity was confined to nerve fibers and clusters of primitive-appearing cells in the fetal adrenal, and to nerve fibers and ganglion cells of the adult adrenal medulla; adrenal chromaffin cells were negative. In PNS neuroectodermal tumors, there was NGFR expression in tumor cells of 6 of 11 neuroblastomas and 6 of 6 ganglioneuroblastomas or ganglioneuromas. Thirteen of thirty-five CNS PNETs showed NGFR positivity. In most CNS

PNETs, NGFR was restricted to scattered single or small groups of cells, but two tumors with astroglial differentiation showed much more extensive immunoreactivity. Most ASTRs (11 of 14) and all ependymomas (3 of 3) were intensely NGFR positive.

In an earlier observation, MED-L cells with the 75kD low-affinity nerve growth factor receptor (p75NGFR) and MED-H cells with the proto-oncogene tropomyosin receptor kinase product (p140trk) were isolated selectively from a parent MED-3 cell line derived from cerebellar MED by panning, and the interaction of NGF with these cell lines was analyzed [49]. NGF treatment induced neuronal differentiation, growth inhibition, and tyrosine phosphorylation of p140trk in MED-H cells, but not in MED-L cells. The cells of MEDs express the functional NGFR, p140trk, which regulates their differentiation and growth.

In another study, positron emission tomography (PET) with the amino acid tracer L-[1-C-11]-tyrosine was evaluated in 27 patients with primary and recurrent brain tumors [50]. Patients underwent either static (n=14) or dynamic PET (n=13), with quantification of protein synthesis rate (PSR) and tumor-to-background ratio. Findings were compared with histopathological findings. Primary brain tumor was proved in 22 patients histologically, as well as metastatic cancer of unknown origin, primary non-Hodgkin lymphoma, meningioma, atypical infarction, and vasculitis in one patient each. At PET, 20 of 22 primary tumors, the metastasis, and non-Hodgkin lymphoma were correctly depicted. A false-positive finding was obtained with the infarction, and the meningioma and vasculitis were not depicted. The calculated sensitivity was 92%; specificity, 67%; and accuracy, 89%. There were no statistically significant relationships between histologic findings, PSR, and tumor-to-background ratio. The results strongly suggested that L-[1-C-11]-tyrosine is a valid tracer for early diagnosis of brain tumors and allowed quantification of PSR. PSR was further measured in human brain tumors using L-[1-(11)C]-tyrosine PET, and the PSR was compared to histopathological parameters of intratumoral cell proliferation and protein synthesis [51]. The authors observed 20 patients who had a positive brain tumor biopsy and who also underwent PET analysis. Formalin fixed, paraffin tissue sections were stained employing the MoAB MIB-1, targeted against the core Ki-67 antigen, and nucleolar organizer regions (NORs) were measured as argyrophilic NORs (AgNORs). The PSR was determined using a kinetic model. PSR (in nmol/ml/min) ranged from 0.44 to 1.99 (mean 0.97), Ki-67 labeling indices ranged from 0.9% to 33.5% (mean 9.5%) and AgNOR area (in mm^2/cm^2) ranged from 0.13 to 0.85. No relationship was found between PSR and Ki-67 labeling neither index nor AgNOR area. These results suggest that the PSR and the intratumoral proliferation, as measured by Ki-67, are two independent processes.

Deregulation of telomerase, a ribonucleoprotein polymerase that compensates progressive loss of telomeric $(TTAGGG)_n$ repeats during DNA replication, has been suggested to facilitate tumorigenesis and cellular immortality by providing unlimited proliferation capacity for cancer cells [52]. The relationship between tumor proliferation activity and *in situ* expression of the telomerase RNA component was investigated in 46 human grade I to IV ASTRs. Heterogeneously distributed telomerase RNA expression was detected from all of the tumor samples as well as from normal human brain tissue. However, expression of telomerase RNA was significantly increased in highly malignant tumors (p=0.024) and in tumors that showed increased proliferation activity determined by MIB-1 immunohistochemistry (p=0.014). Interestingly, increased telomerase RNA levels were observed in a subgroup of grade II ASTRs that showed significant increase in proliferation activity (p=0.047), indicating that the telomerase RNA component is already up-regulated in the early stages of ASTR pathogenesis. Telomeric repeat amplification assays revealed telomerase activity in 4/6 GBMs and in 1 rapidly proliferating grade II ASTR. These results suggest that increased tumor proliferation activity triggers telomerase activation *via* mechanisms that involve increased production of the RNA component of telomerase.

Abnormal p53 detected by immunocytochemistry has been identified to be a predictor of poor disease outcome in a variety of human malignant neoplasms, including brain tumors [53-55). The role of p53 alteration in the pathogenesis of intracranial neuroectodermal tumors was observed by Ng and co-workers [56]. Formalin fixed, paraffin sections of 196 brain tumors were employed in the study. The results demonstrated up to 40% immunoreactivity (presence of p53 alteration) in high grade ASTRs (AA and GBM). p53 alterations were also detected in 11% of well differentiated ASTRs. The extent of tumor cell immunolabeling also increased from the low to high grade ASTRs. Only rare cases of oligodendrogliomas and MEDs showed positive immunoreactivity, whereas ependymomas and choroid plexus tumors were uniformly negative. It seems that p53 alterations play a role in the immunophenotype progression of ASTR cells from low to high grade, as reported by us in a previous study [57]. Small, anaplastic ASTR cells were the predominant cell type expressing aberrant p53 protein.

Glioblastoma multiforme (GBM), the most malignant neoplasm of the human CNS, develops rapidly *de novo* (primary glioblastoma) or through malignant cellular IP progression from low-grade or anaplastic ASTR (so-called secondary glioblastoma) [58]. It was recently reported that mutations of the p53 gene are present in more than two-thirds of secondary glioblastomas, but rarely occur in primary GBMs, suggesting the presence of divergent genetic pathways [59]. Primary and secondary GBMs were screened by immunohistochemistry for murine double minute 2 (MDM2) overexpression and by differential PCR for gene amplification. Tumor cells immunoreactive to MDM2 were found in 15/29 primary GBMs, but in only 3/27 secondary glioblastomas ($p=0.0015$). MDM2 amplification occurred in 2 primary GBMs, but in none of the secondary GBMs. Only 1/15 primary GBMs overexpressing MDM2 contained a p53 mutation. These results suggest that MDM2 overexpression with or without gene amplification constitutes a molecular mechanism of escape from p53-regulated growth control, operative in the evolution of primary GBMs that typically lack p53 mutations.

In another article, p53 and MDM2 oncoprotein expression was evaluated in paraffin-embedded tissues from 61 patients with CNS gliomas (53 ASTRs and 8 oligodendrogliomas) and related to proliferation-associated markers [*i.e.* proliferating cell nuclear antigen (PCNA), Ki-67, and nuclear organizer regions (NORs], as well as epidermal growth factor receptor (EGFR) [60]. The authors employed a library of MoABs including PC-10, MIB-1, DO-1, 1B1O and EGFR 113 and the colloid silver nitrate (AgNOR) technique. MDM2 and p53 were co-expressed in 28% of the glioma cases. A p53-positive/MDM2-negative cellular IP was observed in 15% and a p53-negative/MDM2-positive IP in 20% of cases. There was a positive correlation of p53 and MDM2 expression with grade and proliferation indices. Univariate analysis in the group of diffuse astrocytomas showed that older age, high histological grade, high PCNA labeling index and high AgNOR score were associated with reduced overall survival ($p<0.05$). p53 labeling index, Ki-67 labeling index, AgNOR score, as well as tumor location and grade influenced disease-free survival ($p<0.05$), whereas the only parameters affecting post-relapse survival were histologic grade and Ki-67 labeling index ($p<0.1$). Multivariate analysis revealed that age, radiotherapy, PCNA labeling index and p53 labeling index were the independent predictors of overall survival. p53, Ki-67, MDM2, and

EGFR labeling indices, as well as grade and type of therapy were independent predictors of disease-free survival, and grade was the only independent predictor of post-relapse survival. The authors concluded that p53 and MDM2 labeling indices, as well as EGFR and proliferation marker (PCNA and Ki-67) expression represent useful indicators of overall and disease-free survival in diffuse ASTR patients.

Formalin fixed, paraffin embedded sections of 84 oligodendrogliomas (63 primary tumors, 21 recurrences), 21 GBMs with oligodendroglial growth pattern (15 primaries, 6 recurrences) and 17 mixed gliomas was observed for the presence of mutations in exons 5-9 by means of single stranded conformation polymorphism (SCCP), temperature gradient gel electrophoresis (TGGE) and direct DNA sequencing. In parallel, p53 protein accumulation was determined by means of immunocytochemistry [61]. The percentage of mutations was found to be higher than previously reported (6/44 grade II oligodendrogliomas, 4/19 grade III oligodendrogliomas, 4/15 glioblastomas). In four cases, the mutations lead to distinct changes in the primary or secondary structure of the protein (cysteine ==> tyrosine, proline ==> leucine) and were associated with marked accumulation of p53 protein. A significant correlation between p53 protein accumulation and TP53 gene aberrations was found ($p<0.001$), although p53 protein accumulation was detected more often than TP53 gene anomalies, indicating that factors other than TP53 gene mutation may also lead to p53 oncoprotein accumulation in brain tumor cells. A significant correlation was found for p53 protein accumulation and tumor grade, but not TP53 gene mutations. In conclusion, evaluation of p53 protein accumulation reflected the clinical course of oligodendrogliomas better than the mere presence of TP53 gene mutations.

The *c-myc* protein, which has been reported as a transcription factor having an unclear but apparent dual role in promoting cell proliferation and PCD, may be related to the relative absence of necessary growth factors for producing growth arrest [62]. The gene encoding p53 has been described as the most commonly disrupted gene in human neoplasms, suggesting a tumor-suppressor function for wild-type p53 [63-68]. High levels of p53 are associated with arrest of the cell cycle in G_1, which allows for necessary repairs to be carried out following DNA damage and hypoxia [69]. If the damage cannot be repaired, cell death by apoptosis is triggered. Mutations of the p53 gene lead to a loss of this critical DNA integrity and cell cycle monitoring function, which allows cells with damaged DNA to proliferate, obviously key in the production of neoplastically transformed cells. The bcl-2 family of proteins can inhibit (bcl-XL and Mcl-1) or induce (bax, bcl-XS, bcl-XL and bad) PCD in several cell systems [70-72]. Bcl-2, a 25-26 kD protein, has been described in mitochondria, the nuclear envelope, and in the endoplastic reticulum. Recent data suggests that the activity of bcl-2 is regulated by a 21 kD protein bax, with extensive amino acid homology to bcl-2 [73]. Bax is a homodimer capable of forming heterodimers with bcl-2. Bad is another protein that can interact with bcl-2. It has homology to bcl-2 within the homology domains BH1 and BH2. In mammalian cells, the bad protein is able to selectively heterodimerize with bcl-2 and bcl-XL, but not with other bcl-2 family related proteins. When bad is in a heterodimer with bcl-XL, it displaces bax from bcl-XL and promotes apoptosis.

Recently published evidence has emphasized the importance of PCD or apoptosis in the maintenance of tissue homeostasis and pathogenesis in the growth and progression of human neoplasms. This study, analyzed in breast cancer (BC), the significance of apoptosis in relation to the expression of p53 and bcl-2 proteins, tissue proliferation (defined by Ki-67 expression), hormone receptors, and tumor grade [74]. Immunocytochemistry was performed for p53, bcl-2, estrogen receptor, progesterone receptor, and Ki-67 expression. Mutant p53 protein was detected using a mutant specific ELISA. Immunoreactivity of p53 significantly correlated with the presence of mutant p53 protein detected by ELISA (r=0.654, p=0.00001). An inverse correlation was observed between *bcl-2* expression and the extent of apoptosis (r=-0.33369, p=0.01912). The extent of apoptosis directly correlated with p53 protein accumulation (r=0.485, p=0.00041), Ki-67 immunoreactivity (r=0.435, p=0.001), histopathological grade (r=0.492, p=0.0003), BC size (r=0.326, p=0.023) and lymph node status (r=0.287, p=0.047). A direct correlation was also observed between p53 expression and Ki-67 immunoreactivity (r=0.623, p=0.0002). There was no statistically significant association between estrogen and progesterone receptor status and apoptosis. In addition, the TNM stage of the disease correlated with immunoreactivity of p53 (r=0.572, p=0.00012) and Ki-67 (r=0.3744, p=0.00818). Bcl-2, by inhibiting apoptosis, may cause a shift in tissue kinetics towards the preservation of genetically aberrant cells, thereby facilitating tumor progression. These results imply that rapidly proliferating tumors appear to have a high "cell turnover state" in which there may be an increased chance of apoptosis among the proliferating cells. The ability of apoptosis to also occur in the presence of mutant p53 protein suggests the existence of at least two p53-dependent apoptotic pathways, one requiring activation of specific target genes and the other independent of it.

Genetic observations have provided new insights into the regulation of developmental organization of PCD. During the development of the nematode *Caenorhabditis elegans*, two genes related to PCD were identified: ced3 and ced4 (two potential tumor suppressor genes), as well as, an inhibitor, a cell protector gene named ced9 [75-77]. The ced9 gene is homologous to the bcl-2 proto-oncogene, discovered as a gene associated with a frequent translocation breakpoint in some B cell leukemias [78, 79]. The ced3 gene encodes a cysteine protease that is homologous to the interleukin-1β-converting enzyme (ICE) [80]. During the last few years, a number of novel genes involved in apoptosis, belonging to the ICE/ced-3 family and others, have been discovered: mouse Nedd 2 [81, 82], Ich-1, an ICE/ced-3 related gene that encodes both positive and negative regulators [83], TX/Ich-2/ICE$_{rel}$-II [84], the gene encoding CPP32, a novel human apoptotic protein with homology to the mammalian Il-1β-converting enzyme (85, Mch2 and Mch3 (86, ICE$_{rel}$ II and ICE$_{rel}$ III (87, ICE-LAP3 and ICE-LAP6 [88, 89], and MACH, a novel MORT1/FADD-interacting protease involved in CD95/*FasR*/APO-1, and TNF receptor-induced PCD [90]. There is evidence that ICE family members are also auto-proteolytic, and are able to process one another's substrates, such as poly-ADP ribose polymerase (PARP), lamins, etc. [91-93].

Cadherins are Ca^{2+}-dependent cell adhesion molecules that play an important role in tissue formation and morphogenesis in multicellular organisms. In recent years, there have been reports of cadherin involvement in tumor invasion and metastasis [94]. Twenty-two surgical specimens and some cultured cells were studied by immunohistochemical methods. No significant difference was observed in patients with AA, whereas decreased expression of N-cadherin was detected at the time of recurrence in those with GBM. In these groups, cerebrospinal fluid dissemination was found, and contralateral cerebral metastases and extracranial metastases were observed. It seems that decreased N-cadherin expression identified time of recurrence correlates with tumor invasion and dissemination of cerebrospinal fluid.

Desmosomes represent major intercellular adhesive junctions at basolateral membranes of epithelial cells and in other tissues [95]. They mediate direct cell-cell contacts and provide anchorage sites for intermediate filaments important for the maintenance of tissue architecture. There is increasing evidence now that desmosomes in addition to a simple structural function have new roles in tissue morphogenesis and differentiation. Transmembrane glycoproteins of the cadherin superfamily of Ca^{2+}-dependent cell-cell adhesion molecules which mediate direct intercellular interactions in desmosomes appear to be of central importance in this respect. The complex network of proteins forming the desmosomal plaque associated with the cytoplasmic domain of the desmosomal cadherins, however, is also involved in junction assembly and regulation of adhesive strength.

Together with microtubules and actin microfilaments, approximately 11 nm wide, intermediate filaments (IFs) constitute the integrated, dynamic filament network present in the cytoplasm of metazoan cells. This network is critically involved in division, motility and other cellular processes [96]. While the structures of microtubules and microfilaments are known in atomic detail, IF architecture is presently much less understood. The elementary 'building block' of IFs is a highly elongated, rod-like dimer based on an α-helical coiled-coil structure. Assembly of cytoplasmic IF proteins, such as vimentin, begins with a lateral association of dimers into tetramers and gradually into the so-called unit-length filaments (ULFs). Subsequently ULFs start to anneal longitudinally, ultimately yielding mature IFs after a compaction step. The assembly of nuclear lamins, however, starts with a head-to-tail association of dimers. Recently, X-ray crystallographic data were obtained for several fragments of the vimentin dimer. Based on the dimer structure, molecular models of the tetramer and the entire filament are now a possibility.

Tenascins (TNs) are a family of extracellular matrix glycoproteins. The first member of this family to be recognized, tenascin-C (TN-C), is known to be expressed in various tumors, including human ASTRs. Tenascin-X (TN-X) is the latest member of the TN family to be reported, and its expression in tumor tissues has not yet been examined [97]. Expression of TN-X in glioma cell lines and human ASTRs was reported using immunoblot analysis employing anti-mouse TN-X antibodies. The expression pattern of TN-C and TN-X was also observed immunohistochemically in a series of 32 human ASTRs and tissue sections from five normal brains. Expression of TN-X was upregulated to a higher degree in low-grade ASTRs than in high-grade ASTRs. TN-X was mainly localized in the perivascular stroma around tumor vessels, and weakly expressed in the intercellular spaces among tumor cells. In contrast, TN-C was more strongly expressed in the intercellular spaces and in tumor vessels in high-grade ASTRs (AAs and GBMs) than in low-grade ASTRs. In the tissues expressing both TNs, the distribution of TN-X was often reciprocal to that of TN-C. These findings indicate that the expression of TN-C and TN-X in ASTRs is different, and that these glycoproteins could be involved in neovascularization in different manners.

Recent *in vitro* studies of the EGFR family have revealed complex signaling interactions involving the production of ligand-mediated heterodimers synergistic for the transformation of cells *in vitro* [98] and growth factors have been well established as necessary during the process of neoplastic transformation [99-102]. In a series of 70 patients with childhood MED, immunocytochemistry and Western blotting analysis were conducted to characterize the expression patterns of all four EGFR family members (EGFR, HER-2, HER-3, and HER-4), as well as heregulin-α, a ligand for the HER-3 and HER-4 receptors. The majority of MED cases expressed two or more receptor proteins; coexpression of the HER2 and HER4 receptors occurred in 54%. Expression of heregulin-α was detected in 31% of the tumor cases observed by the authors. To investigate whether co-expression results in receptor heterodimerization, immunoprecipitation of protein extracts from primary tumors was conducted and various patterns of receptor interaction were observed, including that between HER-2 and HER-4. In multivariate 25-year survival analysis with clinicopathological disease features, no individual receptor or heregulin-α achieved significance. In contrast, when considered together in the multivariate model, co-expression of HER-2 and HER-4 demonstrated independent prognostic significance (p=0.006). These data suggest the hypothesis that HER2-HER4 receptor heterodimerization is of particular biological significance in MED, demonstrating the potential clinical significance of EGFR family heterodimerization in human neoplastic cells. The authors also analyzed expression of the AP-2 transcription factor implicated in the positive regulation of HER-2 and HER-3 gene transcription in malignant cells and found an association between AP-2 expression and not only HER-2 and HER-3, but also HER-4 levels in primary MEDs/PNETs.

The neurofibromatosis 2 (NF2) gene-encoded protein (merlin), may function as a molecular link between the cytoskeleton and the plasma membrane [103]. Merlin is thought to play a crucial role as a tumor suppressor not only in hereditary NF2-related tumors, but also in sporadic tumors such as Schwannomas, meningiomas and gliomas. Using a merlin-expression vector system, specific antiserum against merlin was produced. Subsequently, the intracellular distribution of merlin in cultured glioma cells was observed, and merlin expression was further investigated in 116 human brain tumors. Immunofluorescence microscopy revealed that merlin was localized beneath the cell membrane and concentrated at cell-to-cell adhesion sites, where actin filaments are densely associated with plasma membrane. By immunohistochemistry, none of the Schwannomas from neither NF2 patients nor sporadic cases showed any immunoreactivity, while normal Schwann cells of cranial nerves were immunopositive. In meningiomas, merlin expression was frequently detected in the meningothelial subtype (8/10), but no expression could be detected in either the fibrous or the transitional variant. Most normal astrocytes were negative; however, reactive astrocytes often expressed merlin. Glioblastomas and AAs were found to be strongly positive, and focal positive staining was observed in fibrillary and pilocytic ASTRs. Thus, the loss of merlin appears to be integral to Schwannoma formation and the differential pathogenesis of meningioma subtypes. However, merlin alterations do not appear to play a critical role in neither the tumorigenesis nor the malignant transformation of neoplastic astrocytes.

Chang and co-workers have chemically characterized the gangliosides of the Daoy cell line in order to establish a model system for the study of ganglioside metabolism of human MEDs/PNETs [104]. Cells comprising MEDs/PNETs contain a high concentration of gangliosides (143±13nmol LBSA/10^8 cells). The major species have been structurally confirmed to be GM2 (65.9%), GM3 (13.0%), and GD1a (10.3%). Isolation of individual gangliosides homogeneous in both carbohydrate and ceramide moieties by reversed-phase HPLC and analysis by negative-ion fast atom bombardment collisionally activated dissociation tandem mass spectrometry have allowed the authors to unequivocally characterize ceramide structures. In the case of GM2, 10 major ceramide subspecies were identified: d18:1-hC16:0, d18:1-C16:0, d18:0-C16:0, d18:1-C18:0, d18:1-C20:0, d18:1-C22:0, d18:2-C24:1, d18:1-C23:1, d18:1-C24:1, and d18:1-C24:0. Taken together with previous studies, these findings in human MED cells support the view that high expression and marked heterogeneity of ceramide structure are general characteristics of tumor gangliosides, molecules which are shed by tumor cells and are biologically active *in vivo*.

While the number of reports on macrophage infiltration of gliomas is increasing, the extent and mechanisms of macrophage recruitment remain unclear [105]. To investigate whether monocyte chemoattractant protein-1 (MCP-1) plays a role in this process, *in situ* hybridization was performed for 22 GBMs, one AA and 4 grade II fibrillary ASTRs and reverse transcription-polymerase chain reaction was performed in 13 GBMs, one AA and three grade II ASTRs. High levels of MCP-1 mRNA were detectable in most GBMs, while a lower level was detected in grade II ASTRs. Many tumor-associated macrophages were observed by immunohistochemistry within most GBM cases, while the grade II ASTRs contained a lower number of infiltrating macrophages. The positive correlation between MCP-1 level and abundance of macrophagic infiltration suggests that MCP-1 has a role in the recruitment of macrophages to the site of the neoplasm. By combining *in situ* hybridization and immunohistochemistry, high levels of MCP-1 mRNA were shown both in tumor cells and within the tumor-associated macrophages. Reactive astrocytes and microglia along the boundary of the tumors also expressed MCP-1. In areas with T lymphocyte infiltration, larger numbers of MCP-1-positive cells with an enhanced level of expression were identified. The authors proposed that the mechanism of macrophage recruitment is, at least partly, affected by constitutive expression and T cell-mediated up-regulation of MCP-1 in tumor cells, as well as the tumor infiltrating macrophages. The production of MCP-1 by these macrophages establishes a positive amplification circuit for macrophage recruitment in gliomas.

In the last two decades, significant advances have been made in the identification of the soluble angiogenic factors, insoluble extracellular matrix (ECM) molecules and receptor signaling pathways that mediate control of angiogenesis [106]. The question remains how the endothelial cells are capable of integrating these chemical signals with mechanical cues from their *in situ* tissue microenvironment so as to produce functional capillary networks that exhibit specialized form as well as function [107]. These observations have revealed that ECM governs whether an endothelial cell will switch between growth, differentiation, motility, or apoptosis programs in response to a soluble stimulus based on its ability to mechanically resist cell tractional forces and thereby produce cell and cytoskeletal distortion. Transmembrane integrin receptors play a pivotal role in this mechanochemical transduction process because they both organize a cytoskeletal signaling complex within the focal adhesion and preferentially focus mechanical forces on this site. All three molecular filaments within the internal cytoskeleton (*i.e.* microfilaments, microtubules, and intermediate filaments) also contribute to the cell's structural and functional response to mechanical stress through their role as discrete support elements. A similar form of mechanical control also has been shown to be involved in the regulation of contractility in vascular smooth muscle cells and cardiac myocytes. The mechanism by which cells perform mechanochemical transduction and the implications of these findings for morphogenetic control are still not clear yet.

Experimental tumors of the CNS were observed with antibodies to quinolinate to assess the cellular distribution of this endogenous neurotoxin [108]. In advanced F98 and RG-2 GBMs and E367 neuroblastomas in the striatum of rats, variable numbers of quinolinate immunoreactive cells were observed in and around the tumors, with the majority being present within tumors, rather than the brain parenchyma. The stained cells were morphologically variable, including round, complex, rod-shaped, and sparsely dendritic cells. Neuroblastoma and glioma cells were unstained, as were neurons, astrocytes, oligodendrocytes, ependymal cells, endothelial cells, and cells of the choroid plexus and leptomeninges. GFAP immunoreactivity was strongly elevated in astrocytes surrounding the tumors. Dual labeling immunohistochemistry with antibodies to quinolinate and GFAP demonstrated that astrocytes and the cells containing quinolinate immunoreactivity were morphologically disparate and preferentially distributed external and internal to the tumors, respectively, and no dual labeled cells were observed. Lectin histochemistry with Griffonia simplicifolia B4 isolectin and Lycopersicon esculentum lectin demonstrated numerous phagocytic macrophages and reactive microglia in and around the tumors, whose distribution was similar to that of quinolinate immunoreactive cells, although they were much more numerous. Dual labeling studies with antibodies to quinolinate and the lectins demonstrated partial co-distribution of these markers, with most double-labeled cells having the morphology of phagocytes. The present findings suggest the possibility that quinolinate may serve a functional role in a select population of inflammatory cell infiltrates during the host's immune response to primary brain neoplasms.

CANCER TESTIS ANTIGENS AS TARGETS

During the last decade, the aberrant expression of normal testicular proteins in neoplastically transformed cells became common knowledge. Cancer/testis-antigens (CTAs) represent a novel family of immunogenic proteins. The MAGE genes were initially analyzed from melanomas and turned out to have an almost exclusively neoplasm specific expression pattern. CTAs, were detected by serological screening of recombinant cDNA expression libraries. CTAs (e.g. members of the MAGE gene family) are a distinct class of differentiation antigens that have received much attention for being potential targets of human cancer vaccines for T lymphocyte based or receptor specific and directed immunotherapy because of their broad expression in various neoplasms [109, 110]. The first member, MAGE-A1, of the MAGE gene family was discovered and characterized as genes encoding melanoma antigens [110]. During the last decade, 23 human and 12 mouse MAGE genes have been isolated and characterized in various mammalian neoplasms [111]. Numerous gene homologues to MAGE-A1 have been identified on the Xq28, Xp21,3 Xq26, and Xp11.23 and are classified as MAGE-A, -B, -C and -D [112-116]. Previous observations have characterized the MAGE-A subfamily as: (a) they were not present in normal cells except for testis (primitive germ cells, spermatogonia) and placenta [117]; and (b) some antigens encoded by the gene family are presented by the human leukocyte antigen (HLA) [118]. These results suggest that immunoreaction against MAGE proteins could be expected to affect only neoplastically transformed cells (activation or derepression of normally silent CT genes) but not normal cells because testis and placenta lack HLA expression [119, 120]. Melanoma antigens (MAGE) are regarded as inducing tumor-specific immune response and thought to be potential therapeutical agents for anti-neoplastic immunotherapy [121, 122]. Hence, experimental vaccination with MAGE-A peptide provoked neoplasm regression in melanoma patients without significant side effects [109]. The XAGE-1 gene consists of 4 exons and is located on chromosome Xp11.21-Xp11.22. The full length cDNA contains 611 bp and predicts a protein of 16,300 mol. weight, with a potential transmembrane domain at NH_2 terminus [123]. XAGE-1 shares homology with GAGE/PAGE proteins in the COOH terminal. The XAGE-1b antigen, codes for a putative protein of 81 amino acids, harboring a functional bipartite nuclear localization signal and a C-terminal acidic transcription-activation-like domain. XAGE-1b has been shown to have a 50% homology with members of the GAGE family, at least on the nucleotide level [124].

Recently, a new CTA, NY-ESO-1 (one of the ten gene or gene families encoding CTAs), has been identified on the basis of spontaneous antibody responses to NAMs [125]. NY-ESO-1 appears to be one of the most immunogenic antigens known to date, with spontaneous immune responses observed in 50% of patients with NY-ESO-1 expressing neoplams, inducing both a humoral immune response and specific $CD8^+$ cytotoxic T lymphocyte immunoreactivity [126-128]. Immunity to NY-ESO-1 is clearly antigen dependent, disappearing with neoplasm removal or regression [129, 130].

A new member of CT genes, named OY-TES-1, was isolated and defined to be the human homologue of proacrosin binding protein sp32 precursor, which was initially found in the mouse, guinea pig, and pig [131]. OY-TES-1, containing ten exons, maps to chromosome 12p12-p13, with Southern blot analysis suggesting that there are two OY-TES-1-related genes in the human genome. OY-TES-1 mRNA was expressed only in the testis when normal tissues were observed for its presence. However, OY-TES-1 mRNA was detected in various neoplastically transformed cells, including bladder, breast, lung, liver, and colon cancers. Ono et al. deomstrated through a serological survey of 362 cancer patients the presence of anti-OY-TES-1 antibody in twenty-five of these patients. In healthy individuals (n=20), OY-TES-1 sera reactivity was not identified, which indicates that these results show that the OY-TES-1 antigen is immunogenic in the course human neoplastic disease [132].

This expression pattern might contribute to the genetic instability of neoplastically transformed cells. Over the past few years, more than 200 research articles have appeared in the literature concerning CTAs [128]. It has become obvious that CTAs can and will be used for the diagnosis and microstaging of various human neoplasms [129]. Thus far, we have never seen authors writing about specific antigen families all arrive at the same conclusion, except in the case of CTAs, in which all authors have concluded that these antigens could and should be employed for more individualized, antigen targeted and specific anti-neoplastic immunotherapy.

Our immunocytochemical observations have detected the presence and cellular localization of the MAGE-1 CTA, employing anti-MAGE-1 MoAB, only in anaplastic, high grade ASTRs (100%) and in GBMs. The immunoreactivity was always heterogeneous, showing a cytoplasmic pattern and loosely grouped cells with similar staining characteristics being detected within the cellular and hormonal microenvironment of the ASTRs. MAGE-1 was not expressed in the lowest grade, pilocytic ASTR cases. The two cases of pure anaplastic ASTRs demonstrated expression of MAGE-1, located in the cytoplasm of neoplastically transformed cells. The staining intensity in this ASTR subtype was high (A and B) and the number of total cells positively stained ranged from (+) to (++). In the case of the mixed ASTR with primitive neuroectodermal tumor (PNET) elements, MAGE-1 was also present, but with a lower intensity (B) although a similar proportion of ASTR tumor cells exhibited immunoreactivity (++). No staining for PNET elements was identified. High intensity staining (A,B) in well over 50% of the total cell number (+++) was observed in the anaplastic oligo-astrocytoma and other anaplastic ASTRs. MAGE-1 immunoreactivity was of greatest intensity (A) in the four cases of GBM observed by us. A high proportion (over 50%) of the total cell number reacted positively (+++). Extensive immunocytochemical observations performed by our group have confirmed the expression of the MAGE family of peptides in numerous neoplastically transformed cell types including breast and lung carcinomas, and malignant melanomas. As expected, only some differentiating cells of the normal testis tissue, employed as positive tissue control in our immunohistochemical study reacted positively with the anti-MAGE-1 MoAB, while the other normal human tissues, including the postnatal thymus tissue demonstrated no detectable presence of MAGE-1 CT antigen (negative tissue controls).

Detection of Cancer/Testis Antigens in Various Malignant Neoplasms and their Therapeutic Significance

It has become obvious that CTAs can be used for the diagnosis and microstaging of human neoplasms, as well as the population screening of smokers to show an increased risk for lung cancer in their own individual lifetimes and by extension, clearly showing the truly damaging effects of smoking. Thus far, we have never seen authors writing about specific antigen families all arrive at the same conclusion, except in the case of CTAs, in which all authors have concluded that these antigens could and should be used for antigen targeted and specific anti-neoplastic immunotherapy.

The expression of CTAs has also been examined in human brain tumors [133]. Meningiomas were found to express only HOM-TES-14/SCP-1. SSX-4 was found to be the only CT gene expressed in oligodendrogliomas and it was also expressed in oligoastrocytomas and astrocytomas. Astrocytoma cells proved to be the most positive for HOM-TES-14/SCP-1 and SSX-4, with expression of HOM-TES-85, SSX-2 and MAGE-3 also defined in these tumors. MAGE-3 was detected only in grade IV astrocytomas, while the expression of the other CT genes showed no clear correlation with histological grade. Sixty percent of astrocytomas analyzed were found to express at least one CT gene, 21% expressed two CT genes, and 8% coexpressed three CT genes. These authors, like many others in relation to other neoplasms, concluded that a majority of oligoastrocytomas and astrocytomas might be amenable to CTA directed, specific immunotherapeutic interventions.

There has been observation of the expression of CTAs in cryo-preserved cutaneous T cell lymphoma (CTCL) tissues, including mycosis fungoides, pleomorphic cutaneous T-cell lymphoma, Sezary's syndrome (SS), and a non-malignant entity (small plaques parapsoriasis, SPP). The authors used a panel of eleven CT antigens (MAGE-1, MAGE-C1, MAGE-3, BAGE, GAGE, SSX-1, SSX-2, SSX4, SCP-1, NY-ESO-1 and TS85) (HOM-Tes-85), with mRNA expression for SCP-1 being identified in MF and pleomorphic CTCL patients but not in the small plaques parapsoriasis. SS patients demonstrated a more heterogeneous antigen expression pattern, including GAGE, MAGE-1, MAGE-3, MAGE-C1, NY-ESO-1 and TS85. Haffner *et al.* emphasized that CTAs could provide defined targets for antigen-based vaccination and CTA-directed immunotherapy in a high percentage of cases with CTCL. The authors also suggested that SCP-1 antigen expression might serve as an additional diagnostic indicator in early and clinically indistinct lesions suspicious for cutaneous T-cell lymphoma [134].

Another recent article by Mashino and co-workers analyzed the expression of six CT genes including NY-ESO-1, LAGE-1, SCP-1, SSX-1, SSX-2, and SSX-4 in gastrointestinal and breast carcinomas using reverse transcription-polymerase chain reaction [135]. Relatively high expression of SCP-1 and SSX-4 was described in gastric carcinoma, LAGE-1 and NY-ESO-1 in esophageal carcinoma, and SCP-1 in breast carcinoma. Frequent synchronous expression with MAGE was identified, including LAGE-1 in esophageal carcinoma, SSX-4 in gastric carcinoma, and SCP-1 in breast carcinoma. Immunocytochemical analysis of the neoplasms expressing both MAGE-4 and NY-ESO-1 genes demonstrated differences in the distribution between MAGE-4 and NY-ESO-1 in serial sections. The authors suggested that NY-ESO-1, LAGE-1, SCP-1 and SSX-4, in addition to MAGE, genes may be promising candidates for NAM directed immunotherapy. The group of Mashino also added that polyvalent cancer vaccines may indeed be useful for cases of gastrointestinal and breast carcinomas with heterogeneous CTA gene expression profiles.

CTAs are also expressed in a high percentage in hepatocellular carcinomas. In 30 hepatocellular carcinomas, mRNA expression of SSX-1, SSX-2, SSX-4, SSX-5, SCP-1, and NY-ESO-1 has been described, with limited expressions of these genes being detected in few non-neoplastically transformed liver tissues [136].

Synovial sarcomas are high-grade, extremely malignant mesenchymal neoplasms with two, biphasic (BSS) and monophasic (MSS) variants that carry a pathognomonic cytogenetic alteration, t(X;18), involving the SYT gene on chromosome 18 and one of several SSX genes on chromosome X, usually SSX1 or SSX2, a translocation characteristically involving t(X; 18) to (p11.2; q11.2) between SYT and SXX [137]. A recent study analyzed the expression of three CTAs, NY-ESO-1, MAGE-A1 and MAGE-C1 (CT7), through the use of immunocytochemistry, employing three MoABs, ES121 (anti-NY-ESO-1), MA454 (anti-MAGE-A1) and CT7-33 (anti-CT7), in synovial sarcomas [138]. The results suggested that NY-ESO-1 is highly expressed in a homogeneous pattern in synovial sarcomas of both morphologic variants and both translocation types, making these neoplasms an attractive target for NY-ESO-1 antigen-based, and directed immunotherapy.

In the search for biomarkers for early lung cancer detection and possible receptor targeted immunotherapy, the frequencies of the expressional activation of MAGE-A1, MAGE-A3, and MAGE-B2 genes in non-small cell lung cancers (NSCLCs) were observed by Jang *et al.* [139]. Expression of these genes was evaluated by reverse transcription-PCR (RT-PCR) in 20 primary NSCLC samples, with corresponding normal lung tissues, and in 20 bronchial brush specimens from former smokers without lung cancer. mRNA *in situ* hybridization was done to confirm the gene expression pattern at the cellular level. Among the twenty primary NSCLC samples analyzed, 14 expressed MAGE-A1 and 17 expressed both MAGE-A3 and MAGE-B2 while a substantial number of normal lung tissues adjacent to NSCLC also had detectable levels of MAGE expression, specifically 65% for MAGE-A1, 75% for MAGE-A3, and 80% for MAGE-B2. The activation of MAGE-A1, MAGE-A3, and MAGE-B2 genes was found to be common not only in NSCLC, but also in bronchial epithelium with severe carcinogenic insult. I agree with the authors that these results suggest that MAGE genes may be activated during the earliest stages of lung carcinogenesis, but more significantly, I feel that these genes should not only be considered as specific targets for lung cancer therapy, but that lung cancer prevention could be carried out *via* the population screening of smokers.

Since it has been both demonstrated and is now common knowledge that the MAGE genes are expressed in a wide variety of human neoplasms but only in the mitotic spermatogonia (germ cells) and in the primary spermatocytes in the normal testis, Aubry *et al.* chose to examine the expression of MAGE-A4 in a panel of testicular germ cell tumors [121]. Classical seminomas uniformly and specifically expressed MAGE-A4 while anaplastic seminomas and NSGCTs were negative for this antigen. MAGE-A4 was also present in the fetal precursors of the stem germ cells from 17 weeks of gestation onward, which is in agreement with the fact that CIS can arise from prespermatogonia in the fetus. These results reveal that the MAGE-A4 antigen can be considered a specific marker for normal premeiotic germ cells and germ cell neoplasms and can in fact be employed as immunocytochemical markers to characterize classical seminomas.

The MAGE-3 gene is present in a variety of neoplasms, including lung cancer, but not in normal tissues except for the testis and placenta [140]. The scientific aim of a recent observation by Eifuku and co-workers was to clarify whether HLA-A2 restricted MAGE-3 peptide (FLWGPRALV) was a lung cancer associated antigen recognizable by cytotoxic, $CD8^+$ T lymphocytes (CTL). MAGE-3-derived peptide-specific CTL were induced from the peripheral blood mononuclear cells (PBMC) of HLA-A0201-positive healthy donors and the regional lymph node lymphocytes (RLNL) of HLA-A2-positive patients with lung cancer by multiple stimulations with peptide-pulsed HLA-A0201-positive antigen-presenting cells. The lymphocytes stimulated with MAGE-3 peptide produced an antigen directed, specific lysis of Epstein-Barr virus-transformed B cells (EBV-B) pulsing with MAGE-3 peptide. Stronger and specific activity for MAGE-3-presenting targets was found after the second antigenic stimulation, and the activity increased with every repeated stimulation. The peptide-specific activity was inhibited by the addition of MoABs against MHC class I and HLA-A2. Such CTL also recognized established tumor cell lines expressing both HLA-A2 and MAGE-3 in an MHC class I-restricted manner, but did not recognize tumor cell lines that did not express HLA-A2 or MAGE-3. These results suggest that the MAGE-3 peptide could be used as a potential target for antigen directed, specific immunotherapy for HLA-A2 patients with lung cancer [140].

As neoplastically transformed cells spread beyond their primary site, they undergo changes in their gene expression that may be detectable and useful for microstaging of neoplastic disease [141]. The CT antigens like MAGE 1-3, NY-ESO-1, SSX 1-5, and others are potential NAMs for microstaging melanoma. One CTA, CTp11, was shown to be expressed by metastasizing melanoma cell lines but not by nonmetastasizing variants. It was found that CTp11 tended to be expressed by primary melanomas. There was a statistically significant difference in the distribution of the expression of CTp11 and NY-ESO-1 in melanoma from different stages of progression. The authors concluded that NY-ESO-1 may be a prognostically significant CTA, detecting of more advanced neoplastic disease and CTp11 of less advanced disease.

Today it is well known that HLA-A*0201 melanoma patients can frequently develop a CTL response to the CT antigen NY-ESO-1. In a study by Romero et al., the relative antigenicity and in vitro immunogenic effectivity of natural and modified NY-ESO-1 peptide sequences was analyzed [142]. The results revealed that, although suboptimal for binding to the HLA-A*0201 molecule, peptide NY-ESO-1 157-165 is, among natural sequences, very efficiently recognized by specific CTL clones derived from three melanoma patients. In contrast, peptides NY-ESO-1 157-167 and NY-ESO-1 155-163, which bind very strongly to HLA-A*0201, are recognized less efficiently. Substitution of peptide NY-ESO-1 157-165 COOH-terminal C with a number of other amino acids resulted in a significantly increased binding to HLA-A*0201 molecules as well as in an increased CTL recognition, although variable at the clonal level. Among natural peptides, NY-ESO-1 157-165 and NY-ESO-1 157-167 exhibited good in vitro immunogenicity, whereas peptide NY-ESO-1 155-163 was poorly immunogenic. The fine specificity of interaction between peptide NY-ESO-1 C165A, HLA-A*0201, and T lymphocyte receptor was also analyzed at the molecular level employing a series of variant peptides containing single alanine substitutions. I agree with the authors that the results submitted in this article will have significant implications for the further development of NY-ESO-1 peptide based vaccines and for the monitoring of either natural or vaccine-induced NY-ESO-1 specific CTL responses in neoplasm patients.

The identification and characterization of L552S, an over-expressed, alternatively spliced isoform of XAGE-1 was reported in lung adenocarcinoma [143]. Genomic sequence analysis has revealed that L552S and XAGE-1 are alternatively spliced isoforms, and expression of both L552S and XAGE-1 isoforms are present in lung adenocarcinoma. L552S was shown to be expressed at levels greater than 10-fold in lung adenocarcinomas compared with the highest expression level found in all normal tissues tested. L552S was present in both early and late stages of lung adenocarcinoma development, but it was not detected in large cell carcinoma, small cell carcinoma, or atypical lung neuroendocrine carcinoid. Immunocytochemical analysis employing affinity purified L552S polyclonal antibodies demonstrated specific nuclear staining in lung adenocarcinoma samples. Furthermore, antibody responses to recombinant L552S protein were observed lung pleural effusion fluids of lung cancer patients. These results strongly imply that the L552S protein is a strong immunogen and the authors suggested that it could be employed as a vaccine target for lung cancer [143].

In recent experiments of suppression subtractive hybridization, comparing mRNA expression profiles of common nevocellular nevi and melanoma metastases, was employed to identify new potential markers of melanoma progression [131]. The metastatic melanoma tissues contained XAGE-1b. Expression of XAGE-1b in normal tissues was mainly restricted to testis, while placenta and brain were sporadically positive. In general, expression of XAGE-1b was much more prominent than expression of the longer XAGE-1 transcript, isolated from Ewing's sarcoma. In the different stages of melanocytic tumor progression, expression was exclusively seen in melanoma metastases, while all tested common and atypical nevi as well as primary melanomas were negative. Upregulation of receptor expression after treatment with demethylating agent 5-aza-2'-deoxycytidine was identified in only one of four human melanoma cell lines tested. After transfection of XAGE-1 gene into COS cells, the corresponding protein could direct the coupled fluorescent protein to the nucleus, showing a distinct speckled staining aspect. These experimental data imply the nuclear CT associated XAGE-1b to be a marker for late melanocytic tumor progression [131].

An extensive review of the expression of the SSX genes in a variety of human tumors has been provided by Tureci et al. [144]. The authors assessed the expression of SSX-1, -2, -3, -4 and -5 using RT-PCR in a sample of 325 tumors of various histological origins. The expression of at least one of the SSX family members was found to be most frequent in cancers of the head and neck, followed by ovarian cancer, malignant melanoma, lymphoma, colorectal cancer and breast cancer while some leukemias, leiomyosarcomas, seminomas and thyroid cancers were found not to express any SSX gene. These findings further illustrate the amenability of CTAs for use in the targeting of various antigen specific immunotherapeutical approaches.

Extensive immunocytochemical observations performed by our group have confirmed the expression of the MAGE family of peptides in numerous neoplastically transformed tissues including breast and lung carcinomas, malignant melanomas and childhood astrocytomas. Of particular significance is the absence of these markers on the surface of neoplastically non-transformed cells in normal tissues examined employinging the same protocol, further substantiating the prevailing conclusions in regards to the specificity of the CTAs to genetically dedifferentiated populations of neoplastic cells and the distinct and very enticing possibility for their targeting in various immunotherapeutic approaches.

CONCLUSION

It has become clear that immunohistochemistry has revitalized morphological methods in cancer research and clinical oncology. As detailed in the foregoing discussion, the importance of this technique lies not only in its use in basic research focused on the mechanisms and regulatory steps in carcinogenesis, but also in its use in the more accurate diagnosis of neoplasia, including the functional differential diagnosis and staging of brain tumors. It has become clear that the evaluation of the expression of molecular markers of progression, invasion and metastasis should be employed routinely in the establishment of differential diagnosis and to aid in the determination of the most appropriate treatment regimen. The analysis of the IP expression profile of brain tumors of various stages has shed light on many possible NAAs that could be used as targets in fourth-modality immunotherapeutical approaches. It comes as no surprise, that the scientific conferences of the past decade demonstrated great interest in immunohistochemistry since this technique has allows researchers to delve into the molecular biological aspects of cancer, without sacrificing the tangible utility and beauty of morphology. The development of this technique to its present place in research, diagnostics and therapy, of course, could not have been possible without the discovery of monoclonal antibodies, one of the most important scientific discoveries of the twentieth century. The next 20 years will hopefully be increasingly dominated by the development of individualized "cocktails" of conjugated antibody molecules, targeting multiple antigens, as the main line of non-toxic and efficacious therapy of human cancer, especially in the treatment of residual and metastatic disease. With the advances made relevant to the genetic and molecular mechanisms of carcinogenesis it appears increasingly likely that etio-pathologic treatment will become a reality – that the treatment of cancer will be directed towards the etiology of the disease rather than just the symptoms and manifestations of the underlying pathologic process.

REFERENCES

[1]   Kleinman GM, Zagzag D, Miller DC: Diagnostic use of immunohistochemistry in neuropathology. *Neurosurg Clin N Am* 5(1): 97-126, 1994.

[2]   Miller CW, Simon K, Aslo A, Kok Y, Yokota J, Buys ChCm, Terada M, Koeffler HP: p53 mutations in human lung tumors. *Cancer Research* 52: 1695-1698, 1992.

[3]   Szymas J: Diagnostic immunohistochemistry of tumors of the central nervous system. Folia Neuropathol 32: 209-214 1994.

[4] Husgafvel-Pursiainen K, Ridanpaa M, Anttila S, Vainio H: p53 and ras gene mutations in lung cancer: implications for smoking and occupational exposures. *J Occup Environ Med* 37: 68-76, 1995.

[5] Taylor CR: Quality assurance and standardization in immunohistochemistry. A proposal for the annual meeting of the Biological Stain Commission, June, 1991. *Biotech Histochem* 67: 110-117, 1992.

[6] Kawajiri K, Eguchi H, Nakachi K, Sekiya T, Yamamoto M: Association of CYP1A1 germ line polymorphisms with mutations of the p53 gene in lung cancer. *Cancer Res* 56: 72-76, 1996.

[7] Soetrisno E, Tjahjadi G: Pathological aspects of brain tumors. Gan To Kagaku Ryoho 27s(2): 274-278, 2000.

[8] Kernohan JW, Mabon RF, Svien HJ, et al: A simplified classification of gliomas. *Proc Staff Meet Mayo Clin* 24: 71-75, 1949.

[9] Kernohan JW, Sayre GP: Tumors of the central nervous system. In: *Atlas of Tumor Pathology*, Section 10, Vols 35 & 37. Washington DC. Armed Forces Institute of Pathology, 1952.

[10] Kleihues P, Burger PC, Scheithauer BW: *Histological typing of tumors of the central nervous system.* New York: Springer-Verlag, 1993.

[11] Daumas-Duport C, Scheithauer B, O'Fallon J, Kelly P: Grading of astrocytomas. A simple and reproducible method. *Cancer* 62: 2152-2165, 1988.

[12] Schmitt HP, Oberwittler C: Computer-aided classification of malignancy in astrocytomas: II. The value of categorically evaluated histologic and non-histologic features for a numerical classifier. *Analytical Cell Pathol* 4: 409-419, 1992.

[13] Karak AK, Singh R, Tandon PN, Sarkar C: A comparative survival evaluation and assessment of interclassification concordance in adult supratentorial astrocytic tumors. *Pathol Oncol Res* 6(1): 46-52, 2000.

[14] Godard S, Getz G, Delorenzi M, Farmer P, Kobayashi H, Desbaillets I, Nozaki M, Diserens AC, Hamou MF, Dietrich PY, Regli L, Janzer RC, Bucher P, Stupp R, de Tribolet N, Domany E, Hegi ME: Classification of human astrocytic gliomas on the basis of gene expression: a correlated group of genes with angiogenic activity emerges as a strong predictor of subtypes. *Cancer Res* 63(20): 6613-6625, 2003.

[15] Shai R, Shi T, Kremen TJ, Horvath S, Liau LM, Cloughesy TF, Mischel PS, Nelson SF: Gene expression profiling identifies molecular subtypes of gliomas. *Oncogene* 22(31): 4918-4923, 2003.

[16] Steiner G, Shaw A, Choo-Smith LP, Abuid MH, Schackert G, Sobottka S, Steller W, Salzer R, Mantsch HH: Distinguishing and grading human gliomas by IR spectroscopy. *Biopolymers* 72(6): 464-471, 2003.

[17] Son EI, Kim IM, Kim DW, Yim MB, Kang YN, Lee SS, Kwon KY, Suh SI, Kwon TK, Lee JJ, Kim DS, Kim SP: Immunohistochemical analysis for histopathological subtypes in pediatric medulloblastomas. *Pathol Int* 53(2): 67-73, 2003.

[18] Ellison D: Classifying the medulloblastoma: insights from morphology and molecular genetics. *Neuropathol Appl Neurobiol* 28(4): 257-82, 2002.

[19] Perry A: Medulloblastomas with favorable versus unfavorable histology: how many small blue cell tumor types are there in the brain? Adv Anat Pathol 9(6): 345-50, 2002.

[20] Ellison D: Classifying the medulloblastoma: insights from morphology and molecular genetics. *Neuropathol Appl Neurobiol* 28(4): 257-82, 2002.

[21] Rojiani AM, Dorovini-Zis K: Glomeruloid vascular structures in glioblastoma multiforme: an immunohistochemical and ultrastructural study. *J Neurosurg* 85: 1078-1084, 1996.

[22] Cairncross JG, Mattes MJ, Beresford HR, Albino AP, Houghton AN, Lloyd KO, Old LJ: Cell surface antigens of human astrocytoma defined by mouse monoclonal antibodies: identification of astrocytoma subsets. *Proc Natl Acad Sci* USA 79: 5641-5645, 1982.

[23] Rettig WJ, Nishimura H, Yenamandra AK, Seki T, Obata F, Beresford HR, Old LJ, Silver J: Differential expression of the human Thy-1 gene in rodent-human somatic cell hybrids. *J Immunol* 138: 4484-4489, 1987.

[24] Bodey B, Bodey B Jr, Gröger AM, Siegel SE, Kaiser HE: Clinical and prognostic significance of Ki-67 and proliferating cell nuclear antigen expression in childhood primitive neuroectodermal brain tumors. *Anticancer Res* 17: 189-196, 1997.

[25] Bodey B, Bodey B Jr, Siegel SE, Kaiser HE: Immunophenotypical analysis and immunobiology of childhood brain tumors. *Anticancer Res* 19: 2973-2992, 1999.

[26] Bodey B, Bodey B Jr, Siegel SE: Immunophenotypical (IP) differential diagnosis and immunobiology of childhood primary brain tumors. A decade of experience. *Int J Pediatric Hematol/Oncol* 6: 65-84, 1998.

[27] Bodey B, Taylor CR, Siegel SE, Kaiser HE: Immunocytochemical observation of multidrug resistance (MDR - p170) glycoprotein expression in human osteosarcoma cells. The clinical significance of MDR protein overexpression. *Anticancer Res* 15:2461-2468, 1995.

[28] Strojnik T, Lah TT, Zidanik B: Immunohistochemical staining of cathepsins B, L and stefin A in human hypophysis and pituitary adenomas. *Anticancer Res* 25: 587-594; 2005.

[29] Karim A, McCarthy K, Jawahar A, Smith D, Willis B, Nanda A: Differential cyclooxygenase-2 enzyme expression in radiosensitive versus radioresistant glioblastoma multiforme cell lines. *Anticancer Res* 25: 675-679; 2005.

[30] Purow BW, Haque RM, Noel MW, Su Q, Burdick MJ, Lee J, Sundaresan T, Pastorino S, Park JK, Mikolaenko I, Maric D, Eberhart CG, Fine HA: Expression of Notch-1 and its ligands, Delta-like-1 and Jagged-1, is critical for glioma cell survival and proliferation. *Cancer Res* 65: 2353-2363; 2005.

[31] Braun S, Pantel K: Diagnosis and clinical significance of disseminated tumor cells in bone marrow. *Dtsch Med Wochenschr* 125: 1237-1239, 2000.

[32] Vogel I, Kalthoff H: Disseminated tumour cells. Their detection and significance for prognosis of gastrointestinal and pancreatic carcinomas. *Virchows Archiv* 439: 109-117, 2001.

[33] Keene SA, Demeure MJ: The clinical significance of micrometastases and molecular metastases. *Surgery* 129: 1-5, 2001.

[34] Rampaul RS, Miremadi A, Pinder SE, Lee A, Ellis IO: Pathological validation and significance of micrometastasis in sentinel nodes in primary breast cancer. *Breast Cancer Research* 3: 113-116, 2001.

[35] Shi S-R, Key ME, Kalra KL: Antigen retrieval in formalin fixed, paraffin-embedded tissues: an enhancement method for immunohistochemical staining based on microwave oven heating of tissue sections. *J Histochem Cytochem* 39: 741-748, 1991.

[36] Shi S-R, Cote C, Kalra KL, Taylor CR, Tandon AK: A technique for retrieving antigens in formalin-fixed, routinely acid-decalcified, celloidin-embedded human temporal bone sections for immunohistochemistry. *J Histochem Cytochem* 40: 787-792, 1992.

[37] Key ME, Shi S-R, Kalra KL: *Antigen retrieval in formalin fixed tissues using microwave energy.* US Patent # 5,244,787; 14 September 1993.

[38] Beckstead JH: Improved antigen retrieval in formalin-fixed, paraffin-embedded tissues. *Appl Immunohistochem* 2: 274-281, 1994.

[39] Cuevas EC, Bateman AC, Wilkins BS, Johnson PA, Williams JH, Lee AH, Jones DB, Wright DH: Microwave antigen retrieval in immunocytochemistry: a study of 80 antibodies. *J Clin Pathol* 47: 448-452, 1994.

[40] Chen T, Zhang D, Shi S-R, Taylor CR: Antigen retrieval pretreatment: microwaving procedures and alternative heating methods. *BioLink* 4: 2, 1995.

[41] Shi SR, Cote RJ, and Taylor CR: Antigen retrieval techniques: current perspectives. *J Histochem Cytochem* 49: 931-937, 2001.

[42] Shi SR, Cote RJ, and Taylor CR: Antigen retrieval immunohistochemistry: past, present and future. *J Histochem Cytochem* 45: 327-343, 1997.

[43] Jay V, Edwards V, Halliday W, Rutka J, Lau R: "Polyphenotypic" tumors in the central nervous system: problems in nosology and classification. *Pediatr Pathol Lab Med* 17: 369-389, 1997.

[44] Beckmann MJ, Prayson RA: A clinicopathologic study of 30 cases of oligoastrocytoma including p53 immunohistochemistry. *Pathology* 29: 159-164, 1997.

[45] Krouwer HG, van Duinen SG, Kamphorst W, van der Valk P, Algra A: Oligoastrocytomas: a clinicopathological study of 52 cases. *J Neurooncol* 33: 223-238, 1997.

[46] Hirose T, Schneithauer BW, Lopes MB, Gerber HA, Altermatt HJ, VandenBerg SR: Ganglioglioma: an ultrastructural and immunohistochemical study. *Cancer* 79: 989-1003, 1997.

[47] Haapasalo J, Mennander A, Helen P, Haapasalo H, Isola J: Ultrarapid Ki-67 immunostaining in frozen section interpretation of gliomas. *J Clin Pathol* 58: 263-268; 2005.

[48] Baker DL, Molenaar WM, Trojanowski JQ, Evans AE, Ross AH, Rorke LB, Packer RJ, Lee VM, Pleasure D: Nerve growth factor receptor expression in peripheral and central neuroectodermal tumors, other pediatric brain tumors, and during development of the adrenal gland. *Am J Pathol* 139: 115-122, 1991.

[49] Kokunai T, Sawa H, Tamaki N: Functional analysis of trk proto-oncogene product in medulloblastoma cells. *Neurol Med Chir* 36: 796-804, 1996.

[50] Pruim J, Willemsen AT, Molenaar WM, van Waarde A, Paans AM, Heesters MA, Go KG,Visser GM, Franssen EJ, Vaalburg W: Brain tumors: L-[1-C-11]tyrosine PET for visualization and quantification of protein synthesis rate. *Radiology* 197: 221-226, 1995.

[51] de Wolde H, Pruim J, Mastik MF, Koudstaal J, Molenaar WM:Proliferative activity in human brain tumors: comparison of histopathology and L-[1-(11)C]tyrosine PET. *J Nucl Med* 38: 1369-1374, 1997.

[52] Sallinen P, Miettinen H, Sallinen SL, et al: Increased expression of telomerase RNA component is associated with increased cell proliferation in human astrocytomas. *Am J Pathol* 150: 1159-1164, 1997.

[53] Kyritsis AP, Bondy ML, Hess KR , et al: Prognostic significance of p53 immunoreactivity in patients with glioma. *Clin Cancer Res* 1: 1617-1622, 1995.

[54] Korshunov AG, Sycheva RV: An immunohistochemical study of the expression of the oncoprotein p53 in astrocytic gliomas of the cerebral hemispheres. *Arkh Patol* 58: 37-42, 1996.

[55] Bhattacharjee MB, Bruner JM: p53 protein in pediatric malignant astrocytomas: a study of 21 patients. *J Neurooncol* 32: 225-233, 1997.

[56] Ng HK, Lo SY, Huang DP, Poon WS: Paraffin section p53 protein immunohistochemistry in neuroectodermal tumors. *Pathology* 26: 1-5, 1994.

[57] Bodey B, Gröger AM, Bodey B Jr, Siegel SE, Kaiser HE: Immunocytochemical detection of p53 protein expression in various childhood astrocytoma subtypes: Significance in tumor progression. *Anticancer Res* 17: 1187-1194, 1997.

[58] Biernat W, Kleihues P, Yonekawa Y, Ohgaki H: Amplification and overexpression of MDM2 in primary (de novo) glioblastomas. *J Neuropathol Exp Neurol* 56: 180-185, 1997.

[59] Watanabe K, Tachibana O, Sata K, Yonekawa Y, Kleihues P, Ohgaki H: Overexpression of the EGF receptor and p53 mutations are mutually exclusive in the evolution of primary and secondary glioblastomas. *Brain Pathol* 6: 217-223, 1996.

[60] Korkolopoulou P, Christodoulou P, Kouzelis K, Hadjiyannakis M, Priftis A, Stamoulis G, Seretis A, Thomas-Tsagli E: MDM2 and p53 expression in gliomas: a multivariate survival analysis including proliferation markers and epidermal growth factor receptor. *Br J Cancer* 75: 1269-1278, 1997.

[61] Hagel C, Laking G, Laas R, Scheil S, Jung R, Milde-Langosch K, Stavrou DK: Demonstration of p53 protein and TP53 gene mutations in oligodendrogliomas. *Eur J Cancer* 32A: 2242-2248, 1996.

[62] Packham G, Cleveland J: c-Myc and apoptosis. Biochim Biophys Acta 1242: 11-28, 1995.

[63] Clarke AR, Purdie CA, Harrison DJ, Morris RG, Bird CC, Hooper ML, Wyllie AH: Thymocyte apoptosis induced by p53-dependent and independent pathways. *Nature* 362: 849-852, 1993.

[64] Strasser A, Harris AW, Jacks T, Cory S: DNA damage can induce apoptosis in proliferating lymphoid cells via p53-independent mechanisms inhibitable by Bcl-2. *Cell* 79: 329-339, 1994.

[65] Glickman JN, Yang A, Shahsafaei A, McKeon F, Odze RD: Expression of p53 related protein p63 in the gastrointestinal tract and in esophageal metaplastic and neoplastic disorders. *Hum Pathol* 32: 1157-1165, 2001.

[66] Bodey B, Gröger AM, Bodey B JR, Siegel SE, Kaiser HE: Immunocytochemical detection of p53 protein expression in various childhood astrocytoma subtypes: Significance in tumor progression. *Anticancer Res* 17: 1187-1194, 1997.

[67] Bodey B, Bodey B JR, Gröger AM, Luck JV, Siegel SE, Taylor CR, Kaiser HE: Immunocytochemical detection of the p170 multidrug resistance (MDR) and the p53 tumor suppressor gene proteins in human breast cancer cells: Clinical and therapeutical significance. *Anticancer Res* 17: 1311-1318, 1997.

[68] Fuchs EJ, McKenna KA, Bedi A: p53-dependent DNA damage-induced apoptosis requires Fas-APO-1-independent activation of CPP321. *Cancer Res* 57: 2550-2554, 1997.

[69] Graeber TG, Osmanian C, Jacks T, Housman DE, Koch CJ, Lowe SW, Giaccia AJ: Hypoxia-mediated selection of cells with diminished apoptotic potential in solid tumors. *Nature* 379: 88-91, 1996.

[70] Naumowski L, Clearly ML: Bcl-2 inhibits apoptosis associated with terminal differentiation of HL-60 myeloid leukemia cells. *Blood* 83: 2261-2266, 1994.

[71] Reed JC: Regulation of apoptosis by bcl-2 family proteins and its role in cancer and chemoresistance. *Curr Opin Oncol* 7: 541-546, 1995.

[72] Haldar S, Basu A, Croce CM: Bcl-2 is the guardian of microtubule integrity. *Cancer Res* 57: 229-233, 1997.

[73] Oltvai Z, Milliman C, Korsmeyer SJ: Bcl-2 heterodimerizes in vivo with a conserved homolog Bax that accelerates programmed cell death. *Cell* 74: 609-619, 1993.

[74] Pillai MR, Kesari AL, Chellam VG, Madhavan J, Nair P, Nair MK: Spontaneous programmed cell death in infiltrating duct carcinoma: association with p53, BCL-2, hormone receptors and tumor proliferation. *Pathol Res Pract* 194: 549-557, 1998.

[75] Yuan J, Horvitz HR: The Caenorhabditis elegans genes ced-3 and ced-4 act cell autonomously to cause programmed cell death. *Dev Biol* 138: 33-41, 1990.

[76] Hengartner MO, Ellis RE, Horvitz HR: Caenorhabditis elegans gene ced-9 protects cells from programmed cell death. *Nature* 356: 494-499, 1992.

[77] Steller H: Mechanisms and genes of cellular suicide. *Science* 267: 1445-1448, 1995.

[78] Reed JC: Bcl-2 and the regulation of programmed cell death. *J Cell Biol* 124: 1-6, 1994.

[79] Pourzand C, Rossier G, Reelfs O, Borner C, Tyrrell RM: The overexpression of bcl-2 inhibits UVA-mediated immediate apoptosis in rat 6 fibroblasts: evidence for the involvement of bcl-2 as an antioxidant. *Cancer Res* 57: 1405-1411, 1997.

[80] Alnermi ES, Livingston DJ, Nicholson DW, Salvesen G, Thornberry NA, Wong WW, Yuan J: Human ICE/CED-3 protease nomenclature. *Cell* 87: 171, 1996.

[81] Kumar S, Kinoshita M, Noda M, Copeland NG, Jenkins NA: Induction of apoptosis by the mouse Nedd 2 gene, which encodes a protein similar to the product of the Caenorhabditis elegans cell death gene ced-3 and the mammalian IL-1β-converting enzyme. *Genes Dev* 8: 1613-1626, 1994.

[82] Sinkovics JG: Malignant lymphoma arising from natural killer cells: report of the first case in 1970 and newer developments in the FasL-->FasR system. *Acta Microbiol Immunol Hung* 44: 295-303, 1997.

[83] Wang L, Miura M, Bergeron B, Zhu H, Yuan J: Ich-1, an ICE/Ced-3 related gene, encodes both positive and negative regulators of programmed cell death. *Cell* 78: 739-750, 1994.

[84] Kamens J, Paskind M, Hugunin M, Talanian RV, Allen H, Banach D, Bump N, Hackett M, Johnston CG, Li P, Mankovich JA, Terranova M, Ghayur T: Identification and characterization of ICH-2, a novel member of the interleukin-1β-converting enzyme family of cysteine proteases. *J Biol Chem* 270: 15250-15256, 1995.

[85] Fernandes-Alnemri T, Litwack G, Alnemri ES: CPP32, a novel human apoptotic protein with homology to Caenorhabditis elegans cell death protein Ced-3 and mammalian interleukin-1β-converting enzyme. *J Biol Chem* 269: 30761-30764, 1995.

[86] Fernandes-Alnemri T, Litwack G, Alnemri ES: Mch2, a new member of the apoptotic Ced-3/ICE cysteine protease gene family. *Cancer Res* 55: 2737-2742, 1995.

[87] Munday NA, Vaillancourt JP, Ali A, Casano FJ, Miller DK, Molineaux SM, Yamin TT, Yu VL, Nicholson DW: Molecular cloning and pro-apoptotic activity of ICErelII and

ICErelIII members of the ICE/Ced-3 family of cysteine proteases. *J Biol Chem* 270: 15870-15876, 1995.

[88] Duan H, Chinnaiyan AM, Hudson P, Wing JP, He WW, Dixit VM: ICE-LAP3, a novel mammalian homologue of of the Caenorhabditis elegans cell death protein Ced-3 is activated during Fas- and tumor necrosis factor-induced apoptosis. *J Biol Chem* 271: 1621-1625, 1996.

[89] Duan H, Orth K, Chinnaiyan AM, Poirier GG, Froelich CJ, He WW, Dixit VM: ICE-LAP6, a novel member of the ICE-Ced-3 gene family, is activated by the cytotoxic T cell protease granzyme B. *J Biol Chem* 271: 16720-16724, 1996.

[90] Boldin MP, Goncharov TM, Goltsev YV, Wallach D: Involvement of MACH, a novel MORT1/FADD-interacting protease, in Fas/APO-1 and TNF receptor-induced cell death. *Cell* 85: 803-815, 1996.

[91] Lazebnik YA, Kaufmann SH, Desnoyers S, Poirier GG, Earnshaw WC: Cleavage of poly(ADP-ribose) polymerase by a proteinase with properties like ICE. *Nature* 371: 346-347, 1994.

[92] Nicholson DW, Ali A, Thornberry NA, Vaillancourt JP, Ding CK, Gallant M, Gareau Y, Griffin PR, Labelle M, Lazebnik YA: Identification and inhibition of the ICE/CED-3 protease necessary for mammalian apoptosis. *Nature* 376: 37-43, 1995.

[93] Sorensen CM: Apoptosis or planning a death. *Biomedical Products* (September, 1996 issue), pp 38-39, 1996.

[94] Asano K, Kubo O, Tajika Y, Huang MC, Takakura K, Ebina K, Suzuki S: Expression and role of cadherins in astrocytic tumors. *Brain Tumor Pathol* 14: 27-33, 1997.

[95] Huber O: Structure and function of desmosomal proteins and their role in development and disease. *Cell Mol Life Sci* 60: 1872-1890, 2003.

[96] Strelkov SV, Herrmann H, Aebi U: Molecular architecture of intermediate filaments. *Bioessays* 25: 243-251, 2003.

[97] Hasegawa K, Yoshida T, Matsumoto K, Katsuta K, Waga S, Sakakura T: Differential expression of tenascin-C and tenascin-X in human astrocytomas. *Acta Neuropathol* (Berl) 93: 431-437, 1997.

[98] Gilbertson RJ, Perry RH, Kelly PJ, Pearson AD, Lunec J: Prognostic significance of HER2 and HER4 coexpression in childhood medulloblastoma. *Cancer Res* 57: 3272-3280, 1997.

[99] Aaronson SA: Growth factors and cancer. *Science* 254: 1146-1153; 1991.

[100] Engebraaten O, Bjerkvig R, Humphrey PA, Bigner SH, Bigner DD, Laerum OD: Effect of EGF, bFGF, NGF and PDGF(bb) on cell proliferative, migratory and invasive capacities of human brain-tumour biopsies in vitro. *Int J Cancer* 53: 209-214, 1993.

[101] Chicoine MR, Madsen CL, Silbergeld DL: Modification of human glioma locomotion in vitro by cytokines EGF, bFGF, PDGFbb, NGF, and TNFβ. Neurosurg 36: 1165-1171, 1995.

[102] U HS, Espiritu OD, Kelley PY, Klauber MR, Hatton JD: The role of the epidermal growth factor receptor in human gliomas: I. The control of cell growth. *J Neurosurg* 82: 841-846, 1995.

[103] Hitotsumatsu T, Iwaki T, Kitamoto T, Mizoguchi M, Suzuki SO, Hamada Y, Fukui M, Tateishi J: Expression of neurofibromatosis 2 protein in human brain tumors: an immunohistochemical study. *Acta Neuropathol* 93: 225-232, 1997.

[104] Chang F, Li R, Noon K, Gage D, Ladisch S: Human medulloblastoma gangliosides. *Glycobiology* 7: 523-530, 1997.

[105] Leung SY, Wong MP, Chung LP, Chan AS, Yuen ST: Monocyte chemoattractant protein-1 expression and macrophage infiltration in gliomas. *Acta Neuropathol* 93: 518-527, 1997.

[106] Guo P, Imanishi Y, Cackowski FC, Jarzynka MJ, Tao HQ, Nishikawa R, Hirose T, Hu B, Cheng SY: Up-regulation of angiopoietin-2, matrix metalloprotease-2, membrane type 1 metalloprotease, and laminin 5 gamma 2 correlates with the invasiveness of human glioma. *Am J Pathol* 166: 877-890, 2005.

[107] Ingber DE: Mechanical signaling and the cellular response to extracellular matrix in angiogenesis and cardiovascular physiology. *Circ Res* 91: 877-887, 2002.

[108] Moffett JR, Els T, Espey MG, Walter SA, Streit WJ, Namboodiri MA: Quinolinate immunoreactivity in experimental rat brain tumors is present in macrophages but not in astrocytes. *Exp Neurol* 144: 287-301, 1997.

[109] Boon T, Old LJ: Tumor antigens. *Curr Opin Immunol* 9: 681-683, 1997.

[110] Bruggen P van der, Traversari C, Chomez P et al.: A gene encoding an antigen recognized by cytolytic T lymphocytes on a human melanoma. *Science* 254: 1643-1647, 1991.

[111] Boel P, Wildmann C, Sensi ML et al.: BAGE: a new gene encoding an antigen recognized on human melanomas by cytolytic T lymphocytes. *Immunity* 2: 167-175, 1995.

[112] Ma Z, Khatlani TS, Li L et al.: Molecular cloning and expression analysis of feline melanoma antigen (MAGE) obtained from a lymphoma cell line. *Vet Immunol Immunopathol* 83(3-4): 241-252, 2001.

[113] Weiser TS, Ohnmacht GA, Guo ZS et al.: Induction of MAGE-3 expression in lung and esophageal cancer cells. *Ann Thorac Surg* 71: 295-301; discussion 301-302, 2001.

[114] Chomez P, De Backer O, Bertrand M et al.: An overview of the MAGE gene family with the identification of all human members of the family. *Cancer Res* 61: 5544-5551, 2001.

[115] Ohman Forslund K, Nordqvist K: The melanoma antigen genes--any clues to their functions in normal tissues? *Exp Cell Res* 265: 185-194, 2001.

[116] De Plaen E, Arden K, Traversari C et al.: Structure, chromosomal localization, and expression of 12 genes of the MAGE family. *Immunogenetics* 40: 360-369, 1994.

[117] Rogner Uc, Wilke K, Steck E, Korn B, Poutska A: The melanoma antigen (MAGE) family is clustered in the chromosomal band Xq28. *Genomics* 29: 725-731, 1995.

[118] Lurquin C, De Smet C, Brasseur F et al.: Two members of th human MAGEB gene family loacted in Xp21.3 are expressed in tumors of various histological origins. *Genomics* 46: 397-408, 1997.

[119] Lucas S, De Smet C, Arden KC, Viars CS, Lethe B, Lurquin C, Boon T: Identification of a new MAGE gene with tumor-specific expression by representational difference analysis. *Cancer Res* 58: 743-752, 1998.

[120] Pold M, Zhou J, Chen GL et al.: Identification of a new, unorthodox member of the MAGE gene family. *Genomics* 59: 161-167, 1999.

[121] Aubry F, Satie AP, Rioux-Leclercq N et al.: MAGE-A4, a germ cell specific marker, is expressed differentially in testicular tumors. *Cancer* 92: 2778-2785, 2001.

[122] Gillespie AM, Coleman RE: The potential of melanoma antigen expression in cancer therapy. *Cancer Treat Rev* 25: 219-227, 1999.

[123] Chen Y-T, Old LJ: Cancer-testis antigens: targets for cancer immunotherapy. *Cancer J from Scientific American* 5: 16-17, 1999.

[124] Marchand M, Baren N Van, Weynants P et al.: Tumor regressions observed in patients with metastatic melanoma treated with an antigenic peptide encoded by gene MAGE-3 and presented by HLA-A1. *Int J Cancer* 80: 219-230, 1999.

[125] De Backer O, Arden KC, Boretti M et al.: Characterization of the GAGE genes that are expressed in various human cancers and in normal testis. *Cancer Res* 59: 3157-3165, 1999.

[126] Van Den Eynde B, Peeters O, De Backer O et al.: A new family of genes coding for an antigen recognized by autologous cytolytic T lymphocytes. *J Exp Med* 182: 689-698, 1995.

[127] Chen ME, Lin SH, Chung LW, Sikes RA: Isolation and characterization of PAGE-1 and GAGE-7. New genes expressed in the LNCaP prostate cancer progression model that share homology with melanoma-associated antigens. *J Biol Chem* 273: 17618-17625, 1998.

[128] Brinkmann U, Vasmatzis G, Lee B et al.: PAGE-1, an X chromosoma-linked GAGE-like gene that is expressed in normal and neoplastic prostata, testis and uterus. *Proc Natl Acad Sci USA* 95: 10757-10762, 1998.

[129] Brinkmann U, Vasmatzis G, Lee B, Pastan I: Novel genes in the PAGE and GAGE family of tumor antigens found by homology walking in the dbEST database. *Cancer Res* 59: 1445-1448, 1999.

[130] Liu XF, Helman LJ, Yeung C et al.: XAGE-1, a new gene that is frequently expressed in Ewing's sarcoma. *Cancer Res* 60: 4752-4755, 2000.

[131] Zendman AJ, Van Kraats AA, Den Hollander AI et al.: Characterization of XAGE-1b, a short major transcript of cancer/testis-associated gene XAGE-1, induced in melanoma metastasis. *Int J Cancer* 97: 195-204, 2002.

[132] Ono T, Kurashige T, Harada N: Identification of proacrosin binding protein sp32 precursor as a human cancer/testis antigen. *Proc Natl Acad Sci USA* 98: 3282-3287, 2001.

[133] Sahin U, Koslowski M, Tureci O et al.: Expression of cancer testis genes in human brain tumors. *Clin Cancer Res* 6: 3916-3922, 2000.

[134] Haffner AC, Tassis A, Zepter K et al.: Expression of cancer/testis antigens in cutaneous T cell lymphomas. *Int J Cancer* 97: 668-670, 2002.

[135] Mashino K, Sadanaga N, Tanaka F et al.: Expression of multiple cancer-testis antigen genes in gastrointestinal and breast carcinomas. *Br J Cancer* 85: 713-720, 2001.

[136] Chen CH, Chen GJ, Lee HS et al.: Expressions of cancer-testis antigens in human hepatocellular carcinomas. *Cancer Lett* 164: 189-195, 2001.

[137] Clark J, Rocques PJ, Crew AJ et al.: Identification of novel genes, SYT and SSX, involved in the t(x;18) (p11.2;q11.2) translocation found in human synovial sarcoma. *Nat Genet* 7: 502-508, 1994.

[138] Jungbluth AA, Antonescu CR, Busam KJ et al.: Monophasic and biphasic synovial sarcomas abundantly express cancer/testis antigen NY-ESO-1 but not MAGE-A1 or CT7. *Int J Cancer* 94: 252-256, 2001.

[139] Jang SJ, Soria JC, Wang L et al.: Activation of melanoma antigen tumor antigens occurs early in lung carcinogenesis. *Cancer Res* 61: 7959-7963, 2001.

[140] Eifuku R, Takenoyama M, Yoshino I et al.: Analysis of MAGE-3 derived synthetic peptide as a human lung cancer antigen recognized by cytotoxic T lymphocytes. *Int J Clin Oncol* 6: 34-39, 2001.

[141] Goydos JS, Patel M, Shih W: NY-ESO-1 and CTp11 expression may correlate with stage of progression in melanoma. *J Surg Res* 98: 76-80, 2001.

[142] Romero P, Dutoit V, Rubio-Godoy V et al.: CD8+ T-cell response to NY-ESO-1: relative antigenicity and in vitro immunogenicity of natural and analogue sequences. *Clin Cancer Res* 7: 766s-772s, 2001.

[143] Wang T, Fan L, Watanabe Y, Mcneill P et al.: L552S, an alternatively spliced isoform of XAGE-1, is over-expressed in lung adenocarcinoma. *Oncogene* 20: 7699-7709, 2001.

[144] Tureci O, Chen Yt, Sahin U et al.: Expression of SSX genes in human tumors. *Int J Cancer* 77: 19-23, 1998.

In: Leading Topics in Cancer Research
Editor: Lee P. Jeffries, pp. 35-72

ISBN 1-60021-332-4
© 2007 Nova Science Publishers, Inc.

Chapter 2

GENE SILENCING IN TUMORS: THE ROLE OF THE RAS ASSOCIATION DOMAIN FAMILY 1 GENE IN CARCINOGENESIS

Reinhard Dammann [*]

AG Tumorgenetik der Medizinischen Fakultät,
Martin-Luther-Universität Halle-Wittenberg, Germany

ABSTRACT

Epigenetic silencing of tumor suppressor genes plays an important role in the pathogenesis of human cancer. Especially, hypermethylation of the promoter regions of cancer-related genes is often observed in tumors. Recently, a novel tumor suppressor gene, which was termed Ras association domain family 1 (RASSF1A) gene was characterized by its frequent epigenetic silencing in human tumors. RASSF1 consists of two main variants (RASSF1A and RASSF1C), which are transcribed from distinct CpG island promoters. Aberrant methylation of the RASSF1A promoter region is one of the most frequent epigenetic inactivation events detected in human cancer and leads to silencing of RASSF1A. Silencing of RASSF1A was commonly observed in primary tumors including lung, breast, pancreas, kidney, liver, cervix, nasopharyngeal, prostate, thyroid and other cancers. Moreover, RASSF1A methylation was frequently detected in body fluids including blood, urine, nipple aspirates, sputum and bronchial alveolar lavages. Inactivation of RASSF1A was associated with an advanced tumor stage (e.g. bladder, brain, prostate, gastric tumors) and poor prognosis (e.g. lung, sarcoma and breast cancer). Detection of aberrant RASSF1A methylation may serve as a diagnostic and prognostic marker. The functional analyses of RASSF1A reveal an involvement in apoptotic signaling, microtubule stabilization and mitotic progression. The tumor suppressor RASSF1A may act as a negative Ras effector inhibiting cell growth and

[*] Correspondence: AG Tumorgenetik der Medizinischen Fakultät, Martin-Luther-Universität Halle-Wittenberg, Magdeburger Straße 2, 06097 Halle/Saale, Germany; Tel: 49-345-557-4537; Fax: 49-345-557-4293; E-mail: reinhard.dammann@medizin.uni-halle.de

inducing cell death. Thus, RASSF1A represents a tumor suppressor gene, which is frequently epigenetically silenced in the pathogenesis of human cancers.

ABBREVIATIONS

RASSF   Ras-association domain family;
NORE   novel Ras effector;
LOH   loss of heterozygosity;
RA domain   RalGDS/AF6 Ras-association domain;
aa   amino acid;
5-aza-CdR   5-aza-2'-deoxycytidine;
SV40   simian virus 40;
EBV   Epstein-Barr virus;
HPV   human papilloma virus,
ATM   ataxia telangiectasia mutated;
DAG   diacylglycerol;
C1   protein kinase C conserved region 1;
SCC   squamous cell carcinoma;
AC   adenocarcinoma;
SCLC   small cell lung cancer;
NSCLC   non-small cell lung cancer.

INTRODUCTION

Epigenetic silencing of tumor suppressor gene promoters plays a fundamental role in the etiology of cancer [85]. Inactivation of cancer-related genes is mediated through remodeling of chromatin structure, which is correlated to changes in DNA methylation and histone modifications. Gene promoters are often located in CpG-rich DNA regions, so called CpG islands [17]. Active promoters are associated with unmethylated CpG islands and open chromatin structure for transcription regulators (Figure 1). Whereas inactive promoters are in a repressed chromatin structure and the CpGs are hypermethylated (Figure 1). Acetylation of lysines at histones H3 leads to active chromatin and deacetylation is correlated with a repressed chromatin structure [81]. Methylation of histone lysine 9 residue of histone H3 is associated with promoters of inactive genes (Figure 1). Methyl-CpG binding proteins (MBPs) provide a link between methylated DNA and hypoacetylated histones by recruiting histone deacetylases [86, 136]. DNA methyltransferases, which are responsible for the maintenance of methylated DNA and necessary for the establishment of newly methylated promoters, were shown to be associated with proteins including Rb, E2F1, histone deacetylases and a transcriptional repressor [55, 148, 151]. It has been proposed the DNA methylation may be directed by alterations in the chromatin structure [16]. Several studies indicate an altered DNA methylation pattern when components of the chromatin-remodeling system, such as SNF2 like factors were mutated [37, 61, 80]. In *Neurospora crassa* and in *Arabidopsis thaliana*, it has been shown that a repressive chromatin modification, like histone H3 lysine 9

(H3-K9) methylation can direct DNA methylation [78, 170]. In vertebrate, it has been reported that Suv39h-mediated H3-K9 methylation directs DNA methylation to major satellite repeats at pericentric heterochromatin [112]. It has been shown that methylated CpG sites attract methyl CpG binding proteins (MBPs) that interact with the co-repressor complex Sin3 including histone deacetylases [86, 136, 138]. Other studies indicate that DNA methyltransferase and MBP interact with histone methlytransferase [56, 57]. In cancer cells, aberrant DNA methylation may maintain the repressed epigenetic state. This may lead to silencing of tumor suppressor genes, which is irreversible since the presence of an active DNA demethylase in mammalian cells is not evident. It has been shown that the heterochromatin protein 1 (Hp1) isoforms bind to methylated H3-K9 residues [11, 107, 135]. Recently, a link between the Suv39h-Hp1 histone methylation system and the DNA methyltransferase 3b in mammals was demonstrated [112]. Thus Hp1 and MBD may be responsible to lock and maintain the repressed chromatin together with the DNA methyltransferases in silenced cells (Figure 1).

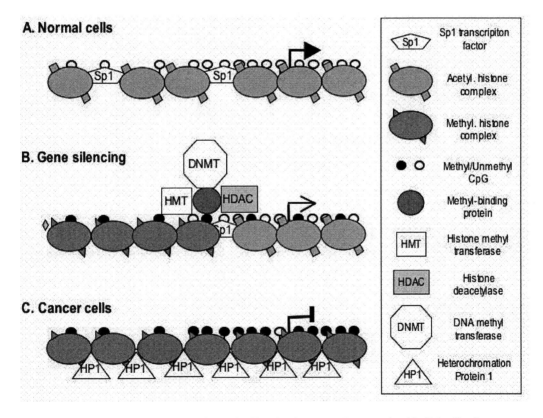

Figure 1. Model of the progressive epigenetic silencing in cancer. In normal epithelial cells, the promoter is transcriptionally active and histones are acetylated and CpGs island is unmethylated (white dots). The open chromatin structure allows binding of the transcription factor Sp1. In senescent cells, silencing is associated with histone deacetylation and methylatio, which is accomplished by histone deacetylase (HDAC) and histone methyltransferase (HMT), respectively. The repressed chromatin structured triggers the *de novo* methylation of CpGs (black dots) by DNA methyl transferase (DNMT). In cancer cells, the inactive state is locked and maintained by Methyl-CpG binding domain proteins (MBD) and heterochromatin protein 1 (Hp1).

In a model of aging and cancer it has been postulated that an age-related CpG island methylation of tumor suppressor genes leads to a hyperproliferative epithelium, but further hypermethylation needs to occur for tumor formation [77]. It has been suggested that a dramatic stop in transcription is the critical precursor in cancer, which is followed by *de novo* methylation and ends with a complete cessation of gene expression [27, 187]. Recent studies have demonstrated that the CpG islands of the Rb, p16, VHL, APC, MLH1 and BRCA1 genes are frequently methylated in a variety of human cancers, but are largely methylation-free in the corresponding normal tissues [4, 85]. It is remarkable that as many, if not more, tumor suppressor genes are silenced by promoter hypermethylation as they are by coding-region mutations. Therefore, epigenetic silencing of tumor suppressor genes plays a key role in human carcinogenesis. Recently, the novel tumor suppressor RASSF1A was identified, which is frequently inactivated in a variety of human cancers. Silencing of RASSF1A is one of the most common epigenetic events, which occurs in the pathogenesis of human tumors.

IDENTIFICATION AND CHARACTERIZATION OF *RASSF1*

Loss of the short arm of chromosome 3 is the earliest and most common alteration, which occurs in the pathogenesis of lung cancer. Several distinct regions are lost, including 3p12, 3p14, 3p21 and 3p24-25 [99]. In these segments, the van Hippel-Lindau disease (*VHL*) gene at 3p25 [87], the gene *FHIT* at 3p14.2 [167], and the *DUTT1/ROBO1* gene at 3p12 [206] have been identified. At segment 3p21.3 heterozygous and homozygous deletions have been described in several cancer cell lines and in primary lung tumors [95, 99, 172, 197, 198, 209]. Allelic loss at 3p21.3 is not limited to lung cancer indicating that this segment may encode a general tumor suppressor. Other tumors with 3p21 involvement include head and neck cancer, renal cell carcinoma, bladder cancer, female genital tract tumors and breast cancer [99]. The region of minimum homozygous deletion at 3p21.3 was narrowed to a fragment of 120 kb using several cancer cell lines [158].

Recently, we and others have cloned the RASSF1 gene from the common homozygous deletion area at 3p21.3 [30, 113]. RASSF1 was isolated through the interaction with the human DNA excision repair protein XPA in a yeast two-hybrid screen [30]. The 1.7 kb cDNA matched the sequences of the minimum homozygous deletion region of 120 kb [158] that may contain the tumor suppressor gene at 3p21.3. The C-terminus of RASSF1 shows high homology (ca. 55% identity) to the murine Ras-effector protein Norel [190] and encodes a Ras-association domain (Figure 2). Therefore, the gene has been termed Ras-association domain family 1 gene [30]. Homology searches and additional cDNA screenings revealed the presence of seven alternatively spliced transcripts: RASSF1A, RASSF1B, RASSF1C, RASSF1D, RASSF1E, RASSF1F and RASSF1G [30, 34]. The two major forms RASSF1A and RASSF1C are transcribed from two distinct CpG island promoters, which are approximately 3.5 kb apart (Figure 2). Both transcripts have four common exons (3 to 6) at their 3' end (Figure 2). These exons encode the RA domain (R194 to S288) [141]. RASSF1A has two 5' exons, designated 1α and 2αβ. The cDNA is 1.9 kb long and contains an ORF of 340 amino acids (aas) with a calculated MW of 38.8 kDa. The N-terminus (H52 to C101) of RASSF1A has high homology to a cysteine-rich diacylglycerol/phorbol ester-binding (DAG) domain, also known as the protein kinase C conserved region (C1), which contains a central

C1 zinc finger [137]. RASSF1A is expressed in all normal tissues tested by Northern blot analysis, but was missing in several cancer cell lines [30]. Transcript RASSF1C is 1.7 kb long and transcription initiates in exon 2γ located at the CpG island C (Figure 2). The cDNA encodes a 270 aas protein with an MW of 31.2 kDa. The protein sequence translated from the first exon 2γ has no significant similarity to any known protein. RASSF1C is transcribed in all normal tissue and cancer cells tested [30]. The aa sequence W125 to K138 (WETPDLSQAEIEQK) of RASSF1A matches a putative ATM kinase phosphorylation consensus motif and in a peptide with this sequence serine is effectively phosphorylated *in vitro* [98]. Recent data show that RASSF1A interacts with the microtubule and stabilizes the cytoskeleton and centrosome [121]. The microtubule association and stabilization domain (MAS) was located at the C-terminus (194 to 288) of RASSF1A (Figure 2).

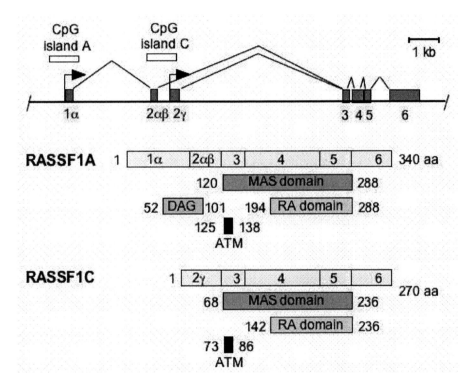

Figure 2. Map of the RASSF1 gene. The two promoters of RASSF1 (arrows) are located in CpG islands (open squares). Two major isoforms (RASSF1A and RASSF1C) are made by alternative promoter usage and splicing of the exons (black boxes). The cDNA of RASSF1A is 1.9 kb long and contains an ORF of 340 amino acids (aas) with a calculated MW of 38.8 kDa. Transcript RASSF1C is 1.7 kb long and initiates in exon 2γ located at the CpG island C. The cDNA encodes a 270 aas protein with a MW of 31.2 kDa. The protein domains are indicated as: DAG, diacylglycerol/phorbol ester binding domain; RA, RalGDS/AF6 Ras-association domain; and ATM, putative ATM phosphorylation site consensus sequence; MAS, microtubule association and stabilization domain.

The expression of RASSF1A and RASSF1C have been analyzed in a variety cell lines and tissues. In all normal cells both forms, RASSF1A and RASSF1C, are highly expressed [30]. RASSF1A expression is missing in several cancer cell lines including non-small cell lung cancer (NSCLC), small cell lung cancer (SCLC), breast carcinoma, nasopharyngeal carcinoma, renal cell carcinoma, and thyroid carcinoma [18, 30-32, 42, 122, 154]. In contrast, RASSF1C was expressed in all analyzed samples without homozygous deletion of 3p21.3 [18, 30-32, 154]. Loss of expression was correlated with hypermethylation of the CpG island of the RASSF1A promoter [1, 30]. In addition, reversion of the epigenetic silencing by treatment with a DNA methylation inhibitor, 5-aza-2'-deoxycytidine (5-aza-CdR), leads to re-expression of RASSF1A in various cancer cell lines [8, 18, 19, 30, 32, 122, 154].

METHYLATION OF RASSF1A IN HUMAN TUMORS

Epigenetic silencing of tumor suppressor genes by aberrant methylation is a fundamental inactivation mechanism of cancer-related genes in the pathogenesis of human cancer [66, 85]. Promoter hypermethylation of RASSF1A was frequently detected in primary human tumors and this methylation was correlated with several additional observations (Table 1). In bladder cancer, high frequency of RASSF1A methylation was observed and was correlated with advanced tumor stage and poor prognosis [21, 45, 108, 126]. In brain cancer, RASSF1A methylation was often detected in neuroblastoma, astrocytoma, glioblastoma and medulloblastoma, however it was less frequent found in benign tumors [8-10, 60, 68, 73, 118, 123, 145, 212, 215]. In benign ganglioneuroma, RASSF1A methylation was not observed [212]. Aberrant methylation of RASSF1A was rarely detected in gallbladder carcinoma and chronic cholecystitis, but was frequently observed in bile duct carcinoma and ampullary carcinoma [169, 185]. Methylation of RASSF1A was frequently found in breast cancer and in serum of breast cancer patients [1, 18, 23, 32, 49, 70, 102, 111, 131, 133]. In cervical cancer, RASSF1A promoter methylation was found in certain tumor types (Table 1) [1, 28, 92, 105, 216]. Kuzmin et al. (2003) have reported an inverse correlation between methylation of RASSF1A and human papilloma virus infection. In cholangiocarcinoma, 65 to 69% of RASSF1A promoter hypermethylation were observed [201, 211]. In colorectal carcinoma, RASSF1A methylation was less frequently found [110, 189, 194, 208, 214]. Interestingly, RASSF1A methylation occurs significantly in colorectal carcinoma with K-ras wild type [152, 188]. In 52% of esophageal squamous cell carcinoma, RASSF1A methylation was reported and correlated with an advanced tumor stage [103]. In gastric cancer, RASSF1A hypermethylation was more frequently found in the advanced tumor stage and in EBV positive carcinoma (Table 1); however, RASSF1A methylation was rarely detected in non-carcinoma tumor samples [19, 74, 88-90, 171]. In head and neck cancer, RASSF1A methylation frequency is less than 20% [40, 65, 69, 125]. Dong el al. 2003 have reported an inverse correlation between RASSF1A methylation and HPV infection (Table 1). In hepatocellular carcinoma, intensive RASSF1A methylation was detected and methylation was also found in adjacent non-cancerous tissue, cirrhosis and hepatitis [109, 155, 216, 217]. In Hodgkins' lymphoma, 65% of RASSF1A methylation was reported [134]. Several reports have investigated the methylation status of RASSF1A in renal cell carcinoma and kidney tumors [13, 42, 43, 62, 132, 173, 214]. In papillary renal cell carcinoma, RASSF1A was frequently inactivated (Table 1). Intensive methylation (>70%) of RASSF1A was reported in small cell lung cancer (SCLC). In non small cell lung cancer (NSCLC), RASSF1A hypermethylation is common and correlated with impaired prognosis and with starting smoking under age 18 [1, 18, 30, 31, 47, 70, 76, 96, 97, 115, 124, 128, 145, 174, 179, 181,

183, 196, 210, 218]. In malignant mesothelioma, 32% of RASSF1A inactivation was found and correlated with the presence of SV40 [180, 182]. In melanoma, frequent RASSF1A methylation was reported in several studies [58, 72, 147, 168]. Reifenberger et al. (2004) observed that tumors with RASSF1A methylation additionally carried BRAF and NRAS mutations, suggesting a synergistic effect of these aberrations on melanoma growth. In less than 30% of multiple myeloma cases, RASSF1A methylation was found [59, 139, 157]. In nasopharyngeal carcinoma, aberrant RASSF1A methylation was frequently (> 50%) observed [22, 106, 122, 178, 202, 203] and occurred in 39% of EBV associated nasopharyngeal carcinoma (Table 1). In 40% of osteosarcoma, hypermethylation of RASSF1A occurred [117]. In ovarian cancer frequent RASSF1A methylation was demonstrated in several studies [1, 36, 38, 146, 214] and also detected in granulosa cell tumors [38]. In endocrine tumors of the pancreas, the frequency of RASSF1A inactivation was higher compared to pancreatic adenocarcinoma (83% versus 64%) [33, 75]. We have reported an inverse correlation between RASSF1A silencing and K-ras mutation in pancreatic cancer. In pediatric tumors, RASSF1A methylation was found in Wilms' tumor, medulloblastoma, retinoblastoma, rhabdomyosarcoma, neuroblastoma, hepatoblastoma, leukemia, pancreatoblastoma, adrenocortical carcinoma and lymphoma [46, 64, 194, 200]. In hereditary pheochromocytoma, RASSF1A methylation was more common compared to the sporadic tumors [8, 35]. In prostate cancer, high frequency of RASSF1A methylation was reported in several studies and correlated with an advanced Gleason score (Table 1) [52, 82, 91, 104, 120, 127, 162, 204, 205]. However, methylation was also observed in several non-carcinoma specimen from matched tumor-normal samples and in benign prostatic hyperplasia. RASSF1A methylation was detected in different entities of soft tissue sarcoma, including leiomyosarcoma [156]. In testicular germ cell tumors, most studies have detected that RASSF1A methylation occurs frequently [71, 93, 100, 101]. Interestingly, RASSF1A methylation occurred more often in cisplatin-resistant tumors (Table 1). In thyroid cancer, RASSF1A hypermethylation was frequently detected in the more aggressive carcinomas [154, 207]. In papillary thyroid cancer, an inverse correlation between RASSF1A methylation and BRAF mutation was reported (Table 1).

In general, RASSF1A methylation frequency is higher in cancer cell lines compared to the primary tumors. These additional changes could be attributed to *de novo* methylation, which occurs when cells are kept in culture [5, 84, 163]. In cell lines with an inactivated RASSF1A gene treatment with 5-aza-CdR reactivated the expression of RASSF1A (Table 1). In principal, methylation of RASSF1A is rarely detected in normal tissue, however methylation was also found in some non-cancerogenous tissue specimen. For instance RASSF1 methylation was detected in adjacent normal tissue of prostate, kidney, thyroid and liver cancer patients (Table 1). This methylation may represent infiltration of tumor cells into normal tissue or a field defect leading to carcinogenesis.

When quantitative methylation analysis was applied to determine the methylation level of RASSF1A in breast, prostate and thyroid tissue no significant methylation was detected in non-neoplastic tissue [111, 207, 213]. Recently, hypermethylation of several cancer-related genes (e.g. p16, MGMT, DAP-kinase, RASSF1A, COX2 and RARß) was detected in histologically negative bronchial margins of resected NSCLC [63]. This hypermethylation may represent a field defect of preneoplastic changes that occurs early in carcinogenesis or may be related to aging [77, 195].

Table 1. RASSF1A methylation in primary human tumors

Tumor entity	Methylation	Ref.	Remarks
Bladder cancer	60% (33/55)	[108]	Inactivation of RASSF1A was correlated with advanced tumor stage
	35% (34/98)	[126]	RASSF1A methylation correlated with parameters of poor prognosis
	48% (19/40)	[21]	RASSF1A methylation was more frequent in cases with LOH at 3p21.3 (73%) compared to cases without LOH (13%; p=0.007). RASSF1A methylation was found in 50% (7/14) of urine samples; no false positives.
Bladder cancer	51% (23/45)	[45]	RASSF1A hypermethylation was found in all pathological grades and stages of bladder cancer and in patients of all ages; in 87% (39/45) of the cases hypermethylation of RASSF1A, APC or p14^{ARF} could be detected in urine of the bladder cancer patients.
Biliary tract cancer	0% (0/50)	[169]	Gallbladder carcinoma; No methylation of RASSF1A was detected in chronic cholecystitis
	11% (1/9)	[185]	Gallbladder carcinoma
	30% (7/23)	[185]	Bile duct carcinoma
	40% (2/5)	[185]	Ampullary carcinoma
Brain cancer	55% (37/67)	[8]	Neuroblastoma; RASSF1A was reexpressed after treatment with 5-aza- CdR in neuroblastoma cell lines
	54% (25/46)	[73]	Glioma
	100% (5/5)	[73]	Medulloblastoma
	10% (1/10)	[73]	Schwannoma (benign)
	17% (2/12)	[73]	Meningioma (benign)
	79% (27/34)	[123]	Epigenetic inactivation by biallelic hypermethylation represents the primary mechanism of RASSF1A inactivation in medulloblastoma.
	93% (41/44)	[118]	Medulloblastoma; in 57% of the cases a total methylation was detected; methylation in all histopathological and clinical disease subtypes100% (11/11) in medulloblastoma cell lines and RASSF1A was reexpressed after treatment with 5-aza-CdR
	57% (36/63)	[68]	Glioma; RASSF1A methylation increased with tumor grade (40% grade II, 53% grade III, 63% grade IV); no association between RASSF1A and BLU methylation; 100% (7/7) in glioma cell lines; reexpression of RASSF1A suppressed the growth of glioma cell line.
	57% (12/21)	[10]	Glioblastoma; a tendency for a longer time to progression for patients with methylated RASSF1A promoter was observed; 50% (13/26) in serum samples
	57% (16/28)	[145]	Glioblastoma; 50% in serum; high correlation between methylation in tumor and serum was observed (Spearman test p=0.0001)

Table 1. RASSF1A methylation in primary human tumors (Continued)

Tumor entity	Methylation	Ref.	Remarks
Brain cancer	55%	[9]	Neuroblastoma; RASSF1A promoter hypermethylataion was more frequent in neuroblastomas with SLIT2 promoter methylation (p= 0.32); inverse relationship between SLIT2 and RASSF1A promoter hypermethylation in Wilms tumor (p= 0.09); no associations with clinicopathological features
	70% (37/53)	[215]	Astrocytoma; RASSF1C was completely unmethylated
	32% (13/14)	[60]	Glioblastoma
	70% (39/56)	[212]	Neuroblastoma; RASSF1A methylation was not found in benign ganglioneuromas; RASSF1A methylation was associated with age($>$1; $p<0.01$), high-risk disease ($p<0.016$) and poor survival ($p<0.001$)
Breast cancer	62% (28/45)	[32]	RASSF1A was reexpressed after treatment with 5-aza-CdR in breast cancer cell lines
	9% (4/44)	[1]	
	49% (19/39)	[18]	
	56% (20/36)	[111]	RASSF1A methylation was detected in epithelial hyperplasia, but not in normal tissue
	58% (54/93)	[23]	
	65% (11/17)	[70]	Invasive breast cancer
	42% (5/12)	[70]	Ductal carcinoma in-situ
	62% (8/13)	[49]	Lobular carcinoma in-situ
	84% (16/19)	[49]	Invasive lobular cancer
	70% (19/27)	[49]	Invasive breast cancer
	75%	[49]	Ductal carcinoma in-situ
	23% (n=26)	[133]	Serum DNA from primary breast cancer patients: patients with methylated RASSF1A and/or APC serum DNA was strongly associated with poor outcome, with a relative risk for death of 5.7 ($p<0.001$); 80% (n=10) in serum DNA from recurrent breast cancer patients.
	56% (14/25)	[131]	Primary breast cancer, additional analyses of metastases : 78% (7/9) bone; 67% (4/6) brain; 100% (10/10) lung; higher prevalence of methylation in lymph node metastasis than in primary tumors
	62%	[102]	Hypermethylation in nipple aspirates was detected in matched breast tumor cases
	65% (22/34)	[44]	Methylation of RASSF1A was only detected in serum DNA of breast cancer patients with methylated tumor
Cervix cancer	0% (0/22)	[1]	
	30% (10/33)	[216]	Squamous cell carcinoma; 41 % hypermethylation among the group of SCC with 3p21 allelic loss whereas only 21% of SCC with retention of 3p21 demonstrated RASSF1A hypermethylation
	12% (2/17)	[216]	Adenocarcinoma ; no correlation between RASSF1A hypermethylation and age of patient, HPV genotype, tumor grade or stage was observed
	10% (4/42)	[105]	Squamous cell carcinoma

Table 1. RASSF1A methylation in primary human tumors (Continued)

Tumor entity	Methylation	Ref.	Remarks
Cervix cancer	21% (4/19)	[105]	Adenosquamous carcinoma
	24% (8/34)	[105]	Adenocarcinoma; significant reverse correlation between inactivation of RASSF1A and the presence of high-risk HPV was observed in cervical tumors and cell lines (p<0.04).
	0% (0/31)	[28]	Squamous cell carcinoma
	12% (10/82)	[92]	Uterine cervical cancer
Cholangio-carcinoma	69% (9/13)	[201]	Expression of RASSF1A in nine cases with promoter methylation indicated reduced expression compared to normal livers.
	65% (47/72)	[211]	Methylation of RASSF1A was more common in extrahepatic than intrahepatic cholangiocarcinoma (p=0.003)
Colorectal cancer	12% (3/26)	[214]	
	20% (45/222)	[188]	RASSF1A methylation occurs predominatly in K-ras wild type colorectal carcinomas (P=0.023)
	45% (13/29)	[194]	RASSF1A was reexpressed after treatment with 5-aza-CdR in a colon cancer cell line
	20% (25/122)	[189]	Sporadic colorectal cancer; data suggest that folate and alcohol intake may be associated with changes in promoter hypermethylation.
	16% (n=149)	[110]	Colorectal carcinoma
	2% (n=95)	[110]	Colorectal adenoma; methylation of RASSF1A is a late event: RASSF1A is rarely methylated in adenoma but significantly methylated in colorectal carcinoma (p<0.001). CpG island methylation plays a more important role in proximal colon tumorigenesis rather than in distal colon tumorigenesis(10.7% (n=56) right colon vs. 19,4% (n=93) in the left colon).
	81% (39/48)	[152]	Early flat-type colorectal tumor; RASSF1A methylation was also detected in 49% of normal colonic mucosal tissue; K-ras mutations and RASSF1A methylation occurred mutually exclusive
	3% (2/65)	[208]	
Esophageal cancer	52% (25/48)	[103]	SSC; significant correlation between RASSF1A methylation and advanced tumor stage was detected (p=0.009, stage I/II vs. stage III/IV).
Gastric cancer	43% (39/90)	[19]	Inactivation of RASSF1A was correlated with advanced tumor stage
	67% (14/21)	[88]	Epstein-Barr virus-positive carcinoma
	4% (2/56)	[88]	Epstein-Barr virus-negative carcinoma
	26% (8/31)	[171]	No significant correlation between methylation of RASSF1A and clinicopathological characteristics of the tumors was found. 11% of the gastric intestinal metaplasia samples showed hypermethylation.

Table 1. RASSF1A methylation in primary human tumors (Continued)

Tumor entity	Methylation	Ref.	Remarks
Gastric cancer	8% (6/80)	[90]	RASSF1A methylation was found only in gastric cancer. No RASSF1A methylation was observed in gastric adenoma (n=79), intestinal metaplasia (n=57) and chronic gastritis (n=74).
	40%	[74]	Gastrointestinal stromal tumor
	0.4 % (n=268)	[89]	Gastric mucosa samples
Head and neck cancer	8% (6/80)	[65]	
	17% (4/24)	[69]	RASSF1A methylation was higher in poorly differentiated SCC (P<0.005)
	15% (7/46)	[40]	A significant inverse correlation between RASSF1A promoter methylation and HPV infection was found (p=0.038).
	0% (0/32)	[125]	Primary tumors SSC, 26% (5/19) methylation in cancer cell lines
Hepatocellular carcinoma	100% (29/29)	[216]	RASSF1A was less frequently methylated in the adjacent non-cancerous liver tissue (24/29, 83%).
	93% (14/15)	[155]	RASSF1A inactivation by methylation is a frequent event in HCC, but was not detected in adenoma.
	95% (41/43)	[217]	The level of methylation in non-tumor tissue was significantly lower than in the corresponding tumor tissue.
	67% (40/60)	[109]	Hepatocellular carcinoma (HCC)
	9% (2/22)	[109]	Dysplastic nodule (DN); no methylation in 30 liver cirrhosis (LC) and 34 chronic hepatitis (CH): HCC vs.DN p>0.001; HCC vs. LC p<0.001; no correlations with age, sex, stage, survival time.
Kidney cancer	56% (18/32)	[214]	Renal cell carcinoma
	91% (39/43)	[42]	Ectopic re-expression of RASSF1A suppressed growth in vitro
	23% (32/138)	[132]	clear cell renal cell carcinoma; RASSF1A was re-expressed after treatment with 5-aza-CdR in cancer cell lines.
	44% (12/27)	[132]	Papillary renal cell carcinoma
	52% (26/50)	[13]	Kidney tumor; RASSF1 methylation was detected in urine DNA
	100% (6/6)	[13]	Papillary kidney tumor; association of RASSF1A hypermethylation and papillary tumors was statistically significant (p=0.022)
	44% (19/43)	[13]	Non-papillary renal cell carcinoma
	45%	[43]	Kidney tumors; RASSF1A methylation was detected at a significant higher frequency in papillary tumors (p=0.011) and in high grade tumors (p=0.003).
	46% (23/50)	[43]	Clear cell renal cell carcinoma
	70% (14/20)	[43]	Papillary kidney tumor
	17% (1/6)	[43]	Chromophobe kidney tumor
	14% (1/7)	[43]	Oncocytoma
	60% (3/5)	[43]	Kidney tumor of the collecting duct
	33% (2/6)	[43]	Transitional cell carcinoma of the renal pelvis

Table 1. RASSF1A methylation in primary human tumors (Continued)

Tumor entity	Methylation	Ref.	Remarks
Kidney cancer	40% (20/50)	[173]	Clear cell renal cell carcinoma (RCC); RASSF1A methylation was found in 84% of RCC cell lines
	100% (9/9)	[62]	Papillary kidney tumor; high level of RASSF1A methylation detected
	90% (19/21)	[62]	Clear cell renal cancer
	25% (2/8)	[62]	Oncocytoma
Lung cancer	38% (22/58)	[30]	Non-small cell lung cancer (NSCLC); exogenous expression of RASSF1A inhibited growth of lung cancer cells in vitro and in vivo
	28% (7/25)	[30]	Adenocarcinoma
	58% (8/14)	[30]	Large cell carcinoma
	37% (7/19)	[30]	Squamous cell carcinoma
	79% (22/28)	[31]	Small cell lung cancer (SCLC)
	72% (21/29)	[1]	SCLC
	34% (14/41)	[1]	NSCLC
	30% (32/107)	[18]	NSCLC; methylation of RASSF1A was associated with impaired patient survival (P=0.046)
	32% (35/110)	[174]	RASSF1A methylation correlated with adverse survival of lung adenocarcinoma patients
	71%	[181]	Atypical carcinoids.
	45%	[181]	Typical carcinoids ; methylation frequency of RASSF1A was significantly higher in neuroendocrine tumors than in the NSCLC tumors(p<0.0001); methylation of RASSF1A was higher in SCLC tumors than in bronchial carcinoids (p=0.002)
	36% (107/299)	[183]	Adenocarcinoma; no significant differences in methylation status of RASSF1A between smokers and non-smokers
	37% (72/194)	[183]	Squamous cell carcinoma
	21% (5/24)	[70]	No correlation between tumor stage, location and RASSF1A methylation status in sputum samples of NSCLC patients. 50% (n=8) SCLC showed methylation in sputum.
	42% (42/100)	[47]	In the cases of stage I and II diseases RASSF1A methylation was associated with earlier recurrence (p=0.0247).
	32% (66/204)	[96]	Hypermethylation of the RASSF1A promoter was found to be significantly associated with the age of starting smoking (p=0.001); RASSF1A promoter was found to be associated with a poor prognosis in NSCLC patients at stages 1 and 2 (p=0.02 and 0.01, respectively).
	33% (80/242)	[97]	NSCLC; RASSF1A methylation was not associated with K-ras mutations (p=0.37); RASSF1A methylation more frequently in adenocarcinomas (39%) than in squamous cell carcinomas (26%); the hazard of failure for those with RASSF1A methylation was higher compared with that of those with neither K-ras mutation nor RASSF1A methylated (p=0.01).
	43% (32/75)	[210]	Methylation of RASSF1A was cancer-specific (p<0.05).

Table 1. RASSF1A methylation in primary human tumors (Continued)

Tumor entity	Methylation	Ref.	Remarks
Lung cancer	45%	[115]	NSCLC; the results indicate a trend of inverse relationship between K-ras activation and RASSF1A promoter methylation
	55%	[115]	Adenocarcinoma
	25%	[115]	Large cell carcinoma
	25%	[115]	Squamous cell carcinoma
	34% (17/50)	[144]	NSCLC; 34% in serum of patients, correlation between methylation in tumor and serum was observed (p=0.0001)
	47% (7/15)	[144]	Adenocarcinoma
	40% (4/10)	[144]	Large cell carcinoma
	24% (6/25)	[144]	Squamous cell carcinoma
	30% (32/107)	[218]	NSCLC; additional analysis of bronchial brushes (6%), bronchoalveolar lavage (5%) and oropharyngeal brushes (4%); methylation events more often in smokers
	41% (51/124)	[128]	NSCLC
	45% (14/31)	[179]	NSCLC; methylation detected in 29% (4/14) bronchoalveolar lavage of tumor patients
	52% (12/21)	[179]	Adenocarcinoma
	28% (17/61)	[76]	Adenocarcinoma
	39% (46/119)	[196]	RASSF1A methylation is a significant predictor of a poor 5-year overall survival rate (p<0.0001)
	52% (50/96)	[124]	Adenocarcinoma; RASSF1A methylation was significantly related to starting smoking under age 18
	31% (22/61)	[124]	Squamours cell carcinoma
	39% (28/72)	[175]	Adenocarcinoma; RASSF1A methylation was more frequently observed in AC than in SCC
	13% (6/45)	[175]	Squamours cell carcinoma
	38% (80/209)	[39]	Adenocarcinoma
Lymphoma	65% (34/52)	[134]	Hodgkin's lymphoma; 83% (5/6) in non-Hodgkin lymphoma cell lines; hypermethylation in serum samples: 9% (2/22)
Melanoma	55% (24/44)	[168]	Malignant cutaneous melanoma
	41% (18/44)	[168]	Region upstream from exon 1α of RASSF1A
	50% (22/44)	[168]	Region within exon 1α of RASSF1A
	15% (3/20)	[72]	Primary tumors; hypermethylation of RASSF1A increases during tumor progression
	57% (49/86)	[72]	Metastatic tumors; RASSF1A methylation in 19% (n=6) of plasma from preoperative blood specimen
	53%	[147]	Transcriptional downregulation of RASSF1A does not function as an alternative mechanism to oncogenic BRAF or N-ras mutation in melanomas
	36% (9/25)	[58]	
Mesothelioma	32% (21/66)	[180]	Malignant mesothelioma; inactivation of RASSF1A was correlated with the presence of SV40 in mesothelioma (P=0.022).

Table 1. RASSF1A methylation in primary human tumors (Continued)

Tumor entity	Methylation	Ref.	Remarks
Myeloma	28% (9/32)	[139]	Multiple myeloma; no mutation of RASSF1A and BRAF
	15% (17/113)	[157]	Multiple myeloma
	14% (4/29)	[157]	Monoclonal gammopathie of undetermined significance
	0% (0/56)	[59]	Multiple myeloma; 80% in multiple myeloma cell lines
Naso-pharyngeal carcinoma	67% (14/21)	[122]	Nasopharyngeal (NP) cancer no significant correlation between methylation of RASSF1A and clinical parameters
	50% (8/16)	[178]	RASSF1A methylation was detected in 39% of EBV associated NP brushing samples
	83% (24/29)	[106]	
	67% (20/30)	[22]	Tumor tissue; methylation of RASSF1A in nasopharyngeal swaps (33%), mouth and throat rinsing fluid (37%) and peripheral blood (3%)
	46% (14/30)	[202]	Undifferentiated NP, methylation of RASSF1A in peripheral blood was detected in all samples with methylated tumor
	65%	[203]	Methylation of RASSF1A was detected in 5% (2/41) of serum of patients with nasopharyngeal carcinoma; the plasma DNA concentration was higher in NPC patients than in normal individuals (p=0.175); hpermethylated gene levels in plasma of NPC patients were not correlated with sex, clinical tumor staging, and lymph node status.
Osteosarcoma	40% (4/10)	[117]	RASSF1A not expressed in 83% (5/6) cell lines; treatment of cell lines with 5-aza-2-deoxycytidine reactivated the transcription of RASSF1A, but not that of RASSF1B
Ovarian cancer	10% (2/21)	[1]	
	40% (8/20)	[214]	
	41% (20/49)	[146]	RASSF1A methylation frequency was significantly higher in sporadic ovarian cancer compared to nonmalignant tissue (P=0.01).
	36% (9/25)	[38]	
	50% (25/50)	[36]	Tumor specific methylation of RASSF1A was observed in serum, plasma and peritoneal fluid from cancer patients
	36% (9/25)	[38]	Granulosa cell tumors
Pancreatic carcinoma	64% (29/45)	[33]	Pancreatic adenocarcinomas with K-ras mutation have significantly less RASSF1A methylation and vice versa (p=0.001); methylation was detected in 44% (8/18) of pancreatitis cases
	83% (10/12)	[33]	Endocrine tumors
	75% (36/48)	[75]	Endocrine tumors (ET); tumors larger than 5 cm and those associated with lymph node or hepatic metastases exhibited a higher frequency of methylation at RASSF1A compared with ET's without malignant features
Pediatric tumors	40% (70/175)	[64]	42% in Wilms: tumor, 88% in medulloblastoma, 59% in retinoblastoma 61% rhabdomyosarcoma, 52% neuroblastoma, 19% hepatoblastoma, 18% acute leukemia
	73% (22/30)	[46]	Wilms' tumor

Table 1. RASSF1A methylation in primary human tumors (Continued)

Tumor entity	Methylation	Ref.	Remarks
Pediatric tumors	54% (21/39)	[194]	Wilms' tumor
	67% (16/24)	[200]	Including neuroblastoma, thyroid cancer, hepatocellular carcinoma pancreatoblastoma, adrenocortical carcinoma, Wilms' tumor, Burkitt's lymphoma and T-Cell lymphoma; RASSF1A methylation was detected in 54%, 40% and 9% of buffy coat samples before, during and after treatment
Phaeochromo-cytoma	22% (5/23)	[8]	
	48% (12/25)	[35]	RASSF1A methylation was more common in hereditary tumors (58%) compared to the sporadic tumors (38%)
Prostate cancer	53% (54/101)	[127]	RASSF1A methylation was correlated with clinicopathological features of poor prognosis
	100% (11/11)	[104]	Reintroduction of RASSF1A suppressed the growth of a prostate cancer cell line in vitro
	71% (37/52)	[120]	RASSF1A methylation frequency was higher in more aggressive tumors (p=0.032)
	84% (31/37)	[91]	The methylation frequency of RASSF1A was higher in prostate cancer with high serum PSA (prostate specific antigen) or with high GS(Gleason score) than those with low PSA or GS (p<0.05).
	66% (59/90)	[205]	No correlation between RASSF1A hypermethylation and tumor grade or stage or race of investigated patients was observed; in benign prostate hyperplasia (n=7) no RASSF1A methylation was found
	83% (20/24)	[204]	Frequency of methylation did not differ by tumor grade; 30% (3/10) of RASSF1A methylation was detected in high-grade prostatic intraepithelial neoplasia
	49%	[162]	RASSF1A methylation was found in 19% of benign prostatic hyperplasia
	78% (88/113)	[52]	
	99% (116/117)	[82]	Methylation of RASSF1A was also detected in 93% of benign hyperplasia (BPH) and 100% of intraepithelial neoplasia (HGPIN); methylation levels were significantly higher in prostate cancer than HGPIN and BPH and correlate with advanced tumor stage (p=0.0025)
Soft tissue sarcoma	20% (7/84)	[156]	RASSF1A methylation was more frequent in leiomyosarcoma (39%) compared to malignant fibrous histiocytomas (6%) and liposarcomas (39%); tumor related death of cancer patients with methylated RASSF1A was significantly increased (p=0.037)
Testicular germ cell tumor	22% (20/92)	[100]	80% (8/10) of methylated tumors showed lack or down-regulation of RASSF1A expression.
	40% (4/10)	[71]	Seminomas
	83% (15/18)	[71]	Nonseminomas; RASSF1A methylation was significantly less in seminomas compared to nonseminomas (p=0.0346). RASSF1A methylation occurs early in tumorigenesis

Table 1. RASSF1A methylation in primary human tumors (Continued)

Tumor entity	Methylation	Ref.	Remarks
Testicular germ cell tumor	0% (0/25)	[93]	Testicular germ cell tumors; 100% (3/3) RASSF1A methylation in testicular malignant lymphomas
	36%	[101]	Nonseminoma; 52% in cisplatin resistant tumors vs. 28% in cisplatin sensitive tumors; RASSF1A may serve as a marker for cisplatin resistance; evidence for hypermethylation by cisplatin treatment
Thyroid cancer	71% (27/38)	[154]	RASSF1A methylation was more frequent in more aggressive thyroid carcinomas
	44% (4/9)	[207]	Follicular adenomas
	75% (9/12)	[207]	Follicular thyroid cancer
	20% (6/30)	[207]	Papillary thyroid cancer; in tumor cell lines and in PTCs an inverse correlation of RASSF1A methylation and BRAF mutation was found

Hypermethylation of the RASSF1A promoter and other tumor-related CpG islands were correlated with the exposure to smoke in lung cancer and an earlier age of starting smoking [96, 124, 183, 184]. The effects of dietary folate and alcohol intake on promoter methylation were investigated in patients with sporadic colorectal cancer [189]. Folate supplies a methyl group to convert homocysteine to methionine, which is then converted to S-adenosylmethionine, the methyl donor for a wide variety of biological substrates. Van Engeland et al. (2003) observed that the frequency of RASSF1A methylation is higher (25%) in cancer patients with low methyl donor dietary supplementation (low folate/high alcohol) compared to patients with high folate and low alcohol intake (15%). However, this difference was not significant for RASSF1A and several other tumor suppressor genes [189]. In summary, RASSF1A methylation is one of the most frequent alterations detected in human tumors and may play crucial roles in the initiation, promotion and progression of cancer originating from different tissue.

RASSF1A METHYLATION AS PROGNOSTIC MARKER

Hypermethylation of RASSF1A occurs frequently in different tumor entities and therefore, aberrant RASSF1A promoter methylation is being widely studied as a biomarker for the prognosis of cancer patients. Various publications have demonstrated that the frequency of RASSF1A hypermethylation in different cancer entities is correlated with clinicopathological aspects, including higher grade of tumors or a reduced time of survival (Table 1). An association of hypermethylation of the promoter of RASSF1A with an advanced tumor stage was found in bladder cancer [108] and in gastric cancer [19]. An increasing RASSF1A methylation frequency from grade II to grade IV glioblastoma was reported [68]. In neuroblastoma, RASSF1A methylation was significantly associated with age >1 (p<0.01), high-risk disease (p<0.016) and poor survival (p<0.001)[212]. Kuroki et al. (2003) have demonstrated a significant correlation between RASSF1A hypermethylation and advanced tumor stage in esophageal squamous cell carcinoma (Table 1). In kidney cancer,

RASSF1A methylation was correlated with high grade and papillary tumors [43]. In prostate cancer, RASSF1A methylation was correlated with high serum PSA and high Gleason score [91, 120]. A recent study showed that the methylation level of RASSF1A is correlated with pathologic tumor stage in prostate cancer (p=0.0025) [82]. A poorer prognosis of cancer patients with aberrant RASSF1A was reported in bladder cancer [126] and in prostate cancer [127]. In NSCLC, several studies have significantly associated RASSF1A methylation with poor prognosis (stage 1 and stage 2) and advanced tumor stage [18, 47, 96, 174, 196]. RASSF1A methylation was dominantly detected in lung tumors with vascular invasion or pleural involvement and was observed more frequently in poorly differentiated tumors than in well or moderately differentiated tumors [174]. RASSF1A methylation was more frequently observed in adenocarcinoma than in squamous cell carcinoma [124, 175]. It was reported that RASSF1A methylation was associated with an earlier age at starting smoking [96, 124]. A direct correlation between RASSF1A methylation and an earlier recurrence in NSCLC was reported by Endoh et al. (2003). It was observed that the methylation frequency was higher in metastases or in late states of certain cancer (Table 1). In lymph node metastasis of breast tumors, RASSF1A methylation was detected more frequent than in the primary breast carcinoma and hypermethylation was found in metastases in bone, brain and lung [131]. Schagdarsurengin et al. (2002) reported that RASSF1A methylation was more often in undifferentiated and medullary thyroid carcinomas. Müller et al. (2003) detected impaired outcome for breast cancer patients with methylation of the RASSF1A promoter in serum. Methylation of RASSF1A occurred more frequently in unaffected women at high-risk for breast cancer (Gail model) than in low/intermediate risk women (70% and 29%, respectively; p=0.04) [114]. The risk of a tumor-related death for soft tissue sarcoma patients with methylated RASSF1A was significantly increased [156]. Lee et al. (2004) reported that methylation of the RASSF1A promoter is a late event in colorectal neoplasia. In melanoma, hypermethylation of RASSF1A promoter increased during tumor progression and was more frequent in metastatic melanomas [72]. In contrast to these results, in testicular germ cell tumors [71] and in hepatocellular carcinoma [216] hypermethylation of the promoter of RASSF1A is an early event in tumorigenesis. In testicular germ cell tumors, an association between the resistance towards the chemo-therapeutic agent cisplatin and RASSF1A hypermethylation was observed [101]. Taken together, RASSF1A methylation was often correlated with an advanced tumor stage and poor survival in different tumor entities.

RASSF1A METHYLATION AS A BIOMARKER FOR CANCER PATIENTS

The detection of tumors at early stages requires new approaches for characterization and identification of cancer-specific biomarkers and the establishment of reliable non–invasive methods for the detection of these biomarkers in body fluids. Methylation-specific PCR (MSP) has been used in several pilot studies to amplify cancer cell DNA obtained from bodily fluids and these DNA methylation analyses may serve as a powerful new tool for cancer diagnosis [186]. For example DNA isolated from serum of cancer patients was used to screen for tumors in the liver [199], in the lung [48] and for head and neck cancer [153]. Additionally, aberrant methylation of tumor-related genes was detected in DNA obtained from sputum or bronchial lavages of lung cancer patients [3, 14] and urine of prostate cancer [20] and bladder cancer patients [21, 45].

Several studies have analyzed the hypermethylation of the RASSF1A promoter in distinct bodily fluids. In nasopharyngeal carcinoma, Wong et al. (2003) found a RASSF1A methylation frequency of only 5% using MSP out of sera, whereas 65% of the primary tumors showed hypermethylation. A similar frequency of hypermethylation (3%) of RASSF1A in peripheral blood of nasopharyngeal carcinoma patients was detected by Chang et al. (2003), and additionally hypermethylation of RASSF1A was detected in nasopharyngeal swaps (33%) and mouth and throat rinsing fluids (37%) of cancer patients [22]. In 4 out of 14 (29%) lung cancer patients who showed hypermethylation of RASSF1A, the bronchoalveolar lavages were positive for hypermethylated RASSF1A [179]. Zöchbauer-Müller et al. (2003) found hypermethylation of RASSF1A in bronchial brushes (6%), bronchoalveolar lavages (5%) and oropharyngeal brushes (2%). In serum of patients with NSCLC, Ramirez et al. (2003) detected a high frequency (34%) of RASSF1A methylated DNA and a high correlation between methylation in tumor tissue and serum (p=0.0001). Another study found in 12% of serum DNA from lung cancer patients RASSF1A methylation and the smoking status was positively associated with its methylation [54]. Sputum of lung cancer patients is another body fluid, which was investigated for hypermethylated DNA of tumor suppressor genes [15, 70]. Honorio et al. (2003) found that in 50% of SCLC and in 21% of NSCLC sputum samples a hypermethylation of RASSF1A was detectable. Belinsky et al. (2002) detected only a low frequency of RASSF1A methylation in the sputum of controls. In 50% sera of glioblastoma patients, RASSF1A methylation was observed and this correlated with the RASSF1A inactivation in the tumor tissue [145]. RASSF1A methylation was also investigated in the urine of patients with bladder and kidney cancer [13, 21, 45, 53]. In 19 of 23 (82%) of patients with a RASSF1A methylated bladder cancer, Dulaimi et al. (2004) detected RASS1A hypermethylation in the urine samples. MSP used for detection of a panel of methylated promoters of cancer related genes (APC, RASSF1A and p14) in urine of bladder cancer patients showed 100% specificity and methylation of RASSF1A was not detected in the urine samples of controls [45]. Chan et al. (2003) detected methylation of RASS1A in 7 out of 14 (50 %) urine specimen and all positive probes showed also epigenetic inactivation of RASSF1A in the corresponding primary bladder tumors. In urine samples of patients with kidney tumor, Battagli et al. (2003) found in 25 out of 50 (50%) hypermethylated RASSF1A. Only for a single case, no RASSF1A methylation was detected in the urine despite of a methylated tumor [13]. However, a recent study indicates the RASSF1A is frequently methylated in urine sediments of cancer free individuals [53]. In patients with Hodgkins' lymphoma, hypermethylation of the RASSF1A promoter occurred in two out of 22 (9%) sera, whereas the frequency of hypermethylation in primary tumors was 65% [134]. In 22 samples of breast cancer, a panel of six genes (GSTP1, RARß2, p16, p14, RASSF1A and DAP-kinase) was examined by Krassenstein et al. (2004), and in the corresponding nipple aspirates. At least one gene showed hypermethylation in its promoter region in the tumor samples and methylation of the same gene was detected in 18 out of 22 (82%) nipple aspirates [102]. In sera of breast cancer patients, hypermethylation of cancer-related genes was investigated and methylation of RASSF1A was only detected in serum DNA of cancer patients with a methylated RASSF1A CpG island [44, 133]. Müller et al. (2003) reported that methylation of the RASSF1A promoter was detected in 6 out of 26 (23%) and associated with a worse prognosis and a poor outcome [133]. Recently, hypermethylation of RASSF1A was also detected in tampons of patients with endometrial cancer [51]. RASSF1A methylation was detected in bodily fluids (serum, plasma and peritoneal fluid) of ovarian cancer patients with 100% specificity [36]. Methylation was undetectable in bodily fluids of patients with RASSF1A-unmethylated tumors and in controls. Taken together, RASSF1A hypermethylation is frequently detected in bodily fluids of cancer patients. Different frequencies in DNA methylation could be attributed to various DNA concentrations of disseminating cancer cells in serum, sputum and other bodily fluids compared to the primary tumors and limitations in the sensitivity of the detection system. Methylation analysis of tumor-related genes in easily obtainable bodily fluids is a promising new experimental approach to screen putative cancer patients.

FUNCTION OF RASSF1A AS TUMOR SUPPRESSOR

RASSF1A is involved in several growth regulating and apoptotic pathways and regulates cell proliferation, cellular integrity and cell death (Figure 3). Ectopic expression of RASSF1A in cancer cell lines, which lack endogenous RASSF1A transcription resulted in reduced colony formation and/or anchorage-independent growth in soft agar in lung, kidney, prostate, glioma and nasopharyngeal cancer cell lines [18, 26, 30, 42, 68, 104, 116]. In nude mice, human cancer cells lacking RASSF1A transcription formed larger tumors compared to the same cells expressing exogenous RASSF1A [18, 26, 30, 116]. Mutant RASSF1A had only a reduced growth suppression activity in vivo and in vitro [42, 116]. Ectopic expression of the RASSF1C isoform showed only a modest reduction of cell viability in vitro [83]. However, a recent report indicates that in a renal cancer cell line overexpression of RASSF1C inhibits growth and induces cell cycle arrest [116]. To gain insight into RASSF1A function, expression profiles of cancer cell lines, which re-expressed RASSF1A were generated [2]. Agathanggelou et al. (2004) have characterized several genes (e.g ETS2, Cyclin D3, CDH2, DAPK1, TXN and CTSL) that may represent gene expression targets for RASSF1A. Shivakumar et al. (2002) have reported that RASSF1A can induce cell-cycle arrest by engaging the Rb family cell-cycle checkpoint. E7 papilloma virus protein-expressing cells are resistant to the RASSF1A-induced cell-cycle arrest [161]. RASSF1A also inhibits accumulation of native cyclin D1 (Figure 3) and the RASSF1A-induced growth arrest can be relieved by ectopic expression of cyclins, but not by oncogenic Ras expression [161].

Activated Ras is usually associated with enhanced proliferation, transformation and cell survival (Figure 3). Ras also induces proliferation inhibitory effects [12, 159] and apoptosis [24, 41, 130, 160]. Ras effectors, like RASSF1A, may be specialized to inhibit cell growth and to induce cell death and these inhibitory signaling pathways may need to be inactivated during carcinogenesis. Vos et al. (2000) have shown that RASSF1C binds Ras in a GTP-dependent manner and expression of RASSF1C induced apoptosis. This pro-apoptotic effect of RASSF1 is enhanced by activated Ras and inhibited by dominant negative Ras [191]. Recent data indicate that in colorectal and pancreatic cancer, the inactivation of RASSF1A and activation of Ras are mutual exclusive [33, 152, 188], but in lung cancer this correlation was not significant [97, 144, 174]. In thyroid cancer, RASSF1A methylation occurred significantly when BRAF was not mutated [207].

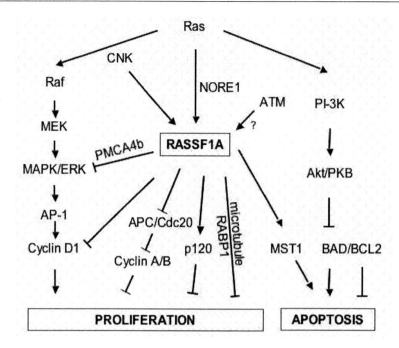

Figure 3. Signaling pathway of RASSF1A-mediated functions. Ras activates cellular proliferation through the MAP-kinase pathway (Raf, MEK, and MAPK/ERK). RASSF1A regulates cellular integrity and proliferation through its interaction with the microtubules, RASSF1A binding protein 1 (RABP1) and CDC20 by inhibiting the anaphase promoting complex and the degradation of cyclin A and B. RASSF1A inhibits the epidermal growth factor dependent activation of Erk through the plasma membrane calmodulin-dependent calcium ATPase 4b (PMCA4b). RASSF1A inhibits the accumulation of cyclin D1 and interacts with the transcription factor p120E4F. Ras inhibits apoptosis by the pathway of the phosphatidylinositol 3 kinase (PI3-K) and stimulates the activity of the protein kinase B Akt (Akt/PKB). Subsequently, Akt inhibits apoptosis induced by members of the Bcl-family (BAD). The RASSF1A tumor suppressor induces apoptosis through its interaction with Ras, the novel Ras effector (NORE1) the connector enhancer of KSR (CNK) and the pro-apoptotic MST1 kinase. The exact role of the ataxia telangiectasia mutated (ATM) kinase is unclear.

Murine models of human cancer may expedite our understanding of carcinogenesis and Rassf1a knockout mice may help to dissect the tumorigenic process involved in the function of Rassf1a. Smith et al. (2002) have created a mouse with a 370 kb deletion of the region homologue to the 3p21.3, which includes Rassf1a. The homozygous deletion of this region is embryonic lethal in mouse [164]. Recently, we have generated Rassf1a-specific knockout mice and consistent with the tumor-suppressive role of RASSF1A, we have observed that these animals were prone to spontaneous and induced carcinogenesis [177]. Interestingly, heterozygous and homozygous Rassf1a knockout mice were significantly more susceptible to spontaneous tumorigenesis ($p<0.05$ and $p<0.001$, respectively) [177]. When heterozygous and homozygous knockout mice were treated with two chemical carcinogens (benzopyrene and urethane), the Rassf1a deficient mice showed increased tumor multiplicity and tumor size compared to the controls [177]. Functional data indicate that Rassf1a knockout embryonic fibroblasts are more sensitive to induced microtubule instability relative to wildtype cells [121]. These functional data and the Rassf1a knockout mice support the tumor suppressor role of RASSF1A observed in cancer.

Another homologue of RASSF1, which encodes a Ras association domain, was characterized in mouse and human and was termed novel Ras effector (NORE1) [176, 190]. Recent data show that the RASSF1A-related Ras effector NORE1 may serve as a Ras-regulated tumor suppressor in lung cancer and melanoma [6, 192] and epigenetic inactivation of NORE1 was detected in several cancers, including lung and kidney cancer [25, 67, 176]. No correlation between RASSF1A methylation and NORE1 inactivation was reported [67], however, in lung cancer hypermethylation of NORE1 occurs preferentially in the context of a wild-type K-ras [76]. Our results indicate that binding of RASSF1A to Ras may require heterodimerization with NORE1, and that RASSF1A binds to Ras only weakly by itself [140]. RASSF1A and NORE1 may function in the same Ras-regulated pathway. Khokhlatchev et al. (2002) showed that RASSF1A and NORE1 interact with the pro-apoptotic kinase MST1, which mediates the apoptotic effect of activated Ras. MST1 is a member of the group II germinal center (protein serine/threonine) kinases and the NORE1/RASSF1-MST1 complex represents a novel Ras-regulated proapoptotic pathway [94]. Praskova et al. (2004) have reported that the MST1 kinase is regulated by robust auto-activation, which is mediated by auto-phosphorylation. Co-expression of RASSF1 and NORE1 suppressed the phosphorylation and therefore the auto-activation of MST1 [142]. Moreover, MST1 activity is stimulated by membrane recruitment and when bound to Ras. Recently, Rabizadeh et al. (2004) have reported that the scaffold protein CNK1 interacts with the tumor suppressor RASSF1A and augments RASSF1A induced cell death. The connector enhancer of KSR (CNK) is a c-Raf1 binding protein, which mediates Ras-induced Raf activation. CNK1 is an interaction partner of RASSF1 and represses growth of dividing cancer cells and initiates apoptosis through the MST1 (or MST2) pathway (Figure 3). However, RASSF1C does not influence CNK1 induced apoptosis [143]. In addition to a pro-proliferating role of CNK1 by activated Ras, CNK1 also participates in a pro-apoptotic pathway through its binding of the RASSF1A-MST complex [143].

In a yeast two-hybrid screen, RASSF1A was identified as a novel interaction partner of PMCA4b, a plasma membrane calmodulin-dependent calcium ATPase [7]. The functionality of the interaction was demonstrated by inhibition of the epidermal growth factor-dependent activation of the Erk pathway when PMCA4b and RASSF1 were coexpressed (Figure 3). In another screen, p120E4F was identified as an interaction partner of RASSF1A [50]. p120E4F is an E1A-regulated transcription factor which interacts with the retinoblastoma protein, p14ARF and p53 and is involved in control of cell cycle arrest near the G1 transition. The G1 cell cycle arrest and S phase inhibition was enhanced by p120E4F in the presence of RASSF1A [50].

Several different groups have reported that RASSF1A is a microtubule-binding protein, which regulates mitotic progression [29, 119, 121, 149, 150, 165, 193]. We have shown that RASSF1A co-localizes with microtubules in interphase and decorates spindles and centrosomes during mitosis [121]. Upon binding to microtubules, RASSF1A has a strong cytoprotective activity against microtubule depolymerization induced by nocodazole *in vivo*. RASSF1A-/- cells were more sensitive against nocodazole induced G2/M arrest than wild type cells [121]. The domain required for both microtubule association and stabilization was mapped to a fragment that contains the Ras association domain. Overexpression of RASSF1A induced mitotic arrest at metaphase with aberrant mitotic cells. These results were confirmed by several other groups [29, 119, 149, 150, 165, 193]. RASSF1 was identified as an interaction partner of the C19ORF5 protein with high similarity to microtubule-associated proteins (MAP1A and MAP1B) [29, 119]. Recently C19ORF was redesignated RASSF1A-binding protein 1 (RABP1) and contains two microtubule-associated protein domains [166]. RABP1 plays an important role in the recruitment of RASSF1A to the spindle poles and in the subsequent RASSF1A-mediated regulation of the APC in mitosis [166]. Dallol et al. (2004) have found that RASSF1A substitutions at codon 65 and 257 perturb the association with microtubules and these mutants are less potent inhibitors of DNA synthesis compared to the wildtype protein. Vos et al. (2004) have shown that a deletion mutant of RASSF1A, which lacks the microtubule association domain of RASSF1 is severely defective for the ability to promote cell cycle arrest and partially inhibits RASSF1A induced cell death. Interestingly, it was also shown that wild type RASSF1A and RASSF1C inhibit genomic instability induced by activated Ras [193]. RASSF1A can regulate microtubule stability and induces G2/M arrest [149, 150]. Song et al. (2004) have reported that RASSF1A regulates mitosis by inhibiting the anaphase promoting complex (APC) through Cdc20 and induces G2-M arrest at pro-metaphase. RASSF1C had no effect on the APC-Cdc20 complex and cell cycle regulation [165]. The N-terminal region of RASSF1A interacts directly with Cdc20; however the C-terminus, which encodes the microtubule association domain is also involved in the inhibition of APC [165]. After interaction with RASSF1A, Cdc20 is inhibited to activate APC and therefore APC is unable to degrade the mitotic cyclins A and B (Figure 3). Inactivation of RASSF1A resulted in the acceleration of mitotic progression and in premature destruction of cyclin A and B [165]. The function of RASSF1A is independent of the protein Emi1 (early mitotic inhibitor 1) and therefore Song et al. (2004) proposed that RASSF1A acts in early prometaphase, before activation of the spindle checkpoint and after Emi1 destruction to prevent the degradation of mitotic cyclins and to delay mitotic progression. Thus, RASSF1A may function as a crucial link between tumor suppression and mitotic cell division through a new mechanism [79, 129]. In summary, RASSF1A induces apoptosis and inhibits cellular proliferation through several pathways (Figure 3). RASSF1A can regulate microtubule stability and control mitotic progression, presumably by modulating centrosomes and spindle function and by regulating the APC complex and accumulation of cyclins A, B and D1.

CONCLUSION

Epigenetic silencing of the RASSF1A tumor suppressor was found in a variety of primary human tumors including, bladder, brain, breast, cervix, colorectal, gastric, liver, kidney, lung, nasopharyngeal, ovarian, pancreatic, prostate and thyroid cancer. RASSF1A silencing was significantly associated with an advanced tumor stage and poorly differentiated tumors. Moreover, hypermethylation of RASSF1A correlated with poor prognosis and impaired survival of the cancer patient. Methylation analysis of the RASSF1A gene could serve as the basis of a diagnostic test for cancer. The observation that RASSF1A inactivation and K-ras activation are mutually exclusive events in the development of certain carcinomas could further pinpoint the function of RASSF1A as a negative effector of Ras. RASSF1A functions as *bona fide* tumor suppressor gene in cancer through several distinct pathways, including apoptosis, genomic and microtubule stability and cell cycle regulation. The exact mechanism of its biological function is complex and may require additional Ras effectors like

NORE1. Understanding the molecular function of RASSF1A may lead to the development of new anticancer drugs and the detection of the aberrant methylation of RASSF1A in patients bodily fluids may serve as promising biomarker for cancer diagnosis. Since *RASSF1A* blocks cell cycle progression the silencing of *RASSF1A* may be a critical step in tumorigenesis. Inactivation of *RASSF1A* may serve as a model for epigenetic CpG island silencing of tumor suppressor genes in cancer pathogenesis. It will be interesting to analyze the influence of inhibitors of DNA methylation and histone deacetylase on the reactivation of the *RASSF1A* gene in silenced cells.

ACKNOWLEDGEMENTS

Data presented in this review were supported by BMBF grant FKZ 01ZZ0104, Land Sachsen-Anhalt, DFG grant DA552-1 to Reinhard Dammann.

REFERENCES

[1]   Agathanggelou, A; Honorio, S; Macartney, DP; Martinez, A; Dallol, A; Rader, J; Fullwood, P; Chauhan, A; Walker, R; Shaw, JA; Hosoe, S; Lerman, MI; Minna, JD; Maher, ER; Latif, F. Methylation associated inactivation of RASSF1A from region 3p21.3 in lung, breast and ovarian tumours. *Oncogene*, 2001, 20, 1509-1518.

[2]   Agathanggelou, A; Bieche, I; Ahmed-Choudhury, J; Nicke, B; Dammann, R; Baksh, S; Gao, B; Minna, JD; Downward, J; Maher, ER; Latif, F. Identification of novel gene expression targets for the Ras association domain family 1 (RASSF1A) tumor suppressor gene in non-small cell lung cancer and neuroblastoma. *Cancer Res*, 2003, 63, 5344-5351.

[3]   Ahrendt, SA; Chow, JT; Xu, LH; Yang, SC; Eisenberger, CF; Esteller, M; Herman, JG; Wu, L; Decker, PA; Jen, J; Sidransky, D. Molecular detection of tumor cells in bronchoalveolar lavage fluid from patients with early stage lung cancer. *J Natl Cancer Inst*, 1999, 91, 332-339.

[4]   Ahuja, N; Li, Q; Mohan, AL; Baylin, SB; Issa, JP. Aging and DNA methylation in colorectal mucosa and cancer. *Cancer Res*, 1998, 58, 5489-5494.

[5]   Antequera, F; Boyes, J; Bird, A. High levels of de novo methylation and altered chromatin structure at CpG islands in cell lines. *Cell*, 1990, 62, 503-514.

[6]   Aoyama, Y; Avruch, J; Zhang, XF. Nore1 inhibits tumor cell growth independent of Ras or the MST1/2 kinases. *Oncogene*, 2004, 23, 3426-3433.

[7]   Armesilla, AL; Williams, JC; Buch, MH; Pickard, A; Emerson, M; Cartwright, EJ; Oceandy, D; Vos, MD; Gillies, S; Clark, GJ; Neyses, L. Novel functional interaction between the plasma membrane Ca2+ pump 4b and the proapoptotic tumor suppressor Ras-associated factor 1 (RASSF1). *J Biol Chem*, 2004, 279, 31318-31328.

[8]   Astuti, D; Agathanggelou, A; Honorio, S; Dallol, A; Martinsson, T; Kogner, P; Cummins, C; Neumann, HP; Voutilainen, R; Dahia, P; Eng, C; Maher, ER; Latif, F. RASSF1A promoter region CpG island hypermethylation in phaeochromocytomas and neuroblastoma tumours. *Oncogene*, 2001, 20, 7573-7577.

[9]   Astuti, D; Da Silva, NF; Dallol, A; Gentle, D; Martinsson, T; Kogner, P; Grundy, R;
      Kishida, T; Yao, M; Latif, F; Maher, ER. SLIT2 promoter methylation analysis in
      neuroblastoma, Wilms' tumour and renal cell carcinoma. *Br J Cancer*, 2004, 90, 515-
      521.

[10] Balana, C; Ramirez, JL; Taron, M; Roussos, Y; Ariza, A; Ballester, R; Sarries, C;
      Mendez, P; Sanchez, JJ; Rosell, R. O6-methyl-guanine-DNA methyltransferase
      methylation in serum and tumor DNA predicts response to 1,3-bis(2-chloroethyl)-1-
      nitrosourea but not to temozolamide plus cisplatin in glioblastoma multiforme. *Clin
      Cancer Res*, 2003, 9, 1461-1468.

[11] Bannister, AJ; Zegerman, P; Partridge, JF; Miska, EA; Thomas, JO; Allshire, RC;
      Kouzarides, T. Selective recognition of methylated lysine 9 on histone H3 by the HP1
      chromo domain. *Nature*, 2001, 410, 120-124.

[12] Bar-Sagi, D; Feramisco, JR. Microinjection of the ras oncogene protein into PC12 cells
      induces morphological differentiation. *Cell*, 1985, 42, 841-848.

[13] Battagli, C; Uzzo, RG; Dulaimi, E; Ibanez de Caceres, I; Krassenstein, R; Al-Saleem,
      T; Greenberg, RE; Cairns, P. Promoter hypermethylation of tumor suppressor genes in
      urine from kidney cancer patients. *Cancer Res*, 2003, 63, 8695-8699.

[14] Belinsky, SA; Nikula, KJ; Palmisano, WA; Michels, R; Saccomanno, G; Gabrielson, E;
      Baylin, SB; Herman, JG. Aberrant methylation of p16(INK4a) is an early event in lung
      cancer and a potential biomarker for early diagnosis. *Proc Natl Acad Sci U S A*, 1998,
      95, 11891-11896.

[15] Belinsky, SA; Palmisano, WA; Gilliland, FD; Crooks, LA; Divine, KK; Winters, SA;
      Grimes, MJ; Harms, HJ; Tellez, CS; Smith, TM; Moots, PP; Lechner, JF; Stidley, CA;
      Crowell, RE. Aberrant promoter methylation in bronchial epithelium and sputum from
      current and former smokers. *Cancer Res*, 2002, 62, 2370-2377.

[16] Bird, A. DNA methylation patterns and epigenetic memory. *Genes Dev*, 2002, 16, 6-21.

[17] Bird, AP. CpG-rich islands and the function of DNA methylation. *Nature*, 1986, 321,
      209-213.

[18] Burbee, DG; Forgacs, E; Zochbauer-Muller, S; Shivakumar, L; Fong, K; Gao, B;
      Randle, D; Kondo, M; Virmani, A; Bader, S; Sekido, Y; Latif, F; Milchgrub, S;
      Toyooka, S; Gazdar, AF; Lerman, MI; Zabarovsky, E; White, M; Minna, JD.
      Epigenetic inactivation of RASSF1A in lung and breast cancers and malignant
      phenotype suppression. *J Natl Cancer Inst*, 2001, 93, 691-699.

[19] Byun, DS; Lee, MG; Chae, KS; Ryu, BG; Chi, SG. Frequent epigenetic inactivation of
      rassf1a by aberrant promoter hypermethylation in human gastric adenocarcinoma.
      Cancer Res, 2001, 61, 7034-7038.

[20] Cairns, P; Esteller, M; Herman, JG; Schoenberg, M; Jeronimo, C; Sanchez-Cespedes,
      M; Chow, NH; Grasso, M; Wu, L; Westra, WB; Sidransky, D. Molecular detection of
      prostate cancer in urine by GSTP1 hypermethylation. *Clin Cancer Res*, 2001, 7, 2727-
      2730.

[21] Chan, MW; Chan, LW; Tang, NL; Lo, KW; Tong, JH; Chan, AW; Cheung, HY; Wong,
      WS; Chan, PS; Lai, FM; To, KF. Frequent hypermethylation of promoter region of
      RASSF1A in tumor tissues and voided urine of urinary bladder cancer patients. *Int J
      Cancer*, 2003, 104, 611-616.

[22] Chang, HW; Chan, A; Kwong, DL; Wei, WI; Sham, JS; Yuen, AP. Evaluation of
      hypermethylated tumor suppressor genes as tumor markers in mouth and throat rinsing

fluid, nasopharyngeal swab and peripheral blood of nasopharygeal carcinoma patient. *Int J Cancer*, 2003, 105, 851-855.

[23] Chen, CM; Chen, HL; Hsiau, TH; Hsiau, AH; Shi, H; Brock, GJ; Wei, SH; Caldwell, CW; Yan, PS; Huang, TH. Methylation target array for rapid analysis of CpG island hypermethylation in multiple tissue genomes. *Am J Pathol*, 2003, 163, 37-45.

[24] Chen, CY; Liou, J; Forman, LW; Faller, DV. Differential regulation of discrete apoptotic pathways by Ras. *J Biol Chem*, 1998, 273, 16700-16709.

[25] Chen, J; Lui, WO; Vos, MD; Clark, GJ; Takahashi, M; Schoumans, J; Khoo, SK; Petillo, D; Lavery, T; Sugimura, J; Astuti, D; Zhang, C; Kagawa, S; Maher, ER; Larsson, C; Alberts, AS; Kanayama, HO; Teh, BT. The t(1;3) breakpoint-spanning genes LSAMP and NORE1 are involved in clear cell renal cell carcinomas. *Cancer Cell*, 2003, 4, 405-413.

[26] Chow, LS; Lo, KW; Kwong, J; To, KF; Tsang, KS; Lam, CW; Dammann, R; Huang, DP. RASSF1A is a target tumor suppressor from 3p21.3 in nasopharyngeal carcinoma. *Int J Cancer*, 2004, 109, 839-847.

[27] Clark, SJ; Melki, J. DNA methylation and gene silencing in cancer: which is the guilty party? *Oncogene*, 2002, 21, 5380-5387.

[28] Cohen, Y; Singer, G; Lavie, O; Dong, SM; Beller, U; Sidransky, D. The RASSF1A tumor suppressor gene is commonly inactivated in adenocarcinoma of the uterine cervix. *Clin Cancer Res*, 2003, 9, 2981-2984.

[29] Dallol, A; Agathanggelou, A; Fenton, SL; Ahmed-Choudhury, J; Hesson, L; Vos, MD; Clark, GJ; Downward, J; Maher, ER; Latif, F. RASSF1A interacts with microtubule-associated proteins and modulates microtubule dynamics. *Cancer Res*, 2004, 64, 4112-4116.

[30] Dammann, R; Li, C; Yoon, JH; Chin, PL; Bates, S; Pfeifer, GP. Epigenetic inactivation of a RAS association domain family protein from the lung tumour suppressor locus 3p21.3. *Nat Genet*, 2000, 25, 315-319.

[31] Dammann, R; Takahashi, T; Pfeifer, GP. The CpG island of the novel tumor suppressor gene RASSF1A is intensely methylated in primary small cell lung carcinomas. *Oncogene*, 2001, 20, 3563-3567.

[32] Dammann, R; Yang, G; Pfeifer, GP. Hypermethylation of the cpG island of Ras association domain family 1A (RASSF1A), a putative tumor suppressor gene from the 3p21.3 locus, occurs in a large percentage of human breast cancers. *Cancer Res*, 2001, 61, 3105-3109.

[33] Dammann, R; Schagdarsurengin, U; Liu, L; Otto, N; Gimm, O; Dralle, H; Boehm, BO; Pfeifer, GP; Hoang-Vu, C. Frequent RASSF1A promoter hypermethylation and K-ras mutations in pancreatic carcinoma. *Oncogene*, 2003, 22, 3806-3812.

[34] Dammann, R; Schagdarsurengin, U; Strunnikova, M; Rastetter, M; Seidel, C; Liu, L; Tommasi, S; Pfeifer, GP. Epigenetic inactivation of the Ras-association domain family 1 (RASSF1A) gene and its function in human carcinogenesis. *Histol Histopathol*, 2003, 18, 665-677.

[35] Dammann, R; Schagdarsurengin, U; Seidel, C; Trumpler, C; Hoang-Vu, C; Gimm, O; Dralle, H; Pfeifer, GP; Brauckhoff, M. Frequent promoter methylation of tumor-related genes in sporadic and men2-associated pheochromocytomas. *Exp Clin Endocrinol Diabetes*, 2005, 113, 1-7.

[36] de Caceres, I; Battagli, C; Esteller, M; Herman, JG; Dulaimi, E; Edelson, MI; Bergman, C; Ehya, H; Eisenberg, BL; Cairns, P. Tumor cell-specific BRCA1 and RASSF1A hypermethylation in serum, plasma, and peritoneal fluid from ovarian cancer patients. *Cancer Res*, 2004, 64, 6476-6481.

[37] Dennis, K; Fan, T; Geiman, T; Yan, Q; Muegge, K. Lsh, a member of the SNF2 family, is required for genome-wide methylation. *Genes Dev*, 2001, 15, 2940-2944.

[38] Dhillon, VS; Aslam, M; Husain, SA. The contribution of genetic and epigenetic changes in granulosa cell tumors of ovarian origin. *Clin Cancer Res*, 2004, 10, 5537-5545.

[39] Divine, KK; Pulling, LC; Marron-Terada, PG; Liechty, KC; Kang, T; Schwartz, AG; Bocklage, TJ; Coons, TA; Gilliland, FD; Belinsky, SA. Multiplicity of abnormal promoter methylation in lung adenocarcinomas from smokers and never smokers. *Int J Cancer*, 2005, 114, 400-405.

[40] Dong, SM; Sun, DI; Benoit, NE; Kuzmin, I; Lerman, MI; Sidransky, D. Epigenetic inactivation of RASSF1A in head and neck cancer. *Clin Cancer Res*, 2003, 9, 3635-3640.

[41] Downward, J. Ras signalling and apoptosis. *Curr Opin Genet Dev*, 1998, 8, 49-54.

[42] Dreijerink, K; Braga, E; Kuzmin, I; Geil, L; Duh, FM; Angeloni, D; Zbar, B; Lerman, MI; Stanbridge, EJ; Minna, JD; Protopopov, A; Li, J; Kashuba, V; Klein, G; Zabarovsky, ER. The candidate tumor suppressor gene, RASSF1A, from human chromosome 3p21.3 is involved in kidney tumorigenesis. *Proc Natl Acad Sci U S A*, 2001, 98, 7504-7509.

[43] Dulaimi, E; De, C, II; Uzzo, RG; Al-Saleem, T; Greenberg, RE; Polascik, TJ; Babb, JS; Grizzle, WE; Cairns, P. Promoter hypermethylation profile of kidney cancer. *Clin Cancer Res*, 2004, 10, 3972-3979.

[44] Dulaimi, E; Hillinck, J; Ibanez de Caceres, I; Al-Saleem, T; Cairns, P. Tumor suppressor gene promoter hypermethylation in serum of breast cancer patients. *Clin Cancer Res*, 2004, 10, 6189-6193.

[45] Dulaimi, E; Uzzo, RG; Greenberg, RE; Al-Saleem, T; Cairns, P. Detection of bladder cancer in urine by a tumor suppressor gene hypermethylation panel. *Clin Cancer Res*, 2004, 10, 1887-1893.

[46] Ehrlich, M; Jiang, G; Fiala, E; Dome, JS; Yu, MC; Long, TI; Youn, B; Sohn, OS; Widschwendter, M; Tomlinson, GE; Chintagumpala, M; Champagne, M; Parham, D; Liang, G; Malik, K; Laird, PW. Hypomethylation and hypermethylation of DNA in Wilms tumors. *Oncogene*, 2002, 21, 6694-6702.

[47] Endoh, H; Yatabe, Y; Shimizu, S; Tajima, K; Kuwano, H; Takahashi, T; Mitsudomi, T. RASSF1A gene inactivation in non-small cell lung cancer and its clinical implication. *Int J Cancer*, 2003, 106, 45-51.

[48] Esteller, M; Sanchez-Cespedes, M; Rosell, R; Sidransky, D; Baylin, SB; Herman, JG. Detection of aberrant promoter hypermethylation of tumor suppressor genes in serum DNA from non-small cell lung cancer patients. *Cancer Res*, 1999, 59, 67-70.

[49] Fackler, MJ; McVeigh, M; Evron, E; Garrett, E; Mehrotra, J; Polyak, K; Sukumar, S; Argani, P. DNA methylation of RASSF1A, HIN-1, RAR-beta, Cyclin D2 and Twist in in situ and invasive lobular breast carcinoma. *Int J Cancer*, 2003, 107, 970-975.

[50] Fenton, SL; Dallol, A; Agathanggelou, A; Hesson, L; Ahmed-Choudhury, J; Baksh, S; Sardet, C; Dammann, R; Minna, JD; Downward, J; Maher, ER; Latif, F. Identification

of the E1A-regulated transcription factor p120 E4F as an interacting partner of the RASSF1A candidate tumor suppressor gene. *Cancer Res*, 2004, 64, 102-107.

[51] Fiegl, H; Gattringer, C; Widschwendter, A; Schneitter, A; Ramoni, A; Sarlay, D; Gaugg, I; Goebel, G; Muller, HM; Mueller-Holzner, E; Marth, C; Widschwendter, M. Methylated DNA collected by tampons--a new tool to detect endometrial cancer. *Cancer Epidemiol Biomarkers Prev*, 2004, 13, 882-888.

[52] Florl, AR; Steinhoff, C; Muller, M; Seifert, HH; Hader, C; Engers, R; Ackermann, R; Schulz, WA. Coordinate hypermethylation at specific genes in prostate carcinoma precedes LINE-1 hypomethylation. *Br J Cancer*, 2004, 91, 985-994.

[53] Friedrich, MG; Weisenberger, DJ; Cheng, JC; Chandrasoma, S; Siegmund, KD; Gonzalgo, ML; Toma, MI; Huland, H; Yoo, C; Tsai, YC; Nichols, PW; Bochner, BH; Jones, PA; Liang, G. Detection of methylated apoptosis-associated genes in urine sediments of bladder cancer patients. *Clin Cancer Res*, 2004, 10, 7457-7465.

[54] Fujiwara, K; Fujimoto, N; Tabata, M; Nishii, K; Matsuo, K; Hotta, K; Kozuki, T; Aoe, M; Kiura, K; Ueoka, H; Tanimoto, M. Identification of epigenetic aberrant promoter methylation in serum DNA is useful for early detection of lung cancer. *Clin Cancer Res*, 2005, 11, 1219-1225.

[55] Fuks, F; Burgers, WA; Godin, N; Kasai, M; Kouzarides, T. Dnmt3a binds deacetylases and is recruited by a sequence-specific repressor to silence transcription. *Embo J*, 2001, 20, 2536-2544.

[56] Fuks, F; Hurd, PJ; Deplus, R; Kouzarides, T. The DNA methyltransferases associate with HP1 and the SUV39H1 histone methyltransferase. *Nucleic Acids Res*, 2003, 31, 2305-2312.

[57] Fuks, F; Hurd, PJ; Wolf, D; Nan, X; Bird, AP; Kouzarides, T. The methyl-CpG-binding protein MeCP2 links DNA methylation to histone methylation. *J Biol Chem*, 2003, 278, 4035-4040.

[58] Furuta, J; Umebayashi, Y; Miyamoto, K; Kikuchi, K; Otsuka, F; Sugimura, T; Ushijima, T. Promoter methylation profiling of 30 genes in human malignant melanoma. *Cancer Sci*, 2004, 95, 962-968.

[59] Galm, O; Wilop, S; Reichelt, J; Jost, E; Gehbauer, G; Herman, JG; Osieka, R. DNA methylation changes in multiple myeloma. *Leukemia*, 2004, 18, 1687-1692.

[60] Gao, Y; Guan, M; Su, B; Liu, W; Xu, M; Lu, Y. Hypermethylation of the RASSF1A gene in gliomas. *Clin Chim Acta*, 2004, 349, 173-179.

[61] Gibbons, RJ; McDowell, TL; Raman, S; O'Rourke, DM; Garrick, D; Ayyub, H; Higgs, DR. Mutations in ATRX, encoding a SWI/SNF-like protein, cause diverse changes in the pattern of DNA methylation. *Nat Genet*, 2000, 24, 368-371.

[62] Gonzalgo, ML; Yegnasubramanian, S; Yan, G; Rogers, CG; Nicol, TL; Nelson, WG; Pavlovich, CP. Molecular profiling and classification of sporadic renal cell carcinoma by quantitative methylation analysis. *Clin Cancer Res*, 2004, 10, 7276-7283.

[63] Guo, M; House, MG; Hooker, C; Han, Y; Heath, E; Gabrielson, E; Yang, SC; Baylin, SB; Herman, JG; Brock, MV. Promoter hypermethylation of resected bronchial margins: a field defect of changes? *Clin Cancer Res*, 2004, 10, 5131-5136.

[64] Harada, K; Toyooka, S; Maitra, A; Maruyama, R; Toyooka, KO; Timmons, CF; Tomlinson, GE; Mastrangelo, D; Hay, RJ; Minna, JD; Gazdar, AF. Aberrant promoter methylation and silencing of the RASSF1A gene in pediatric tumors and cell lines. *Oncogene*, 2002, 21, 4345-4349.

[65] Hasegawa, M; Nelson, HH; Peters, E; Ringstrom, E; Posner, M; Kelsey, KT. Patterns of gene promoter methylation in squamous cell cancer of the head and neck. *Oncogene*, 2002, 21, 4231-4236.

[66] Herman, JG; Baylin, SB. Gene silencing in cancer in association with promoter hypermethylation. *N Engl J Med*, 2003, 349, 2042-2054.

[67] Hesson, L; Dallol, A; Minna, JD; Maher, ER; Latif, F. NORE1A, a homologue of RASSF1A tumour suppressor gene is inactivated in human cancers. *Oncogene*, 2003, 22, 947-954.

[68] Hesson, L; Bieche, I; Krex, D; Criniere, E; Hoang-Xuan, K; Maher, ER; Latif, F. Frequent epigenetic inactivation of RASSF1A and BLU genes located within the critical 3p21.3 region in gliomas. *Oncogene*, 2004, 23, 2408-2419.

[69] Hogg, RP; Honorio, S; Martinez, A; Agathanggelou, A; Dallol, A; Fullwood, P; Weichselbaum, R; Kuo, MJ; Maher, ER; Latif, F. Frequent 3p allele loss and epigenetic inactivation of the RASSF1A tumour suppressor gene from region 3p21.3 in head and neck squamous cell carcinoma. *Eur J Cancer*, 2002, 38, 1585-1592.

[70] Honorio, S; Agathanggelou, A; Schuermann, M; Pankow, W; Viacava, P; Maher, ER; Latif, F. Detection of RASSF1A aberrant promoter hypermethylation in sputum from chronic smokers and ductal carcinoma in situ from breast cancer patients. *Oncogene*, 2003, 22, 147-150.

[71] Honorio, S; Agathanggelou, A; Wernert, N; Rothe, M; Maher, ER; Latif, F. Frequent epigenetic inactivation of the RASSF1A tumour suppressor gene in testicular tumours and distinct methylation profiles of seminoma and nonseminoma testicular germ cell tumours. *Oncogene*, 2003, 22, 461-466.

[72] Hoon, DS; Spugnardi, M; Kuo, C; Huang, SK; Morton, DL; Taback, B. Profiling epigenetic inactivation of tumor suppressor genes in tumors and plasma from cutaneous melanoma patients. *Oncogene*, 2004, 23, 4014-4022.

[73] Horiguchi, K; Tomizawa, Y; Tosaka, M; Ishiuchi, S; Kurihara, H; Mori, M; Saito, N. Epigenetic inactivation of RASSF1A candidate tumor suppressor gene at 3p21.3 in brain tumors. *Oncogene*, 2003, 22, 7862-7865.

[74] House, MG; Guo, M; Efron, DT; Lillemoe, KD; Cameron, JL; Syphard, JE; Hooker, CM; Abraham, SC; Montgomery, EA; Herman, JG; Brock, MV. Tumor suppressor gene hypermethylation as a predictor of gastric stromal tumor behavior. *J Gastrointest Surg*, 2003, 7, 1004-1014; discussion 1014.

[75] House, MG; Herman, JG; Guo, MZ; Hooker, CM; Schulick, RD; Lillemoe, KD; Cameron, JL; Hruban, RH; Maitra, A; Yeo, CJ. Aberrant hypermethylation of tumor suppressor genes in pancreatic endocrine neoplasms. *Ann Surg*, 2003, 238, 423-431; discussion 431-422.

[76] Irimia, M; Fraga, MF; Sanchez-Cespedes, M; Esteller, M. CpG island promoter hypermethylation of the Ras-effector gene NORE1A occurs in the context of a wild-type K-ras in lung cancer. *Oncogene*, 2004, 23, 8695-8699.

[77] Issa, JP. Aging, DNA methylation and cancer. *Crit Rev Oncol Hematol*, 1999, 32, 31-43.

[78] Jackson, JP; Lindroth, AM; Cao, X; Jacobsen, SE. Control of CpNpG DNA methylation by the KRYPTONITE histone H3 methyltransferase. *Nature*, 2002, 416, 556-560.

[79] Jackson, PK. Linking tumor suppression, DNA damage and the anaphase-promoting complex. *Trends Cell Biol*, 2004, 14, 331-334.

[80] Jeddeloh, JA; Stokes, TL; Richards, EJ. Maintenance of genomic methylation requires a SWI2/SNF2-like protein. *Nat Genet*, 1999, 22, 94-97.

[81] Jenuwein, T; Allis, CD. Translating the histone code. *Science*, 2001, 293, 1074-1080.

[82] Jeronimo, C; Henrique, R; Hoque, MO; Mambo, E; Ribeiro, FR; Varzim, G; Oliveira, J; Teixeira, MR; Lopes, C; Sidransky, D. A quantitative promoter methylation profile of prostate cancer. *Clin Cancer Res*, 2004, 10, 8472-8478.

[83] Ji, L; Nishizaki, M; Gao, B; Burbee, D; Kondo, M; Kamibayashi, C; Xu, K; Yen, N; Atkinson, EN; Fang, B; Lerman, MI; Roth, JA; Minna, JD. Expression of several genes in the human chromosome 3p21.3 homozygous deletion region by an adenovirus vector results in tumor suppressor activities in vitro and in vivo. *Cancer Res*, 2002, 62, 2715-2720.

[84] Jones, PA; Wolkowicz, MJ; Rideout, WM, 3rd; Gonzales, FA; Marziasz, CM; Coetzee, GA; Tapscott, SJ. De novo methylation of the MyoD1 CpG island during the establishment of immortal cell lines. *Proc Natl Acad Sci U S A*, 1990, 87, 6117-6121.

[85] Jones, PA; Baylin, SB. The fundamental role of epigenetic events in cancer. *Nat Rev Genet*, 2002, 3, 415-428.

[86] Jones, PL; Veenstra, GJ; Wade, PA; Vermaak, D; Kass, SU; Landsberger, N; Strouboulis, J; Wolffe, AP. Methylated DNA and MeCP2 recruit histone deacetylase to repress transcription. *Nat Genet*, 1998, 19, 187-191.

[87] Kaelin, WG, Jr.; Maher, ER. The VHL tumour-suppressor gene paradigm. *Trends Genet*, 1998, 14, 423-426.

[88] Kang, GH; Lee, S; Kim, WH; Lee, HW; Kim, JC; Rhyu, MG; Ro, JY. Epstein-barr virus-positive gastric carcinoma demonstrates frequent aberrant methylation of multiple genes and constitutes CpG island methylator phenotype-positive gastric carcinoma. *Am J Pathol*, 2002, 160, 787-794.

[89] Kang, GH; Lee, HJ; Hwang, KS; Lee, S; Kim, JH; Kim, JS. Aberrant CpG island hypermethylation of chronic gastritis, in relation to aging, gender, intestinal metaplasia, and chronic inflammation. *Am J Pathol*, 2003, 163, 1551-1556.

[90] Kang, GH; Lee, S; Kim, JS; Jung, HY. Profile of aberrant CpG island methylation along multistep gastric carcinogenesis. *Lab Invest*, 2003, 83, 519-526.

[91] Kang, GH; Lee, S; Lee, HJ; Hwang, KS. Aberrant CpG island hypermethylation of multiple genes in prostate cancer and prostatic intraepithelial neoplasia. *J Pathol*, 2004, 202, 233-240.

[92] Kang, S; Kim, JW; Kang, GH; Park, NH; Song, YS; Kang, SB; Lee, HP. Polymorphism in folate- and methionine-metabolizing enzyme and aberrant CpG island hypermethylation in uterine cervical cancer. *Gynecol Oncol*, 2005, 96, 173-180.

[93] Kawakami, T; Okamoto, K; Kataoka, A; Koizumi, S; Iwaki, H; Sugihara, H; Reeve, AE; Ogawa, O; Okada, Y. Multipoint methylation analysis indicates a distinctive epigenetic phenotype among testicular germ cell tumors and testicular malignant lymphomas. *Genes Chromosomes Cancer*, 2003, 38, 97-101.

[94] Khokhlatchev, A; Rabizadeh, S; Xavier, R; Nedwidek, M; Chen, T; Zhang, XF; Seed, B; Avruch, J. Identification of a novel Ras-regulated proapoptotic pathway. *Curr Biol*, 2002, 12, 253-265.

[95] Killary, AM; Wolf, ME; Giambernardi, TA; Naylor, SL. Definition of a tumor suppressor locus within human chromosome 3p21-p22. *Proc Natl Acad Sci U S A*, 1992, 89, 10877-10881.

[96] Kim, DH; Kim, JS; Ji, YI; Shim, YM; Kim, H; Han, J; Park, J. Hypermethylation of RASSF1A promoter is associated with the age at starting smoking and a poor prognosis in primary non-small cell lung cancer. *Cancer Res*, 2003, 63, 3743-3746.

[97] Kim, DH; Kim, JS; Park, JH; Lee, SK; Ji, YI; Kwon, YM; Shim, YM; Han, J; Park, J. Relationship of Ras association domain family 1 methylation and K-ras mutation in primary non-small cell lung cancer. *Cancer Res*, 2003, 63, 6206-6211.

[98] Kim, ST; Lim, DS; Canman, CE; Kastan, MB. Substrate specificities and identification of putative substrates of ATM kinase family members. *J Biol Chem*, 1999, 274, 37538-37543.

[99] Kok, K; Naylor, SL; Buys, CH. Deletions of the short arm of chromosome 3 in solid tumors and the search for suppressor genes. *Adv Cancer Res*, 1997, 71, 27-92.

[100] Koul, S; Houldsworth, J; Mansukhani, MM; Donadio, A; McKiernan, JM; Reuter, VE; Bosl, GJ; Chaganti, RS; Murty, VV. Characteristic promoter hypermethylation signatures in male germ cell tumors. *Mol Cancer*, 2002, 1, 8.

[101] Koul, S; McKiernan, JM; Narayan, G; Houldsworth, J; Bacik, J; Dobrzynski, DL; Assaad, AM; Mansukhani, M; Reuter, VE; Bosl, GJ; Chaganti, RS; Murty, VV. Role of promoter hypermethylation in Cisplatin treatment response of male germ cell tumors. *Mol Cancer*, 2004, 3, 16.

[102] Krassenstein, R; Sauter, E; Dulaimi, E; Battagli, C; Ehya, H; Klein-Szanto, A; Cairns, P. Detection of breast cancer in nipple aspirate fluid by CpG island hypermethylation. *Clin Cancer Res*, 2004, 10, 28-32.

[103] Kuroki, T; Trapasso, F; Yendamuri, S; Matsuyama, A; Alder, H; Mori, M; Croce, CM. Promoter hypermethylation of RASSF1A in esophageal squamous cell carcinoma. *Clin Cancer Res*, 2003, 9, 1441-1445.

[104] Kuzmin, I; Gillespie, JW; Protopopov, A; Geil, L; Dreijerink, K; Yang, Y; Vocke, CD; Duh, FM; Zabarovsky, E; Minna, JD; Rhim, JS; Emmert-Buck, MR; Linehan, WM; Lerman, MI. The RASSF1A Tumor Suppressor Gene Is Inactivated in Prostate Tumors and Suppresses Growth of Prostate Carcinoma Cells. *Cancer Res*, 2002, 62, 3498-3502.

[105] Kuzmin, I; Liu, L; Dammann, R; Geil, L; Stanbridge, EJ; Wilczynski, SP; Lerman, MI; Pfeifer, GP. Inactivation of RAS association domain family 1A gene in cervical carcinomas and the role of human papillomavirus infection. *Cancer Res*, 2003, 63, 1888-1893.

[106] Kwong, J; Lo, KW; To, KF; Teo, PM; Johnson, PJ; Huang, DP. Promoter hypermethylation of multiple genes in nasopharyngeal carcinoma. *Clin Cancer Res*, 2002, 8, 131-137.

[107] Lachner, M; O'Carroll, D; Rea, S; Mechtler, K; Jenuwein, T. Methylation of histone H3 lysine 9 creates a binding site for HP1 proteins. *Nature*, 2001, 410, 116-120.

[108] Lee, MG; Kim, HY; Byun, DS; Lee, SJ; Lee, CH; Kim, JI; Chang, SG; Chi, SG. Frequent epigenetic inactivation of rassf1a in human bladder carcinoma. *Cancer Res*, 2001, 61, 6688-6692.

[109] Lee, S; Lee, HJ; Kim, JH; Lee, HS; Jang, JJ; Kang, GH. Aberrant CpG island hypermethylation along multistep hepatocarcinogenesis. *Am J Pathol*, 2003, 163, 1371-1378.

[110] Lee, S; Hwang, KS; Lee, HJ; Kim, JS; Kang, GH. Aberrant CpG island hypermethylation of multiple genes in colorectal neoplasia. *Lab Invest*, 2004, 84, 884-893.

[111] Lehmann, U; Langer, F; Feist, H; Glockner, S; Hasemeier, B; Kreipe, H. Quantitative assessment of promoter hypermethylation during breast cancer development. *Am J Pathol*, 2002, 160, 605-612.

[112] Lehnertz, B; Ueda, Y; Derijck, AA; Braunschweig, U; Perez-Burgos, L; Kubicek, S; Chen, T; Li, E; Jenuwein, T; Peters, AH. Suv39h-mediated histone H3 lysine 9 methylation directs DNA methylation to major satellite repeats at pericentric heterochromatin. *Curr Biol*, 2003, 13, 1192-1200.

[113] Lerman, MI; Minna, JD. The 630-kb lung cancer homozygous deletion region on human chromosome 3p21.3: identification and evaluation of the resident candidate tumor suppressor genes. The International Lung Cancer Chromosome 3p21.3 Tumor Suppressor Gene Consortium. *Cancer Res*, 2000, 60, 6116-6133.

[114] Lewis, CM; Cler, LR; Bu, DW; Zochbauer-Muller, S; Milchgrub, S; Naftalis, EZ; Leitch, AM; Minna, JD; Euhus, DM. Promoter hypermethylation in benign breast epithelium in relation to predicted breast cancer risk. *Clin Cancer Res*, 2005, 11, 166-172.

[115] Li, J; Zhang, Z; Dai, Z; Popkie, AP; Plass, C; Morrison, C; Wang, Y; You, M. RASSF1A promoter methylation and Kras2 mutations in non small cell lung cancer. *Neoplasia*, 2003, 5, 362-366.

[116] Li, J; Wang, F; Protopopov, A; Malyukova, A; Kashuba, V; Minna, JD; Lerman, MI; Klein, G; Zabarovsky, E. Inactivation of RASSF1C during in vivo tumor growth identifies it as a tumor suppressor gene. *Oncogene*, 2004, 23, 5941-5949.

[117] Lim, S; Yang, MH; Park, JH; Nojima, T; Hashimoto, H; Unni, KK; Park, YK. Inactivation of the RASSF1A in osteosarcoma. *Oncol Rep*, 2003, 10, 897-901.

[118] Lindsey, JC; Lusher, ME; Anderton, JA; Bailey, S; Gilbertson, RJ; Pearson, AD; Ellison, DW; Clifford, SC. Identification of tumour-specific epigenetic events in medulloblastoma development by hypermethylation profiling. *Carcinogenesis*, 2004, 25, 661-668.

[119] Liu, L; Amy, V; Liu, G; McKeehan, WL. Novel complex integrating mitochondria and the microtubular cytoskeleton with chromosome remodeling and tumor suppressor RASSF1 deduced by in silico homology analysis, interaction cloning in yeast, and colocalization in cultured cells. *In Vitro Cell Dev Biol Anim*, 2002, 38, 582-594.

[120] Liu, L; Yoon, JH; Dammann, R; Pfeifer, GP. Frequent hypermethylation of the RASSF1A gene in prostate cancer. *Oncogene*, 2002, 21, 6835-6840.

[121] Liu, L; Tommasi, S; Lee, DH; Dammann, R; Pfeifer, GP. Control of microtubule stability by the RASSF1A tumor suppressor. *Oncogene*, 2003, 22, 8125-8136.

[122] Lo, KW; Kwong, J; Hui, AB; Chan, SY; To, KF; Chan, AS; Chow, LS; Teo, PM; Johnson, PJ; Huang, DP. High frequency of promoter hypermethylation of RASSF1A in nasopharyngeal carcinoma. *Cancer Res*, 2001, 61, 3877-3881.

[123] Lusher, ME; Lindsey, JC; Latif, F; Pearson, AD; Ellison, DW; Clifford, SC. Biallelic epigenetic inactivation of the RASSF1A tumor suppressor gene in medulloblastoma development. *Cancer Res*, 2002, 62, 5906-5911.

[124] Marsit, CJ; Kim, DH; Liu, M; Hinds, PW; Wiencke, JK; Nelson, HH; Kelsey, KT. Hypermethylation of RASSF1A and BLU tumor suppressor genes in non-small cell

lung cancer: implications for tobacco smoking during adolescence. *Int J Cancer*, 2005, 114, 219-223.

[125] Maruya, S; Issa, JP; Weber, RS; Rosenthal, DI; Haviland, JC; Lotan, R; El-Naggar, AK. Differential methylation status of tumor-associated genes in head and neck squamous carcinoma: incidence and potential implications. *Clin Cancer Res*, 2004, 10, 3825-3830.

[126] Maruyama, R; Toyooka, S; Toyooka, KO; Harada, K; Virmani, AK; Zochbauer-Muller, S; Farinas, AJ; Vakar-Lopez, F; Minna, JD; Sagalowsky, A; Czerniak, B; Gazdar, AF. Aberrant promoter methylation profile of bladder cancer and its relationship to clinicopathological features. *Cancer Res*, 2001, 61, 8659-8663.

[127] Maruyama, R; Toyooka, S; Toyooka, KO; Virmani, AK; Zochbauer-Muller, S; Farinas, AJ; Minna, JD; McConnell, J; Frenkel, EP; Gazdar, AF. Aberrant promoter methylation profile of prostate cancers and its relationship to clinicopathological features. *Clin Cancer Res*, 2002, 8, 514-519.

[128] Maruyama, R; Sugio, K; Yoshino, I; Maehara, Y; Gazdar, AF. Hypermethylation of FHIT as a prognostic marker in nonsmall cell lung carcinoma. *Cancer*, 2004, 100, 1472-1477.

[129] Mathe, E. RASSF1A, the new guardian of mitosis. *Nat Genet*, 2004, 36, 117-118.

[130] Mayo, MW; Wang, CY; Cogswell, PC; Rogers-Graham, KS; Lowe, SW; Der, CJ; Baldwin, AS, Jr. Requirement of NF-kappaB activation to suppress p53-independent apoptosis induced by oncogenic Ras. *Science*, 1997, 278, 1812-1815.

[131] Mehrotra, J; Vali, M; McVeigh, M; Kominsky, SL; Fackler, MJ; Lahti-Domenici, J; Polyak, K; Sacchi, N; Garrett-Mayer, E; Argani, P; Sukumar, S. Very high frequency of hypermethylated genes in breast cancer metastasis to the bone, brain, and lung. *Clin Cancer Res*, 2004, 10, 3104-3109.

[132] Morrissey, C; Martinez, A; Zatyka, M; Agathanggelou, A; Honorio, S; Astuti, D; Morgan, NV; Moch, H; Richards, FM; Kishida, T; Yao, M; Schraml, P; Latif, F; Maher, ER. Epigenetic inactivation of the RASSF1A 3p21.3 tumor suppressor gene in both clear cell and papillary renal cell carcinoma. *Cancer Res*, 2001, 61, 7277-7281.

[133] Muller, HM; Widschwendter, A; Fiegl, H; Ivarsson, L; Goebel, G; Perkmann, E; Marth, C; Widschwendter, M. DNA methylation in serum of breast cancer patients: an independent prognostic marker. *Cancer Res*, 2003, 63, 7641-7645.

[134] Murray, PG; Qiu, GH; Fu, L; Waites, ER; Srivastava, G; Heys, D; Agathanggelou, A; Latif, F; Grundy, RG; Mann, JR; Starczynski, J; Crocker, J; Parkes, SE; Ambinder, RF; Young, LS; Tao, Q. Frequent epigenetic inactivation of the RASSF1A tumor suppressor gene in Hodgkin's lymphoma. *Oncogene*, 2004, 23, 1326-1331.

[135] Nakayama, J; Rice, JC; Strahl, BD; Allis, CD; Grewal, SI. Role of histone H3 lysine 9 methylation in epigenetic control of heterochromatin assembly. *Science*, 2001, 292, 110-113.

[136] Nan, X; Ng, HH; Johnson, CA; Laherty, CD; Turner, BM; Eisenman, RN; Bird, A. Transcriptional repression by the methyl-CpG-binding protein MeCP2 involves a histone deacetylase complex. *Nature*, 1998, 393, 386-389.

[137] Newton, AC. Protein kinase C. Seeing two domains. *Curr Biol*, 1995, 5, 973-976.

[138] Ng, HH; Zhang, Y; Hendrich, B; Johnson, CA; Turner, BM; Erdjument-Bromage, H; Tempst, P; Reinberg, D; Bird, A. MBD2 is a transcriptional repressor belonging to the MeCP1 histone deacetylase complex. *Nat Genet*, 1999, 23, 58-61.

[139] Ng, MH; Lau, KM; Wong, WS; To, KW; Cheng, SH; Tsang, KS; Chan, NP; Kho, BC; Lo, KW; Tong, JH; Lam, CW; Chan, JC. Alterations of RAS signalling in Chinese multiple myeloma patients: absent BRAF and rare RAS mutations, but frequent inactivation of RASSF1A by transcriptional silencing or expression of a non-functional variant transcript. *Br J Haematol*, 2003, 123, 637-645.

[140] Ortiz-Vega, S; Khokhlatchev, A; Nedwidek, M; Zhang, XF; Dammann, R; Pfeifer, GP; Avruch, J. The putative tumor suppressor RASSF1A homodimerizes and heterodimerizes with the Ras-GTP binding protein Nore1. *Oncogene*, 2002, 21, 1381-1390.

[141] Ponting, CP; Benjamin, DR. A novel family of Ras-binding domains. *Trends Biochem Sci*, 1996, 21, 422-425.

[142] Praskova, M; Khoklatchev, A; Ortiz-Vega, S; Avruch, J. Regulation of the MST1 kinase by autophosphorylation, by the growth inhibitory proteins, RASSF1 and NORE1, and by Ras. *Biochem J*, 2004, 381, 453-462.

[143] Rabizadeh, S; Xavier, RJ; Ishiguro, K; Bernabeortiz, J; Lopez-Ilasaca, M; Khokhlatchev, A; Mollahan, P; Pfeifer, GP; Avruch, J; Seed, B. The scaffold protein CNK1 interacts with the tumor suppressor RASSF1A and augments RASSF1A-induced cell death. *J Biol Chem*, 2004, 279, 29247-29254.

[144] Ramirez, JL; Sarries, C; de Castro, PL; Roig, B; Queralt, C; Escuin, D; de Aguirre, I; Sanchez, JM; Manzano, JL; Margeli, M; Sanchez, JJ; Astudillo, J; Taron, M; Rosell, R. Methylation patterns and K-ras mutations in tumor and paired serum of resected non-small-cell lung cancer patients. *Cancer Lett*, 2003, 193, 207-216.

[145] Ramirez, JL; Taron, M; Balana, C; Sarries, C; Mendez, P; de Aguirre, I; Nunez, L; Roig, B; Queralt, C; Botia, M; Rosell, R. Serum DNA as a tool for cancer patient management. *Rocz Akad Med Bialymst*, 2003, 48, 34-41.

[146] Rathi, A; Virmani, AK; Schorge, JO; Elias, KJ; Maruyama, R; Minna, JD; Mok, SC; Girard, L; Fishman, DA; Gazdar, AF. Methylation profiles of sporadic ovarian tumors and nonmalignant ovaries from high-risk women. *Clin Cancer Res*, 2002, 8, 3324-3331.

[147] Reifenberger, J; Knobbe, CB; Sterzinger, AA; Blaschke, B; Schulte, KW; Ruzicka, T; Reifenberger, G. Frequent alterations of Ras signaling pathway genes in sporadic malignant melanomas. *Int J Cancer*, 2004, 109, 377-384.

[148] Robertson, KD; Ait-Si-Ali, S; Yokochi, T; Wade, PA; Jones, PL; Wolffe, AP. DNMT1 forms a complex with Rb, E2F1 and HDAC1 and represses transcription from E2F-responsive promoters. *Nat Genet*, 2000, 25, 338-342.

[149] Rong, R; Jin, W; Zhang, J; Saeed Sheikh, M; Huang, Y. Tumor suppressor RASSF1A is a microtubule-binding protein that stabilizes microtubules and induces G(2)/M arrest. *Oncogene*, 2004.

[150] Rong, R; Jin, W; Zhang, J; Sheikh, MS; Huang, Y. Tumor suppressor RASSF1A is a microtubule-binding protein that stabilizes microtubules and induces G2/M arrest. *Oncogene*, 2004, 23, 8216-8230.

[151] Rountree, MR; Bachman, KE; Baylin, SB. DNMT1 binds HDAC2 and a new co-repressor, DMAP1, to form a complex at replication foci. *Nat Genet*, 2000, 25, 269-277.

[152] Sakamoto, N; Terai, T; Ajioka, Y; Abe, S; Kobayasi, O; Hirai, S; Hino, O; Watanabe, H; Sato, N; Shimoda, T; Fujii, H. Frequent hypermethylation of RASSF1A in early flat-type colorectal tumors. *Oncogene*, 2004, 23, 8900-8907.

[153] Sanchez-Cespedes, M; Esteller, M; Wu, L; Nawroz-Danish, H; Yoo, GH; Koch, WM; Jen, J; Herman, JG; Sidransky, D. Gene promoter hypermethylation in tumors and serum of head and neck cancer patients. *Cancer Res*, 2000, 60, 892-895.

[154] Schagdarsurengin, U; Gimm, O; Hoang-Vu, C; Dralle, H; Pfeifer, GP; Dammann, R. Frequent epigenetic silencing of the CpG island promoter of RASSF1A in thyroid carcinoma. *Cancer Res*, 2002, 62, 3698-3701.

[155] Schagdarsurengin, U; Wilkens, L; Steinemann, D; Flemming, P; Kreipe, HH; Pfeifer, GP; Schlegelberger, B; Dammann, R. Frequent epigenetic inactivation of the RASSF1A gene in hepatocellular carcinoma. *Oncogene*, 2003, 22, 1866-1871.

[156] Seidel, C; Bartel, F; Rastetter, M; Bluemke, K; Wurl, P; Taubert, H; Dammann, R. Alterations of cancer-related genes in soft tissue sarcomas: Hypermethylation of RASSF1A is frequently detected in leiomyosarcoma and associated with poor prognosis in sarcoma. *Int J Cancer*, 2005, 114, 442-447.

[157] Seidl, S; Ackermann, J; Kaufmann, H; Keck, A; Nosslinger, T; Zielinski, CC; Drach, J; Zochbauer-Muller, S. DNA-methylation analysis identifies the E-cadherin gene as a potential marker of disease progression in patients with monoclonal gammopathies. *Cancer*, 2004, 100, 2598-2606.

[158] Sekido, Y; Ahmadian, M; Wistuba, II; Latif, F; Bader, S; Wei, MH; Duh, FM; Gazdar, AF; Lerman, MI; Minna, JD. Cloning of a breast cancer homozygous deletion junction narrows the region of search for a 3p21.3 tumor suppressor gene. *Oncogene*, 1998, 16, 3151-3157.

[159] Serrano, M; Lin, AW; McCurrach, ME; Beach, D; Lowe, SW. Oncogenic ras provokes premature cell senescence associated with accumulation of p53 and p16INK4a. *Cell*, 1997, 88, 593-602.

[160] Shao, J; Sheng, H; DuBois, RN; Beauchamp, RD. Oncogenic Ras-mediated cell growth arrest and apoptosis are associated with increased ubiquitin-dependent cyclin D1 degradation. *J Biol Chem*, 2000, 275, 22916-22924.

[161] Shivakumar, L; Minna, J; Sakamaki, T; Pestell, R; White, MA. The RASSF1A tumor suppressor blocks cell cycle progression and inhibits cyclin D1 accumulation. *Mol Cell Biol*, 2002, 22, 4309-4318.

[162] Singal, R; Ferdinand, L; Reis, IM; Schlesselman, JJ. Methylation of multiple genes in prostate cancer and the relationship with clinicopathological features of disease. *Oncol Rep*, 2004, 12, 631-637.

[163] Smiraglia, DJ; Rush, LJ; Fruhwald, MC; Dai, Z; Held, WA; Costello, JF; Lang, JC; Eng, C; Li, B; Wright, FA; Caligiuri, MA; Plass, C. Excessive CpG island hypermethylation in cancer cell lines versus primary human malignancies. *Hum Mol Genet*, 2001, 10, 1413-1419.

[164] Smith, AJ; Xian, J; Richardson, M; Johnstone, KA; Rabbitts, PH. Cre-loxP chromosome engineering of a targeted deletion in the mouse corresponding to the 3p21.3 region of homozygous loss in human tumours. *Oncogene*, 2002, 21, 4521-4529.

[165] Song, MS; Song, SJ; Ayad, NG; Chang, JS; Lee, JH; Hong, HK; Lee, H; Choi, N; Kim, J; Kim, H; Kim, JW; Choi, EJ; Kirschner, MW; Lim, DS. The tumour suppressor RASSF1A regulates mitosis by inhibiting the APC-Cdc20 complex. *Nat Cell Biol*, 2004, 6, 129-137.

[166] Song, MS; Chang, JS; Song, SJ; Yang, TH; Lee, H; Lim, DS. The centrosomal protein RAS association domain family protein 1A (RASSF1A)-binding protein 1 regulates

mitotic progression by recruiting RASSF1A to spindle poles. *J Biol Chem*, 2005, 280, 3920-3927.

[167] Sozzi, G; Veronese, ML; Negrini, M; Baffa, R; Cotticelli, MG; Inoue, H; Tornielli, S; Pilotti, S; De Gregorio, L; Pastorino, U; Pierotti, MA; Ohta, M; Huebner, K; Croce, CM. The FHIT gene 3p14.2 is abnormal in lung cancer. *Cell*, 1996, 85, 17-26.

[168] Spugnardi, M; Tommasi, S; Dammann, R; Pfeifer, GP; Hoon, DS. Epigenetic inactivation of RAS association domain family protein 1 (RASSF1A) in malignant cutaneous melanoma. *Cancer Res*, 2003, 63, 1639-1643.

[169] Takahashi, T; Shivapurkar, N; Riquelme, E; Shigematsu, H; Reddy, J; Suzuki, M; Miyajima, K; Zhou, X; Bekele, BN; Gazdar, AF; Wistuba, II. Aberrant promoter hypermethylation of multiple genes in gallbladder carcinoma and chronic cholecystitis. *Clin Cancer Res*, 2004, 10, 6126-6133.

[170] Tamaru, H; Selker, EU. A histone H3 methyltransferase controls DNA methylation in Neurospora crassa. *Nature*, 2001, 414, 277-283.

[171] To, KF; Leung, WK; Lee, TL; Yu, J; Tong, JH; Chan, MW; Ng, EK; Chung, SC; Sung, JJ. Promoter hypermethylation of tumor-related genes in gastric intestinal metaplasia of patients with and without gastric cancer. *Int J Cancer*, 2002, 102, 623-628.

[172] Todd, S; Franklin, WA; Varella-Garcia, M; Kennedy, T; Hilliker, CE, Jr.; Hahner, L; Anderson, M; Wiest, JS; Drabkin, HA; Gemmill, RM. Homozygous deletions of human chromosome 3p in lung tumors. *Cancer Res*, 1997, 57, 1344-1352.

[173] Tokinaga, K; Okuda, H; Nomura, A; Ashida, S; Furihata, M; Shuin, T. Hypermethylation of the RASSF1A tumor suppressor gene in Japanese clear cell renal cell carcinoma. *Oncol Rep*, 2004, 12, 805-810.

[174] Tomizawa, Y; Kohno, T; Kondo, H; Otsuka, A; Nishioka, M; Niki, T; Yamada, T; Maeshima, A; Yoshimura, K; Saito, R; Minna, JD; Yokota, J. Clinicopathological Significance of Epigenetic Inactivation of RASSF1A at 3p21.3 in Stage I Lung Adenocarcinoma. *Clin Cancer Res*, 2002, 8, 2362-2368.

[175] Tomizawa, Y; Iijima, H; Nomoto, T; Iwasaki, Y; Otani, Y; Tsuchiya, S; Saito, R; Dobashi, K; Nakajima, T; Mori, M. Clinicopathological significance of aberrant methylation of RARbeta2 at 3p24, RASSF1A at 3p21.3, and FHIT at 3p14.2 in patients with non-small cell lung cancer. *Lung Cancer*, 2004, 46, 305-312.

[176] Tommasi, S; Dammann, R; Jin, SG; Zhang Xf, XF; Avruch, J; Pfeifer, GP. RASSF3 and NORE1: identification and cloning of two human homologues of the putative tumor suppressor gene RASSF1. *Oncogene*, 2002, 21, 2713-2720.

[177] Tommasi, S; Dammann, R; Zhang, Z; Wang, Y; Liu, L; Tsark, WM; Wilczynski, SP; Li, J; You, M; Pfeifer, GP. Tumor susceptibility of Rassf1a knockout mice. *Cancer Res*, 2005, 65, 92-98.

[178] Tong, JH; Tsang, RK; Lo, KW; Woo, JK; Kwong, J; Chan, MW; Chang, AR; van Hasselt, CA; Huang, DP; To, KF. Quantitative Epstein-Barr virus DNA analysis and detection of gene promoter hypermethylation in nasopharyngeal (NP) brushing samples from patients with NP carcinoma. *Clin Cancer Res*, 2002, 8, 2612-2619.

[179] Topaloglu, O; Hoque, MO; Tokumaru, Y; Lee, J; Ratovitski, E; Sidransky, D; Moon, CS. Detection of promoter hypermethylation of multiple genes in the tumor and bronchoalveolar lavage of patients with lung cancer. *Clin Cancer Res*, 2004, 10, 2284-2288.

[180] Toyooka, S; Pass, HI; Shivapurkar, N; Fukuyama, Y; Maruyama, R; Toyooka, KO; Gilcrease, M; Farinas, A; Minna, JD; Gazdar, AF. Aberrant methylation and simian virus 40 tag sequences in malignant mesothelioma. *Cancer Res*, 2001, 61, 5727-5730.

[181] Toyooka, S; Toyooka, KO; Maruyama, R; Virmani, AK; Girard, L; Miyajima, K; Harada, K; Ariyoshi, Y; Takahashi, T; Sugio, K; Brambilla, E; Gilcrease, M; Minna, JD; Gazdar, AF. DNA methylation profiles of lung tumors. *Mol Cancer Ther*, 2001, 1, 61-67.

[182] Toyooka, S; Carbone, M; Toyooka, KO; Bocchetta, M; Shivapurkar, N; Minna, JD; Gazdar, AF. Progressive aberrant methylation of the RASSF1A gene in simian virus 40 infected human mesothelial cells. *Oncogene*, 2002, 21, 4340-4344.

[183] Toyooka, S; Maruyama, R; Toyooka, KO; McLerran, D; Feng, Z; Fukuyama, Y; Virmani, AK; Zochbauer-Muller, S; Tsukuda, K; Sugio, K; Shimizu, N; Shimizu, K; Lee, H; Chen, CY; Fong, KM; Gilcrease, M; Roth, JA; Minna, JD; Gazdar, AF. Smoke exposure, histologic type and geography-related differences in the methylation profiles of non-small cell lung cancer. *Int J Cancer*, 2003, 103, 153-160.

[184] Toyooka, S; Suzuki, M; Tsuda, T; Toyooka, KO; Maruyama, R; Tsukuda, K; Fukuyama, Y; Iizasa, T; Fujisawa, T; Shimizu, N; Minna, JD; Gazdar, AF. Dose effect of smoking on aberrant methylation in non-small cell lung cancers. *Int J Cancer*, 2004, 110, 462-464.

[185] Tozawa, T; Tamura, G; Honda, T; Nawata, S; Kimura, W; Makino, N; Kawata, S; Sugai, T; Suto, T; Motoyama, T. Promoter hypermethylation of DAP-kinase is associated with poor survival in primary biliary tract carcinoma patients. *Cancer Sci*, 2004, 95, 736-740.

[186] Tsou, JA; Hagen, JA; Carpenter, CL; Laird-Offringa, IA. DNA methylation analysis: a powerful new tool for lung cancer diagnosis. *Oncogene*, 2002, 21, 5450-5461.

[187] Turker, MS. Gene silencing in mammalian cells and the spread of DNA methylation. *Oncogene*, 2002, 21, 5388-5393.

[188] van Engeland, M; Roemen, GM; Brink, M; Pachen, MM; Weijenberg, MP; de Bruine, AP; Arends, JW; van den Brandt, PA; de Goeij, AF; Herman, JG. K-ras mutations and RASSF1A promoter methylation in colorectal cancer. *Oncogene*, 2002, 21, 3792-3795.

[189] van Engeland, M; Weijenberg, MP; Roemen, GM; Brink, M; de Bruine, AP; Goldbohm, RA; van den Brandt, PA; Baylin, SB; de Goeij, AF; Herman, JG. Effects of dietary folate and alcohol intake on promoter methylation in sporadic colorectal cancer: the Netherlands cohort study on diet and cancer. *Cancer Res*, 2003, 63, 3133-3137.

[190] Vavvas, D; Li, X; Avruch, J; Zhang, XF. Identification of Nore1 as a potential Ras effector. *J Biol Chem*, 1998, 273, 5439-5442.

[191] Vos, MD; Ellis, CA; Bell, A; Birrer, MJ; Clark, GJ. Ras uses the novel tumor suppressor RASSF1 as an effector to mediate apoptosis. *J Biol Chem*, 2000, 275, 35669-35672.

[192] Vos, MD; Martinez, A; Ellis, CA; Vallecorsa, T; Clark, GJ. The pro-apoptotic Ras effector Nore1 may serve as a Ras-regulated tumor suppressor in the lung. *J Biol Chem*, 2003, 278, 21938-21943.

[193] Vos, MD; Martinez, A; Elam, C; Dallol, A; Taylor, BJ; Latif, F; Clark, GJ. A role for the RASSF1A tumor suppressor in the regulation of tubulin polymerization and genomic stability. *Cancer Res*, 2004, 64, 4244-4250.

[194] Wagner, KJ; Cooper, WN; Grundy, RG; Caldwell, G; Jones, C; Wadey, RB; Morton, D; Schofield, PN; Reik, W; Latif, F; Maher, ER. Frequent RASSF1A tumour suppressor gene promoter methylation in Wilms' tumour and colorectal cancer. *Oncogene*, 2002, 21, 7277-7282.

[195] Waki, T; Tamura, G; Sato, M; Motoyama, T. Age-related methylation of tumor suppressor and tumor-related genes: an analysis of autopsy samples. *Oncogene*, 2003, 22, 4128-4133.

[196] Wang, J; Lee, JJ; Wang, L; Liu, DD; Lu, C; Fan, YH; Hong, WK; Mao, L. Value of p16INK4a and RASSF1A promoter hypermethylation in prognosis of patients with resectable non-small cell lung cancer. *Clin Cancer Res*, 2004, 10, 6119-6125.

[197] Wei, MH; Latif, F; Bader, S; Kashuba, V; Chen, JY; Duh, FM; Sekido, Y; Lee, CC; Geil, L; Kuzmin, I; Zabarovsky, E; Klein, G; Zbar, B; Minna, JD; Lerman, MI. Construction of a 600-kilobase cosmid clone contig and generation of a transcriptional map surrounding the lung cancer tumor suppressor gene (TSG) locus on human chromosome 3p21.3: progress toward the isolation of a lung cancer TSG. *Cancer Res*, 1996, 56, 1487-1492.

[198] Wistuba, II; Behrens, C; Virmani, AK; Mele, G; Milchgrub, S; Girard, L; Fondon, JW, 3rd; Garner, HR; McKay, B; Latif, F; Lerman, MI; Lam, S; Gazdar, AF; Minna, JD. High resolution chromosome 3p allelotyping of human lung cancer and preneoplastic/preinvasive bronchial epithelium reveals multiple, discontinuous sites of 3p allele loss and three regions of frequent breakpoints. *Cancer Res*, 2000, 60, 1949-1960.

[199] Wong, IH; Lo, YM; Zhang, J; Liew, CT; Ng, MH; Wong, N; Lai, PB; Lau, WY; Hjelm, NM; Johnson, PJ. Detection of aberrant p16 methylation in the plasma and serum of liver cancer patients. *Cancer Res*, 1999, 59, 71-73.

[200] Wong, IH; Chan, J; Wong, J; Tam, PK. Ubiquitous aberrant RASSF1A promoter methylation in childhood neoplasia. *Clin Cancer Res*, 2004, 10, 994-1002.

[201] Wong, N; Li, L; Tsang, K; Lai, PB; To, KF; Johnson, PJ. Frequent loss of chromosome 3p and hypermethylation of RASSF1A in cholangiocarcinoma. *J Hepatol*, 2002, 37, 633-639.

[202] Wong, TS; Tang, KC; Kwong, DL; Sham, JS; Wei, WI; Kwong, YL; Yuen, AP. Differential gene methylation in undifferentiated nasopharyngeal carcinoma. *Int J Oncol*, 2003, 22, 869-874.

[203] Wong, TS; Kwong, DL; Sham, JS; Wei, WI; Kwong, YL; Yuen, AP. Quantitative plasma hypermethylated DNA markers of undifferentiated nasopharyngeal carcinoma. *Clin Cancer Res*, 2004, 10, 2401-2406.

[204] Woodson, K; Gillespie, J; Hanson, J; Emmert-Buck, M; Phillips, JM; Linehan, WM; Tangrea, JA. Heterogeneous gene methylation patterns among pre-invasive and cancerous lesions of the prostate: a histopathologic study of whole mount prostate specimens. *Prostate*, 2004, 60, 25-31.

[205] Woodson, K; Hanson, J; Tangrea, J. A survey of gene-specific methylation in human prostate cancer among black and white men. *Cancer Lett*, 2004, 205, 181-188.

[206] Xian, J; Clark, KJ; Fordham, R; Pannell, R; Rabbitts, TH; Rabbitts, PH. Inadequate lung development and bronchial hyperplasia in mice with a targeted deletion in the Dutt1/Robo1 gene. *Proc Natl Acad Sci U S A*, 2001, 98, 15062-15066.

[207] Xing, M; Cohen, Y; Mambo, E; Tallini, G; Udelsman, R; Ladenson, PW; Sidransky, D. Early occurrence of RASSF1A hypermethylation and its mutual exclusion with BRAF mutation in thyroid tumorigenesis. *Cancer Res*, 2004, 64, 1664-1668.

[208] Xu, XL; Yu, J; Zhang, HY; Sun, MH; Gu, J; Du, X; Shi, DR; Wang, P; Yang, ZH; Zhu, JD. Methylation profile of the promoter CpG islands of 31 genes that may contribute to colorectal carcinogenesis. *World J Gastroenterol*, 2004, 10, 3441-3454.

[209] Yamakawa, K; Takahashi, T; Horio, Y; Murata, Y; Takahashi, E; Hibi, K; Yokoyama, S; Ueda, R; Nakamura, Y. Frequent homozygous deletions in lung cancer cell lines detected by a DNA marker located at 3p21.3-p22. *Oncogene*, 1993, 8, 327-330.

[210] Yanagawa, N; Tamura, G; Oizumi, H; Takahashi, N; Shimazaki, Y; Motoyama, T. Promoter hypermethylation of tumor suppressor and tumor-related genes in non-small cell lung cancers. *Cancer Sci*, 2003, 94, 589-592.

[211] Yang, B; House, MG; Guo, M; Herman, JG; Clark, DP. Promoter methylation profiles of tumor suppressor genes in intrahepatic and extrahepatic cholangiocarcinoma. *Mod Pathol*, 2005, 18, 412-420.

[212] Yang, Q; Zage, P; Kagan, D; Tian, Y; Seshadri, R; Salwen, HR; Liu, S; Chlenski, A; Cohn, SL. Association of epigenetic inactivation of RASSF1A with poor outcome in human neuroblastoma. *Clin Cancer Res*, 2004, 10, 8493-8500.

[213] Yegnasubramanian, S; Kowalski, J; Gonzalgo, ML; Zahurak, M; Piantadosi, S; Walsh, PC; Bova, GS; De Marzo, AM; Isaacs, WB; Nelson, WG. Hypermethylation of CpG islands in primary and metastatic human prostate cancer. *Cancer Res*, 2004, 64, 1975-1986.

[214] Yoon, JH; Dammann, R; Pfeifer, GP. Hypermethylation of the CpG island of the RASSF1A gene in ovarian and renal cell carcinomas. *Int J Cancer*, 2001, 94, 212-217.

[215] Yu, J; Zhang, H; Gu, J; Lin, S; Li, J; Lu, W; Wang, Y; Zhu, J. Methylation profiles of thirty four promoter-CpG islands and concordant methylation behaviours of sixteen genes that may contribute to carcinogenesis of astrocytoma. *BMC Cancer*, 2004, 4, 65.

[216] Yu, MY; Tong, JH; Chan, PK; Lee, TL; Chan, MW; Chan, AW; Lo, KW; To, KF. Hypermethylation of the tumor suppressor gene RASSFIA and frequent concomitant loss of heterozygosity at 3p21 in cervical cancers. *Int J Cancer*, 2003, 105, 204-209.

[217] Zhong, S; Yeo, W; Tang, MW; Wong, N; Lai, PB; Johnson, PJ. Intensive hypermethylation of the CpG island of Ras association domain family 1A in hepatitis B virus-associated hepatocellular carcinomas. *Clin Cancer Res*, 2003, 9, 3376-3382.

[218] Zochbauer-Muller, S; Lam, S; Toyooka, S; Virmani, AK; Toyooka, KO; Seidl, S; Minna, JD; Gazdar, AF. Aberrant methylation of multiple genes in the upper aerodigestive tract epithelium of heavy smokers. *Int J Cancer*, 2003, 107, 612-616.

In: Leading Topics in Cancer Research
Editor: Lee P. Jeffries, pp. 73-93
ISBN 1-60021-332-4
© 2007 Nova Science Publishers, Inc.

Chapter 3

GENETIC TESTING OF WOMEN
AT HIGH-RISK FOR DEVELOPMENT
OF HEREDITARY BREAST CANCER

*Ute Hamann**

German Cancer Research Center, Heidelberg, Germany

ABSTRACT

Breast cancer is the most common malignancy among women. Whereas most breast cancers are sporadic that is, not inherited, some are the result of inherited predisposition. Approximately 5% to 10% of breast cancers develop in individuals who were born with mutations in highly penetrant genes. Women who carry mutations in such genes have increased lifetime risks of developing breast and ovarian cancer. These risks are modified by alterations in other genes and environmental factors, an interaction that is poorly understood at present. The purpose of this review article is to provide an overview of current knowledge with regard to breast cancer susceptibility. It highlights first the genetic basis of hereditary breast cancer syndromes, in particular the role of the two major breast cancer susceptibility genes *BRCA1* and *BRCA2,* secondly the genetic testing with its benefits and limitations, and finally the management options for women with an inherited predisposition with regard to surveillance for the early detection of disease and with regard to prevention.

---

* Correspondence: Ute Hamann, PhD, Associate Professor; German Cancer Research Center; Molecular Genetics of Breast Cancer, B055; Im Neuenheimer Feld 580; D-69120 Heidelberg; Germany; Tel.: 0049/6221/42-2344; Fax: 0049/6221/42-4721; E-mail: u.hamann@dkfz-heidelberg.de

INTRODUCTION

Breast cancer in women is a major public health problem worldwide. Despite inroads that have been made in reducing the mortality of breast cancer, the burden for affected women, their families, and their communities is enormous. Worldwide, it is by far the most commonly diagnosed neoplasm in women, accounting for more than one million new cases of breast cancer each year (Parkin et al., 2005). It is also the primary cause of cancer death among women globally, responsible for more than 400,000 deaths in the year 2002 (Parkin et al., 2005). Breast cancer incidence rates vary at least tenfold between countries. The age-standardized incidence rates (ASR) are high in most developed areas (except for Japan) with a high incidence in Northern America, Australia/New Zealand, Northern, Western, and Southern Europe (ASR 99-62 per 100,000), while incidence is more modest in Eastern Europe, South America, Southern Africa, and Western Asia (ASR 46-33 per 100,000) and low in most of Africa and in most Asia (below 30 per 100,000).

Breast cancer is a multiplex disease caused by the interplay of various non-genetic and genetic factors. Non-genetic factors contributing to disease etiology include age, geographic location, socioeconomic status, family history of breast cancer and reproductive factors (age of menarche, nulliparity, age at first pregnancy, parity, age of menopause) all relating to the estrogen milieu to which the breast is exposed from menarche to the cessation of ovulation at menopause (Pike et al., 1983). Other factors are exogenous hormones (oral contraceptives and hormone replacement therapy), lifestyle factors (alcohol consumption, diet, obesity, physical activity), mammographic density, history of benign breast disease and ionizing radiation (Martin and Weber, 2000; McPherson et al., 2000). The higher prevalence of these risk factors in developed countries explains their higher breast cancer rates compared to those in developing countries.

Among the genetic factors that contribute to disease etiology are highly penetrant susceptibility genes, which confer a high degree of risk to the individual (so-called high penetrance in genetic terms). A hallmark of these genes is their association with multiple occurrences of cancer in a family, in a Mendelian, often autosomal dominant inheritance pattern, a predisposition to earlier onset disease and multiple primary cancers in a single individual, such as bilateral breast cancer, or breast plus ovarian cancer.

HEREDITARY BREAST CANCER

Approximately 5-10% of all breast cancers are hereditary occurring in individuals with mutations in highly penetrant susceptibility genes, which have been inherited through the germline. Inactivation of the second allele of these tumor suppressor genes results in loss of protein function, and in consequence, allows the cell to enter the tumorigenic pathway. Several genes have been identified as causing the different hereditary breast cancer syndromes including *BRCA1*, *BRCA2*, *TP53*, *PTEN*, *MLH1*, *MSH2*, and *STK11* (Table 1).

Table 1. Hereditary Breast Cancer Syndromes

Syndromes	Component Tumors	Gene	Mode of Inheritance
Hereditary breast cancer and ovarian cancer	Breast cancer, ovarian cancer, prostate cancer, pancreatic cancer, Fanconi anemia	*BRCA1* *BRCA2*	Autosomal dominant
Li-Fraumeni	Soft tissue sarcoma, breast cancer, osteosarcoma, leukemia, brain tumors, adrencortical carcinoma	*TP53*	Autosomal dominant
Cowden	Breast cancer, thyroid cancer, endometrial cancer and others	*PTEN*	Autosomal dominant
Muir-Torre	Colon cancer, endometrial cancer, ovarian cancer, pancreatic cancer and others	*MLH1* *MSH2*	Autosomal dominant
Peutz-Jeghers	Colon cancer, breast cancer, ovarian cancer, pancreatic cancer, small bowel cancer	*STK11*	Autosomal dominant
Ataxia telangiectasia	Leukemia, lymphoma, breast cancer	*ATM*	Autosomal recessive

BRCA1: Breast cancer gene 1; *BRCA2*: Breast Cancer gene 2; *PTEN:* Phosphatase and tensin homolog on chromosome 10; *MLH1*: Mut L homolog 1; *MSH2:* Mut S homolog 2; *STK11:* Serine threonine kinase 11.

BRCA1 and *BRCA2*

Germline mutations in two genes, *BRCA1* and *BRCA2,* are the most important ones numerically accounting for 84% of all hereditary breast cancers and probably about 2% of breast cancer cases overall (Ford et al., 1998; Peto et al., 1999). Mutations in these two genes cause site-specific hereditary breast cancer syndrome (HBC) occurring in families in the absence of any other familial occurring malignancy (Lynch 1981) and hereditary breast-ovarian cancer syndrome (HBOC) that occurs in families with ovarian cancer (Lynch et al., 1978). In addition, *BRCA2* is also responsible for Fanconi anemia (Howlett et al., 2002), Wilms´ tumors (Offit et al., 2003), and hereditary pancreatic cancer (Hahn et al., 2003).

Gene Structures and Functions

The *BRCA1* and *BRCA2* genes were cloned in 1994 and 1995, respectively (Miki et al., 1994; Wooster et al., 1995; Tavtigian et al., 1996). Both are reasonable large genes. *BRCA1,* located on chromosome 17q, consists of 22 coding exons, spans about 100 kb of genomic DNA and encodes an 1863 amino acid, 220 kDa protein, while *BRCA2,* located on chromosome 13q, has 26 coding exons, spans about 70 kb and encodes a 3418 amino acid, 384 kDa protein. Both proteins are highly charged nuclear phosphoproteins, which are ubiquitously expressed in human tissues. They have a cell-cycle regulated expression pattern (Chen et al., 1996; Vaughn et al., 1996) showing their highest levels of expression in the testis, thymus and ovaries (Miki et al., 1994; Tavtigian et al., 1996) Extensive research has revealed that BRCA1 and BRCA2 bind and interact with a number of regulatory proteins that enable them to function in multiple cellular processes (Venkitaraman, 2002; Yoshida and Miki, 2004). BRCA1 plays a role in DNA repair, transcriptional regulation, G2-M cell cycle check point control, ubiquitylation of proteins tagging them for degradation by the proteasome, chromatin remodeling around DNA-double strand DNA breaks thereby most probably facilitating DNA repair, and X-chromosome inactivation. The functions of BRCA2 are limited to DNA repair and regulation of cell cleavage and separation (Rudkin and Foulkes, 2005).

Germline Mutations and Founder Effects

So far, more than 1200 deleterious mutations have been identified throughout the length of each of these large genes. An update of mutations reported worldwide is maintained in the Breast Cancer Information Core Web site (BIC database, 2005). The vast majority of mutations are truncating mutations and less than 10% are large-scale genomic rearrangements including deletions, insertions, or duplications of more than 500 kb of DNA (Petrij-Bosch et al., 1997; Swensen et al., 1997; Nordling et al., 1998; Puget et al., 1999). About 10% of sequence variants are of unclear significance and generally are missense mutations.

While the majority of mutations are infrequently observed, certain mutations in *BRCA1* and *BRCA2* have been observed multiple times. Haplotype analysis using intragenic markers has shown that in most breast cancer patients, these recurrent mutations have descended from a common founder. These so called founder mutations tend to become common where there has been a strong reduction in population size and then rapid expansion, or where genetic isolation arises due to geographic or cultural restraints on marriage.

Founder mutations have been identified in various populations. For example in the Eastern European Jewish population, three mutations are commonly found, 185delAG and 5382insC in *BRCA1* and 6174delT in *BRCA2*. These three mutations account for almost all *BRCA1* and *BRCA2* mutations identified in this population. The frequency of these mutations is considerable higher than *BRCA1* and *BRCA2* mutations in other populations. In consequence, they are detected in a high percentage of breast and ovarian cancer families and patients in this population. The prevalence of nonfounder mutations in Jewish women undergoing genetic testing is only 2% (Kauff et al., 2002a). In the Icelandic population, one *BRCA2* mutation, 999del5, also associated with notable prostate cancer risk in some families, is common (Thorlacius et al., 1996). Founder mutations were also found in other populations, such as the Dutch (Petrij-Bosch et al., 1997), Polish (Gorski et al., 2000), Russian (Gayther et al., 1997), Belgian (Peelen et al., 1997), Norwegian (Andersen et al., 1996), Finish (Huusko et al., 1998), Scottish (Liede et al., 2000) and French-Canadian (Tonin et al., 1998) populations.

BRCA1/2-Associated Cancer Risks

Mutations in the *BRCA1* and *BRCA2* genes are responsible for familial clustering in the majority of breast and ovarian cancer families and for about one-half of site-specific breast cancer families (Ford et al., 1998). Detection of *BRCA1* and *BRCA2* mutations is clinically important because of the associated high lifetime risks of developing cancer. It has been estimated that the breast cancer risk associated with *BRCA1* mutations is in the range of 50-80%, and of 40-70% for *BRCA2*, with the range influenced by the study population, higher from studies of affected families, and lower from studies of populations (Ford et al., 1998; Antoniou et al., 2003). The ovarian cancer risk of *BRCA1* mutation carriers is about 40%, exceeding the risk of *BRCA2* carriers at 20%, in a linear function that is less influenced by age (Risch et al., 2001). The ovarian cancer risks associated with specific *BRCA2* mutations differ and are highest for mutations in the central region of the gene, the ovarian cancer cluster region (OCCR). In addition, affected *BRCA1* and *BRCA2* mutation carriers have estimated lifetime risks of 64% and 52% of developing contralateral breast cancer and of 44% and 16% of developing ovarian cancer, respectively (Ford et al., 1994; The Breast Cancer Linkage Consortium 1999). Further, male *BRCA2* carriers have an estimated lifetime risk of 6% of developing breast cancer (Easton et al., 1997). The cancer risks in *BRCA1* carriers are confined largely to breast and ovary, while pancreas, prostate, melanoma and other cancer risks are increased in *BRCA2* carriers (The Breast Cancer Linkage Consortium 1999).

Clinicopathological Characteristics of *BRCA1/2*-Related Breast and Ovarian Cancers

The histopathologic and immunohistochemical features of breast and ovarian cancers arising in patients harboring germline mutations in the *BRCA1* and *BRCA2* genes may be useful in identifying probable mutation carriers (Lakhani et al., 1998; Jacquemier et al., 2001). Several groups have reported that the pathobiology of *BRCA1*-related tumors, and perhaps to a lesser extent that of *BRCA2*-related ones, differs overall from sporadic breast cancer. *BRCA1*-related tumors are usually of high grade, poorly differentiated, and infiltrating ductal carcinomas. An atypical medullary phenotype is also more common in *BRCA1*-related tumors than in matched controls (Lakhani et al., 1998; Chappuis et al., 2000). Immunohistochemical profiling showed that they usually stain negative for estrogen and progesterone receptors, the receptor tyrosine kinase ERBB2 (HER2/neu) and also frequently stain for the basal cytokeratins 5/6, 14 and 17, osteonectin and EGFR, overexpress cyclin E and p53, and underexpress p27 (Lakhani et al., 2002; Korsching et al., 2002; Quenneville et al., 2002; Lakhani et al., 2005). Identifying a phenotype that characterizes *BRCA2*-associated breast tumors has been more difficult. Generally, *BRCA2*-related tumors cannot be readily distinguished from sporadic cancers on a morphological basis (Lakhani et al., 1998). However, there is evidence that overexpression of cyclin D1 may be a useful marker for *BRCA2*-related tumors (Hedenfalk et al., 2001).

BRCA1/2–related ovarian cancers usually are serous papillary carcinomas, although endometroid and clear-cell carcinomas also occur (Moslehi et al., 2000; Lakhani et al., 2004). In contrast, mucinous and borderline tumors are rarely seen in *BRCA1/2* mutation carriers (Gotlieb et al., 1998; Moslehi et al., 2000; Boyd et al., 2000).

Other Breast Cancer Genes

Mutations in other known dominant high-risk genes, such as *TP53, PTEN, MLH1, MSH2*, and *STK11* predisposing to breast cancer tend to be rare and are associated with specific clinical features on which diagnosis is made (Table 1). Mutations in the *TP53* gene cause the Li-Fraumeni syndrome (Lynch 1981), which includes soft tissue and osteosarcomas, brain tumors, adrenal cortical carcinoma and leukemia (Li et al., 1988). *PTEN* mutations are responsible for the development of Cowden´s syndrome, characterized by facial trichelloma, acral keratoses, papillomatous and mucosal lesions and multiple hamartomas with a high risk of benign and malignant tumors of the skin, thyroid, oral mucosa, breast, and endometrium (Brownstein et al., 1978), while mutations in *MLH1, MSH2* cause the Muir-Torre syndrome, including benign and malignant sebaceous tumors, adenocarcinomas of the colon or other cancers observed in the context of hereditary non-polyposis colorectal cancer (HNPCC) (Hall et al., 1994). Mutations in the *STK11* gene are responsible for the Peutz-Jegher syndrome, characterized by gastrointestinal tract hamartomas, skin and mucosal pigmentation, and benign and malignant tumors of the intestinal tract, the pancreas, ovaries, testis, breast and uterus (Spigelman et al., 1989).

Two further genes are associated with breast cancer risk: *ATM* and *CHEK2*. Mutations in *ATM* gene cause Ataxia telangiectasia (AT), an autosomal recessive inherited disorder, characterized by progressive cerebellar ataxia, immunodeficiency, an excessive sensitivity to ionizing radiation and various cancers including cancer of the pancreas, the stomach, bladder, ovary and chronic lymphocytic leukemia (Shiloh 1995). Heterozygote *ATM* carriers have up to a 7-fold increased risk for developing breast cancer (Swift et al., 1987). One *ATM* mutation, 7271 T>G has been shown to be associated with a high risk of breast cancer in a few families (Chenevix-Trench et al., 2002). A mutation in the low penetrance gene *CHEK2* (1100delC) increases the risk of breast cancer by 2-fold in familial *BRCA1/2*-negative breast cancer patients and by 10-fold in men (Meijers-Heijboer et al., 2002).

GENETIC TESTING FOR *BRCA1* AND *BRCA2* MUTATIONS

Although the clinicopathologic characteristics of *BRCA*-associated breast and ovarian cancers have been established, genetic testing for diagnosis and risk prediction was introduced into clinical practice in many diagnostic clinical genetic services. The goal of predictive genetic testing is to identify women with predisposing mutations in the *BRCA1* and *BRCA2* genes prior to the development of cancer. Genetic testing will be relatively easy, fast and cheap only in populations in which a small number of founder mutations has occurred. Examples are the Ashkenazi Jewish, the Polish and the Icelandic populations where one to three founder mutations account for the majority of mutations in cancer families.

Candidates for Genetic Testing

A meaningful application of the genetic test is restricted to women with a high risk of developing cancer, in order to limit the cost of testing in a clinical setting and to direct resources at families likely to benefit most from this health intervention. Women who are at high-risk show certain characteristics, such as having at least three first-degree relatives with breast and/or ovarian cancer, a tendency towards early onset and the presence of bilateral or multifocal carcinomas. Testing of families with a single case of breast or ovarian cancer with no history of the disease on either parental side, even if young, is not useful since the expected number of mutation carriers would be low (Stratton et al., 1997; Eccles et al., 1998; Hamann et al., 2003; Lalloo et al., 2003).

Following a detailed family and personal history assessment, the genetic counsellor, medical geneticist and other health professionals provide the individual with a genetic risk assessment, based on the collected information, and discuss the benefits, limits and risks of genetic testing. The woman then has to decide whether to proceed with genetic testing or not. When deciding to pursue genetic testing she additionally will receive counseling after the testing and follow-up care.

Table 2. Commonly used methods to detect *BRCA1/2* mutations

Method	Advantages and disadvantages
SSCP	Detects 50-95% of all small mutations in DNA fragments < 400 bp
	Rapid, easy to perform
	Low analysis costs
DHPLC	Detects > 96% of all mutations in DNA fragments < 800 bp
	High specificity
	Rapid, easy to perform
	High throughput, automation
	Low analysis costs
	Requires an expansive machine
PTT	Applicable for DNA fragments > 800 bp
	Allows approximate location of the mutation
	Difficult to set up
	Detects only truncating mutations
	High analysis costs
DS	Detects > 99% of all mutations in DNA fragments < 800 bp
	Allows exact location of the mutation
	Allows determination of the mutation type
	High analysis costs

SSCP: Single strand conformation polymorphism analysis; DHPLC: Denaturing high performance liquid chromatography; PTT: Protein truncation test; DS: Direct DNA sequencing.

Methods for *BRCA1* and *BRCA2* Mutation Screening

International studies indicate that the majority of *BRCA1/2* mutations are small sequence alterations, such as point mutations, small insertions and deletions resulting in truncated, non-functional proteins (Couch and Weber, 1996; BIC database, 2005). The methods most widely used by genetic laboratories for the screening of small *BRCA1/2* mutations are based on the polymerase chain reaction (PCR), such as single strand conformational polymorphism analysis (SSCP), denaturing high pressure liquid chromatography (DHPLC), protein truncation test (PTT) and automated DNA sequencing (Hogervorst et al., 1995; Plummer et al., 1995; Hamann et al., 1997; Arnold et al., 1999). For the detection of large genomic rearrangements that are not detected by usual analytical PCR-based screening technologies (Unger et al., 2000), reverse transcriptase polymerase chain reaction (RT-PCR) and Southern blot analysis are mostly applied (Petrij-Bosch et al., 1997). A summary of the most commonly used PCR-based mutation detection methods with their advantages and disadvantages, and representative examples of variants detected by these methods are shown in Table 2 and Figure 1, respectively.

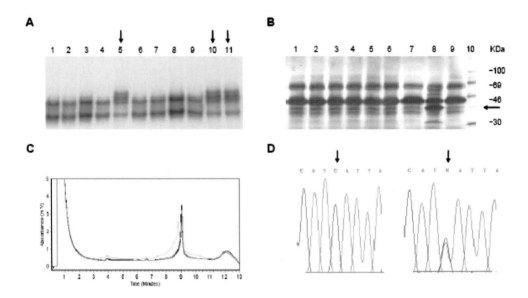

Figure 1. Detection of *BRCA1/2* mutations by SSCP (A), PTT (B), DHPLC (C) and direct DNA sequencing (D). (A) Amplification of *BRCA1* exon 15 from eleven familial breast cancer patients. Wild-type bands: lanes 1-4, 6-9; variant bands: lanes 5, 10, 11. Variant patterns are indicated by an arrow. Direct sequencing of DNA samples of patients 5, 10, and 11 revealed a deleterious *BRCA1* mutation. (B) Amplification of *BRCA1* exon 11 from nine familial breast cancer patients. Wild-type bands: lanes 1-7, 9; variant band: lane 8; protein marker: lane 10. The truncated protein is indicated by an arrow. Direct sequencing of the DNA of patient 8 revealed a deleterious *BRCA1* mutation. (C) Amplification of *BRCA2* exon 14 from one breast cancer patient and three healthy controls. The overlay of chromatograms is displayed. Normal elution pattern (healthy controls): blue, black, and red curves; variant elution pattern (patient): gray curve. Direct sequencing of the patient´s DNA revealed a deleterious *BRCA2* mutation. (D) DNA from a healthy control (left panel) and one familial breast cancer patient with a variant SSCP pattern (right panel) was amplified with *BRCA1* exon 15 primers, purified and sequenced. The sequence of the forward strand is shown. The patient carries a C to A nucleotide change at position 4627, which is indicated by an arrow.

A pedigree of a breast cancer family in which disease is likely to be caused by a *BRCA* mutation is shown in Figure 1A. There are three women in generations I and II affected by breast cancer and all had an age of diagnosis below 40 years. Since mutations transmit cancer risk in an autosomal dominant fashion, the children whose parent is affected by breast cancer have a 50% chance of inheriting the condition. Genetic testing revealed a deleterious *BRCA* germline mutation in the affected parent (Figure 1B). Predictive testing of her two daughters showed that one has inherited the mutation and the other not.

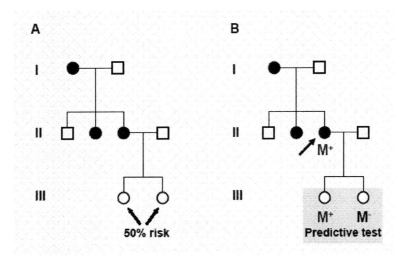

Figure 2. (A) Pedigree of a family which may have the hereditary type of breast cancer. (B) Genetic testing of affected and unaffected family members. Circles are females, squares are males. Filled symbols indicate breast cancer patients. M+: Carriers of a pathogenic *BRCA* mutation; M-: Non-carrier.

Interpretation of Test Results

Genetic testing has two possible outcomes: A negative test result indicates that no deleterious mutation has been identified in either *BRCA1* or *BRCA2* and a positive test result indicates that a deleterious mutation has been identified. However, the obtained result cannot simply be interpreted in the context of a simple positive or negative result. Their interpretation depends upon the following specific scenarios:

Scenario 1: Positive Test Result in Affected Women (Figure 2B)

A positive test result indicates that a clearly pathogenic, usually a truncating *BRCA* mutation has been detected. This result has implications for other family members. Since each of the patient´s siblings and children, regardless of gender, has a 50% chance of having inherited the mutation, patients with a positive test result are encouraged to share their test results with their extended family, in the event that other family members wish to be tested. A positive result in an affected woman is the most useful outcome for the wider family as it gives the family members the option for a definite, meaningful genetic test. This result is informative and reveals that unaffected women harboring pathogenic *BRCA* mutations have increased risks of developing breast and ovarian cancer. It however, cannot predict when, and if at all, these women will develop the disease. A *BRCA1/2* mutation does not inevitably cause cancer. It only increases the likelihood of developing breast and ovarian cancer, but other genetic and environmental factors also contribute to this phenotype. Thus, a positive test result does not necessarily mean that cancer is inescapable. A positive test result has implications on the mutation carrier. It can relieve uncertainty and allow women to make informed decisions with regard to the available management options, including heightened surveillance, preventive strategies including prophylactic surgery and more recently chemoprevention.

Genetic testing can also lead to the identification of sequence variants of uncertain significance that are not known to be common in the population but where the effect of the mutations on the predicted protein is too subtle to know whether it might affect the protein function. These variants are usually missense mutations that substitute one amino acid for another resulting in full-length proteins. The biological significance and clinical implication of these variants can only be determined when functional testing may be possible, which, however will be research-based. Alternatively, other factors can be used to determine the pathogenicity of these variants including the relative frequency of the variants in breast cancer patients and healthy controls and the co-segregation of the variant with disease in the family. If the variant is found in healthy controls and does not segregate with the cancer in the family, it may be of less concern clinically. Further, if the variant was identified in a patient that also harbored a deleterious mutation, then it is less likely to be of clinical significance. This is based on an animal model suggesting that *BRCA1* deficiency is lethal at the embryo stage (Gowen et al., 1996). Since a variant result is often unclear, it is frustrating to both the patient and the health care provider. Genetic testing for the variant in other unaffected family members is generally not recommended, as the results are of no use in guiding clinical management.

Scenario 2: Negative Test Result in Unaffected Women from Families with a Known BRCA1/2 Mutation (Figure 2B)

If a deleterious mutation has been identified within the family, and the unaffected woman receives a negative test result, then this result is true negative: the women did not inherit the mutation. Such a test result is informative and reveals that these women have risks of developing breast and ovarian cancer similar to those of the general population being 10%.

Scenario 3: Negative Test Result in Affected Women

A negative result indicates that a mutation in *BRCA1* or *BRCA2* is not responsible for disease development. However, in this scenario, the result can either be true negative in the sense that there is really no *BRCA1/2* mutation affecting that family, and all cases represent sporadic cases, i.e., that there is no cancer susceptibility in the family. In contrast, the result could also be false negative. Since mutation analysis is not straightforward, the *BRCA1/2* mutation could have been missed. *BRCA1* and *BRCA2* both are large genes, mutations can occur throughout the coding or even non-coding regions of the genes, and there is no single method or combination of methods available for genetic testing that allows the detection of all possible mutations with even the most sensitive methods having a sensitivity of less than 90%. Moreover, since about 10% of mutations are large genomic alterations, these would be missed because they are not detected by the most commonly applied PCR-based screening methods. Additionally, it is possible that i) another gene is responsible for cancer predisposition in that family, ii) multiple genes of lower penetrance are the basis for the clustering of the disease in the family, iii) the cancer susceptibility was not detected in that family because the patient chosen for initial genetic testing represents a sporadic case. Predictive testing of unaffected women from a family without a disease causing mutation is of no clinical use.

Pitfalls of Genetic Testing

In deciding whether to have genetic testing, women must weigh complex information about the potential benefits of testing against the limitations and possible risks of this new technology. There are many reasons why they might decline genetic testing for cancer susceptibility. These include the uncertainty that is associated with a positive test result, psychological distress, concerns about family stress, and concerns about privacy and potential genetic discrimination by employers and insurances (Lerman and Shields, 2004). The potential for stigmatization and discrimination could be specially pronounced for racial or ethnic subgroups in which genetic risk variants are more common. In consequence, to protect women against disadvantages caused by genetic testing, national and international guidelines concerning genetic testing have been developed. These guidelines comprise five main principles: autonomy (the resulting information in highly personal), privacy (the test results are confidential), justice (children and incompetent adults should participate in the decision process), equity (equity of access to genetic testing, testing, information), and quality (specific criteria for test sensitivity, specificity and effectiveness) (Knoppers and Chadwick, 1994).

OPTIONS OF WOMEN HARBORING *BRCA1/2* MUTATIONS

Three options are available for *BRCA1/2* mutation carriers: Intensive surveillance, medical prevention and surgical prevention.

Surveillance for Breast Cancer

Intensive surveillance for breast cancer includes breast self-examination, breast clinical examination, and imaging studies including mammography, ultrasound sonography, and magnetic resonance imaging (MRI) (Smith et al., 2003).

Monthly self-examinations (beginning at age 18-21 years) and semiannual or annual clinical examinations (beginning at age 25-35 years) of the breast are recommended for high-risk women. However, the efficacy of these screening strategies on reduction of mortality from breast cancer remains to be established (Burke et al., 1997; Levavi and Sabah, 2003).

The diagnostic usefulness of mammography is discussed controversially. Annual mammography and clinical examination have been recommended for women 25 to 35 years or older (Burke et al., 1997). However, recent studies have shown that the sensitivity of detecting small tumors in *BRCA1/2* mutation carriers is low implying that mammography does not seem to be the best technique for screening *BRCA1/2* mutation carriers (Goffin et al., 2001; Stoutjesdijk et al., 2001; Levavi and Sabah, 2003). There is evidence that lesions in *BRCA1* carriers are more difficult to detect than those in women with sporadic disease (Goffin et al., 2001). The efficacy of mammography in young women has been questioned, because the young breast is denser than the postmenopausal breast, causing problems in interpretation (Evans and Lalloo, 2002). Although strong evidence for the routine use of mammography for mutation carriers is missing, recommendations suggest that mammography should be offered annually to women 35 years or older who have a moderate to high breast cancer risk (Burke et al., 1997; Evans and Lalloo, 2002).

The diagnostic usefulness of ultrasound sonography for *BRCA1/2* mutation carriers is uncertain, although screening by ultrasound sonography and mammography may be of benefit for high-risk patients (Evans and Lalloo, 2002), Recently, MRI was shown to detect breast cancer at a higher rate than mammography and ultrasound sonography in *BRCA1/2* carriers or those who have a strong family history of disease (Warner et al., 2001). These findings suggest that MRI may be effective for the surveillance of *BRCA1/2* carriers. However, due to the high cost, this screening strategy will not be used on a routine basis.

Surveillance for Ovarian Cancer

Surveillance for ovarian cancer is difficult, owing to the difficulty in detecting tumors at an early stage. Semiannual or annual CA-125 tumor marker level determinations, annual rectovaginal pelvic examination and transvaginal ultrasound with color Doppler (beginning at age 25-35 years) are recommended for women with a high risk of ovarian cancer (NIH consensus conference 1995; Burke et al., 1997). However, data of the efficacy of these screening strategies in reduction of mortality from ovarian cancer remain to be established (NIH consensus conference 1995).

Medical Prevention for Breast Cancer with Tamoxifen

Tamoxifen has been found to reduce the risk of estrogen-receptor positive breast cancer in various prevention studies that recruited women at high breast cancer risk (Fisher et al., 1998; Cuzick et al., 2002). Unfortunately, as yet, there is no evidence about the long-term risk-benefit ratio. Further, there are no doubts on the adverse side effects of Tamoxifen including an increased risk of endometrial cancer and increased risk of deep vein thrombosis (Goel 1998). Tamoxifen as adjuvant therapy in *BRCA1* carriers reduced the risk of contralateral breast cancer (Narod et al., 2000). However, this treatment is rarely applied as adjuvant therapy in *BRCA1*-related cancers because most of these do not express the estrogen receptor.

Medical Prevention for Ovarian Cancer with Oral Contraceptives

A chemopreventive strategy to decrease the risk of ovarian cancer in women is the use of oral contraceptives. Long-term use of oral contraceptives decreased the risk of ovarian cancer in women with *BRCA1* mutations by more than half (Narod et al., 1998). One drawback is that the reduction in ovarian cancer risk may be associated with an increased breast cancer risk (Ursin et al., 1997). Recently, an increase in breast cancer in *BRCA1* mutation carriers using oral contraceptives was reported, which was highest in those who had taken oral contraceptives for five years and more before the age of 40 years (Narod et al., 2002). However, an increased risk was not seen in *BRCA2* mutation carriers taking oral contraceptives. Thus, further studies are needed to clarify the effects of oral contraceptives in *BRCA1/2* mutation carriers.

Surgical Prevention

Prophylactic mastectomy and prophylactic oophorectomy may be the preferred option for some women at high risk. Recent studies however have shown that surgery can greatly reduce the risks for future cancers (Hartmann et al., 1999; Rebbeck et al., 1999; Rebbeck et al., 2002; Kauff et al., 2002b; Rebbeck et al., 2004), although probably not eliminating them completely (Tobacman et al., 1982; Eldar et al., 1984; Mies 1993; Piver et al., 1993). Thus, a thorough assessment before surgery with imaging and after surgery with careful pathological examination for occult malignancy is necessary (Scott et al., 2003). Because the fallopian tubes of mutation carriers have been shown to harbor dysplastic changes and these patients have a high risk of developing tubal cancer (Colgan et al., 2001; Piek et al., 2001; Aziz et al., 2001), it is essential to excise both ovaries as well as fallopian tubes.

Due to the high lethality of ovarian cancer and the inefficacy of current screening methods, prophylactic bilateral oophorectomy is recommended for women from HBOC families at 35 years of age or after child-bearing (NIH consensus conference 1995). Most women with *BRCA1* and *BRCA2* mutations will develop ovarian cancer after the age of 45 years (Lynch et al., 1991; Rubin et al., 1996), however prophylactic oophorectomy should be performed closer to 35 years of age as recommended by this panel, due to the young age of some diagnosed.

CONCLUSION

Genetic testing for inherited breast and ovarian cancer susceptibility is a major advance in modern medical practice. The benefits of predictive testing to determine cancer susceptibility are substantial. However, there are still many difficulties and uncertainties regarding the sensitivity of tests, interpretation of test results and management of women carrying *BRCA1/2* mutations. Therefore in the future, the ultimate goals are the elucidation of the precise role of *BRCA1* and *BRCA2* in breast and ovarian cancer etiology, determination of the clinical significance of sequence variants, identification of other genes and environmental factors that modify hereditary breast and ovarian cancer risks, and the development and validation of better strategies for detection and prevention of cancers in women at high risk. A key to fast and meaningful progress is the design of comprehensive studies and close interactions between laboratory scientists, surgeons, medical oncologists, genetic counselors, gynecologists, and radiologists in a multidisciplinary environment.

REFERENCES

Andersen TI, Borresen AL, Moller P (1996) A common BRCA1 mutation in Norwegian breast and ovarian cancer families? *Am J Hum Genet* 59:486-487.

Antoniou A, Pharoah PD, Narod S, Risch HA, Eyfjord JE, Hopper JL, Loman N, Olsson H, Johannsson O, Borg A, Pasini B, Radice P, Manoukian S, Eccles DM, Tang N, Olah E, Anton-Culver H, Warner E, Lubinski J, Gronwald J, Gorski B, Tulinius H, Thorlacius S, Eerola H, Nevanlinna H, Syrjakoski K, Kallioniemi OP, Thompson D, Evans C, Peto J, Lalloo F, Evans DG, Easton DF (2003) Average risks of breast and ovarian cancer associated with BRCA1 or BRCA2 mutations detected in case series unselected for family history: a combined analysis of 22 studies. *Am J Hum Genet* 72:1117-1130.

Arnold N, Gross E, Schwarz-Boeger U, Pfisterer J, Jonat W, Kiechle M (1999) A highly sensitive, fast, and economical technique for mutation analysis in hereditary breast and ovarian cancers. *Hum Mutat* 14:333-339.

Aziz S, Kuperstein G, Rosen B, Cole D, Nedelcu R, McLaughlin J, Narod SA (2001) A genetic epidemiological study of carcinoma of the fallopian tube. *Gynecol Oncol* 80:341-345.

BIC database (2005) Breast Cancer Information Core (BIC) database. [http://www.nhgri.nih.gov/Intramural_research/Lab_transfer/Bic/].

Boyd J, Sonoda Y, Federici MG, Bogomolniy F, Rhei E, Maresco DL, Saigo PE, Almadrones LA, Barakat RR, Brown CL, Chi DS, Curtin JP, Poynor EA, Hoskins WJ (2000) Clinicopathologic features of BRCA-linked and sporadic ovarian cancer. *JAMA* 283:2260-2265.

Brownstein MH, Wolf M, Bikowski JB (1978) Cowden's disease: a cutaneous marker of breast cancer. *Cancer* 41:2393-2398.

Burke W, Daly M, Garber J, Botkin J, Kahn MJ, Lynch P, McTiernan A, Offit K, Perlman J, Petersen G, Thomson E, Varricchio C (1997) Recommendations for follow-up care of individuals with an inherited predisposition to cancer. II. BRCA1 and BRCA2. Cancer Genetics Studies Consortium. *JAMA* 277:997-1003.

Chappuis PO, Nethercot V, Foulkes WD (2000) Clinico-pathological characteristics of BRCA1- and BRCA2-related breast cancer. *Semin Surg Oncol* 18:287-295.

Chen Y, Farmer AA, Chen CF, Jones DC, Chen PL, Lee WH (1996) BRCA1 is a 220-kDa nuclear phosphoprotein that is expressed and phosphorylated in a cell cycle-dependent manner. *Cancer Res* 56:3168-3172.

Chenevix-Trench G, Spurdle AB, Gatei M, Kelly H, Marsh A, Chen X, Donn K, Cummings M, Nyholt D, Jenkins MA, Scott C, Pupo GM, Dork T, Bendix R, Kirk J, Tucker K, McCredie MR, Hopper JL, Sambrook J, Mann GJ, Khanna KK (2002) Dominant negative ATM mutations in breast cancer families. *J Natl Cancer Inst* 94:205-215.

Colgan TJ, Murphy J, Cole DE, Narod S, Rosen B (2001) Occult carcinoma in prophylactic oophorectomy specimens: prevalence and association with BRCA germline mutation status. *Am J Surg Pathol* 25:1283-1289.

Couch FJ and Weber BL (1996) Mutations and polymorphisms in the familial early-onset breast cancer (BRCA1) gene. Breast Cancer Information Core. *Hum Mutat* 8:8-18.

Cuzick J, Forbes J, Edwards R, Baum M, Cawthorn S, Coates A, Hamed A, Howell A, Powles T (2002) First results from the International Breast Cancer Intervention Study (IBIS-I): a randomised prevention trial. *Lancet* 360:817-824.

Easton DF, Steele L, Fields P, Ormiston W, Averill D, Daly PA, McManus R, Neuhausen SL, Ford D, Wooster R, Cannon-Albright LA, Stratton MR, Goldgar DE (1997) Cancer risks in two large breast cancer families linked to BRCA2 on chromosome 13q12-13. *Am J Hum Genet* 61:120-128.

Eccles DM, Englefield P, Soulby MA, Campbell IG (1998) BRCA1 mutations in southern England. *Br J Cancer* 77:2199-2203.

Eldar S, Meguid MM, Beatty JD (1984) Cancer of the breast after prophylactic subcutaneous mastectomy. *Am J Surg* 148:692-693.

Evans DG and Lalloo F (2002) Risk assessment and management of high risk familial breast cancer. *J Med Genet* 39:865-871.

Fisher B, Costantino JP, Wickerham DL, Redmond CK, Kavanah M, Cronin WM, Vogel V, Robidoux A, Dimitrov N, Atkins J, Daly M, Wieand S, Tan-Chiu E, Ford L, Wolmark N (1998) Tamoxifen for prevention of breast cancer: report of the National Surgical Adjuvant Breast and Bowel Project P-1 Study. *J Natl Cancer Inst* 90:1371-1388.

Ford D, Easton DF, Bishop DT, Narod SA, Goldgar DE (1994) Risks of cancer in BRCA1-mutation carriers. Breast Cancer Linkage Consortium. *Lancet* 343:692-695.

Ford D, Easton DF, Stratton M, Narod S, Goldgar D, Devilee P, Bishop DT, Weber B, Lenoir G, Chang-Claude J, Sobol H, Teare MD, Struewing J, Arason A, Scherneck S, Peto J, Rebbeck TR, Tonin P, Neuhausen S, Barkardottir R, Eyfjord J, Lynch H, Ponder BA, Gayther SA, Zelada-Hedman M (1998) Genetic heterogeneity and penetrance analysis of the BRCA1 and BRCA2 genes in breast cancer families. The Breast Cancer Linkage Consortium. *Am J Hum Genet* 62:676-689.

Gayther SA, Harrington P, Russell P, Kharkevich G, Garkavtseva RF, Ponder BA (1997) Frequently occurring germ-line mutations of the BRCA1 gene in ovarian cancer families from Russia. *Am J Hum Genet* 60:1239-1242.

Goel V (1998) Tamoxifen and breast cancer prevention: what should you tell your patients? *CMAJ* 158:1615-1617.

Goffin J, Chappuis PO, Wong N, Foulkes WD (2001) Re: Magnetic resonance imaging and mammography in women with a hereditary risk of breast cancer. *J Natl Cancer Inst* 93:1754-1755.

Gorski B, Byrski T, Huzarski T, Jakubowska A, Menkiszak J, Gronwald J, Pluzanska A, Bebenek M, Fischer-Maliszewska L, Grzybowska E, Narod SA, Lubinski J (2000) Founder mutations in the BRCA1 gene in Polish families with breast-ovarian cancer. *Am J Hum Genet* 66:1963-1968.

Gotlieb WH, Friedman E, Bar-Sade RB, Kruglikova A, Hirsh-Yechezkel G, Modan B, Inbar M, Davidson B, Kopolovic J, Novikov I, Ben Baruch G (1998) Rates of Jewish ancestral mutations in BRCA1 and BRCA2 in borderline ovarian tumors. *J Natl Cancer Inst* 90:995-1000.

Gowen LC, Johnson BL, Latour AM, Sulik KK, Koller BH (1996) Brca1 deficiency results in early embryonic lethality characterized by neuroepithelial abnormalities. *Nat Genet* 12:191-194.

Hahn SA, Greenhalf B, Ellis I, Sina-Frey M, Rieder H, Korte B, Gerdes B, Kress R, Ziegler A, Raeburn JA, Campra D, Grutzmann R, Rehder H, Rothmund M, Schmiegel W, Neoptolemos JP, Bartsch DK (2003) BRCA2 germline mutations in familial pancreatic carcinoma. *J Natl Cancer Inst* 95:214-221.

Hall NR, Williams MA, Murday VA, Newton JA, Bishop DT (1994) Muir-Torre syndrome: a variant of the cancer family syndrome. *J Med Genet* 31:627-631.

Hamann U, Brauch H, Garvin AM, Bastert G, Scott RJ (1997) German family study on hereditary breast and/or ovarian cancer: germline mutation analysis of the BRCA1 gene. *Genes Chromosomes Cancer* 18:126-132.

Hamann U, Liu X, Bungardt N, Ulmer HU, Bastert G, Sinn HP (2003) Similar contributions of BRCA1 and BRCA2 germline mutations to early-onset breast cancer in Germany. *Eur J Hum Genet* 11:464-467.

Hartmann LC, Schaid DJ, Woods JE, Crotty TP, Myers JL, Arnold PG, Petty PM, Sellers TA, Johnson JL, McDonnell SK, Frost MH, Jenkins RB (1999) Efficacy of bilateral prophylactic mastectomy in women with a family history of breast cancer. *N Engl J Med* 340:77-84.

Hedenfalk I, Duggan D, Chen Y, Radmacher M, Bittner M, Simon R, Meltzer P, Gusterson B, Esteller M, Kallioniemi OP, Wilfond B, Borg A, Trent J (2001) Gene-expression profiles in hereditary breast cancer. *N Engl J Med* 344:539-548.

Hogervorst FB, Cornelis RS, Bout M, van Vliet M, Oosterwijk JC, Olmer R, Bakker B, Klijn JG, Vasen HF, Meijers-Heijboer H (1995) Rapid detection of BRCA1 mutations by the protein truncation test. *Nat Genet* 10:208-212.

Howlett NG, Taniguchi T, Olson S, Cox B, Waisfisz Q, Die-Smulders C, Persky N, Grompe M, Joenje H, Pals G, Ikeda H, Fox EA, D'Andrea AD (2002) Biallelic inactivation of BRCA2 in Fanconi anemia. *Science* 297:606-609.

Huusko P, Paakkonen K, Launonen V, Poyhonen M, Blanco G, Kauppila A, Puistola U, Kiviniemi H, Kujala M, Leisti J, Winqvist R (1998) Evidence of founder mutations in Finnish BRCA1 and BRCA2 families. *Am J Hum Genet* 62:1544-1548.

Jacquemier J, Lidereau R, Birnbaum D, Eisinger F, Sobol H (2001) Assessing the risk of BRCA1-associated breast cancer using individual morphological criteria. *Histopathology* 38:378-379.

Kauff ND, Perez-Segura P, Robson ME, Scheuer L, Siegel B, Schluger A, Rapaport B, Frank TS, Nafa K, Ellis NA, Parmigiani G, Offit K (2002a) Incidence of non-founder BRCA1 and BRCA2 mutations in high risk Ashkenazi breast and ovarian cancer families. *J Med Genet* 39:611-614.

Kauff ND, Satagopan JM, Robson ME, Scheuer L, Hensley M, Hudis CA, Ellis NA, Boyd J, Borgen PI, Barakat RR, Norton L, Castiel M, Nafa K, Offit K (2002b) Risk-reducing salpingo-oophorectomy in women with a BRCA1 or BRCA2 mutation. *N Engl J Med* 346:1609-1615.

Knoppers BM and Chadwick R (1994) The Human Genome Project: under an international ethical microscope. *Science* 265:2035-2036.

Korsching E, Packeisen J, Agelopoulos K, Eisenacher M, Voss R, Isola J, van Diest PJ, Brandt B, Boecker W, Buerger H (2002) Cytogenetic alterations and cytokeratin expression patterns in breast cancer: integrating a new model of breast differentiation into cytogenetic pathways of breast carcinogenesis. *Lab Invest* 82:1525-1533.

Lakhani SR, Jacquemier J, Sloane JP, Gusterson BA, Anderson TJ, van de Vijver MJ, Farid LM, Venter D, Antoniou A, Storfer-Isser A, Smyth E, Steel CM, Haites N, Scott RJ, Goldgar D, Neuhausen S, Daly PA, Ormiston W, McManus R, Scherneck S, Ponder BA, Ford D, Peto J, Stoppa-Lyonnet D, Bignon YJ, Struewing JP, Spurr NK, Bishop DT, Klijn JG, Devilee P, Cornelisse CJ, Lasset C, Lenoir G, Barkardottir RB, Egilsson V, Hamann U, Chang-Claude J, Sobol H, Weber B, Stratton MR, Easton DF (1998) Multifactorial analysis of differences between sporadic breast cancers and cancers involving BRCA1 and BRCA2 mutations. *J Natl Cancer Inst* 90:1138-1145.

Lakhani SR, Manek S, Penault-Llorca F, Flanagan A, Arnout L, Merrett S, McGuffog L, Steele D, Devilee P, Klijn JG, Meijers-Heijboer H, Radice P, Pilotti S, Nevanlinna H,

Butzow R, Sobol H, Jacquemier J, Lyonet DS, Neuhausen SL, Weber B, Wagner T, Winqvist R, Bignon YJ, Monti F, Schmitt F, Lenoir G, Seitz S, Hamman U, Pharoah P, Lane G, Ponder B, Bishop DT, Easton DF (2004) Pathology of ovarian cancers in BRCA1 and BRCA2 carriers. *Clin Cancer Res* 10:2473-2481.

Lakhani SR, Reis-Filho JS, Fulford L, Penault-Llorca F, van de Vijver M, Parry S, Bishop T, Benitez J, Rivas C, Bignon YJ, Chang-Claude J, Hamann U, Cornelisse CJ, Devilee P, Beckmann MW, Nestle-Kramling C, Daly PA, Haites N, Varley J, Lalloo F, Evans G, Maugard C, Meijers-Heijboer H, Klijn JG, Olah E, Gusterson BA, Pilotti S, Radice P, Scherneck S, Sobol H, Jacquemier J, Wagner T, Peto J, Stratton MR, McGuffog L, Easton DF; Breast Cancer Linkage Consortium (2005) Prediction of BRCA1 status in patients with breast cancer using estrogen receptor and basal phenotype. *Clin Cancer Res* 11:5175-5180.

Lakhani SR, van de Vijver MJ, Jacquemier J, Anderson TJ, Osin PP, McGuffog L, Easton DF (2002) The pathology of familial breast cancer: predictive value of immunohistochemical markers estrogen receptor, progesterone receptor, HER-2, and p53 in patients with mutations in BRCA1 and BRCA2. *J Clin Oncol* 20:2310-2318.

Lalloo F, Varley J, Ellis D, Moran A, O'Dair L, Pharoah P, Evans DG (2003) Prediction of pathogenic mutations in patients with early-onset breast cancer by family history. *Lancet* 361:1101-1102.

Lerman C and Shields AE (2004) Genetic testing for cancer susceptibility: the promise and the pitfalls. *Nat Rev Cancer* 4:235-241.

Levavi H and Sabah G (2003) BRCA susceptibility genes--a review of current conservative management of BRCA mutation carriers. *Eur J Gynaecol Oncol* 24:463-466.

Li FP, Fraumeni JF, Jr., Mulvihill JJ, Blattner WA, Dreyfus MG, Tucker MA, Miller RW (1988) A cancer family syndrome in twenty-four kindreds. *Cancer Res* 48:5358-5362.

Liede A, Cohen B, Black DM, Davidson RH, Renwick A, Hoodfar E, Olopade OI, Micek M, Anderson V, De Mey R, Fordyce A, Warner E, Dann JL, King MC, Weber B, Narod SA, Steel CM (2000) Evidence of a founder BRCA1 mutation in Scotland. *Br J Cancer* 82:705-711.

Lynch HT (1981) Genetic heterogeneity and breast cancer: Variable tumor spectra. In: Lynch HT (ed) *Genetics and breast cancer.* Van Nostrand Reinhold, New York, Cincinnati, Atlanta, Dallas, San Francisco, London, Toronto, Melbourne, 134-173.

Lynch HT, Conway T, Lynch J (1991) Hereditary ovarian cancer. Pedigree studies, Part II. *Cancer Genet Cytogenet* 53:161-183.

Lynch HT, Harris RE, Guirgis HA, Maloney K, Carmody LL, Lynch JF (1978) Familial association of breast/ovarian carcinoma. *Cancer* 41:1543-1549.

Martin AM and Weber BL (2000) Genetic and hormonal risk factors in breast cancer. *J Natl Cancer Inst* 92:1126-1135.

McPherson K, Steel CM, Dixon JM (2000) ABC of breast diseases. Breast cancer-epidemiology, risk factors, and genetics. *BMJ* 321:624-628.

Meijers-Heijboer H, van den Ouweland A, Klijn J, Wasielewski M, de Snoo A, Oldenburg R, Hollestelle A, Houben M, Crepin E, van Veghel-Plandsoen M, Elstrodt F, van Duijn C, Bartels C, Meijers C, Schutte M, McGuffog L, Thompson D, Easton D, Sodha N, Seal S, Barfoot R, Mangion J, Chang-Claude J, Eccles D, Eeles R, Evans DG, Houlston R, Murday V, Narod S, Peretz T, Peto J, Phelan C, Zhang HX, Szabo C, Devilee P, Goldgar D, Futreal PA, Nathanson KL, Weber B, Rahman N, Stratton MR, CHEK2-Breast Cancer

Consortium (2002) Low-penetrance susceptibility to breast cancer due to CHEK2(*)1100delC in noncarriers of BRCA1 or BRCA2 mutations. *Nat Genet* 31:55-59.

Mies C (1993) Recurrent secretory carcinoma in residual mammary tissue after mastectomy. *Am J Surg Pathol* 17:715-721.

Miki Y, Swensen J, Shattuck-Eidens D, Futreal PA, Harshman K, Tavtigian S, Liu Q, Cochran C, Bennett LM, Ding W (1994) A strong candidate for the breast and ovarian cancer susceptibility gene BRCA1. *Science* 266:66-71.

Moslehi R, Chu W, Karlan B, Fishman D, Risch H, Fields A, Smotkin D, Ben David Y, Rosenblatt J, Russo D, Schwartz P, Tung N, Warner E, Rosen B, Friedman J, Brunet JS, Narod SA (2000) BRCA1 and BRCA2 mutation analysis of 208 Ashkenazi Jewish women with ovarian cancer. *Am J Hum Genet* 66:1259-1272.

Narod SA, Brunet JS, Ghadirian P, Robson M, Heimdal K, Neuhausen SL, Stoppa-Lyonnet D, Lerman C, Pasini B, de los Rios P, Weber B, Lynch H (2000) Tamoxifen and risk of contralateral breast cancer in BRCA1 and BRCA2 mutation carriers: a case-control study. Hereditary Breast Cancer Clinical Study Group. *Lancet* 356:1876-1881.

Narod SA, Dube MP, Klijn J, Lubinski J, Lynch HT, Ghadirian P, Provencher D, Heimdal K, Moller P, Robson M, Offit K, Isaacs C, Weber B, Friedman E, Gershoni-Baruch R, Rennert G, Pasini B, Wagner T, Daly M, Garber JE, Neuhausen SL, Ainsworth P, Olsson H, Evans G, Osborne M, Couch F, Foulkes WD, Warner E, Kim-Sing C, Olopade O, Tung N, Saal HM, Weitzel J, Merajver S, Gauthier-Villars M, Jernstrom H, Sun P, Brunet JS (2002) Oral contraceptives and the risk of breast cancer in BRCA1 and BRCA2 mutation carriers. *J Natl Cancer Inst* 94:1773-1779.

Narod SA, Risch H, Moslehi R, Dorum A, Neuhausen S, Olsson H, Provencher D, Radice P, Evans G, Bishop S, Brunet JS, Ponder BA (1998) Oral contraceptives and the risk of hereditary ovarian cancer. Hereditary Ovarian Cancer Clinical Study Group. *N Engl J Med* 339:424-428.

NIH consensus conference (1995) Ovarian cancer. Screening, treatment, and follow-up. NIH Consensus Development Panel on Ovarian Cancer. *JAMA* 273:491-497.

Nordling M, Karlsson P, Wahlstrom J, Engwall Y, Wallgren A, Martinsson T (1998) A large deletion disrupts the exon 3 transcription activation domain of the BRCA2 gene in a breast/ovarian cancer family. *Cancer Res* 58:1372-1375.

Offit K, Levran O, Mullaney B, Mah K, Nafa K, Batish SD, Diotti R, Schneider H, Deffenbaugh A, Scholl T, Proud VK, Robson M, Norton L, Ellis N, Hanenberg H, Auerbach AD (2003) Shared genetic susceptibility to breast cancer, brain tumors, and Fanconi anemia. *J Natl Cancer Inst* 95:1548-1551.

Parkin DM, Bray F, Ferlay J, Pisani P (2005) Global cancer statistics, 2002. *CA Cancer J Clin* 55:74-108.

Peelen T, van Vliet M, Petrij-Bosch A, Mieremet R, Szabo C, van den Ouweland AM, Hogervorst F, Brohet R, Ligtenberg MJ, Teugels E, van der Luijt R, van der Hout AH, Gille JJ, Pals G, Jedema I, Olmer R, van Leeuwen I, Newman B, Plandsoen M, van der Est M, Brink G, Hageman S, Arts PJ, Bakker MM, Devilee P (1997) A high proportion of novel mutations in BRCA1 with strong founder effects among Dutch and Belgian hereditary breast and ovarian cancer families. *Am J Hum Genet* 60:1041-1049.

Peto J, Collins N, Barfoot R, Seal S, Warren W, Rahman N, Easton DF, Evans C, Deacon J, Stratton MR (1999) Prevalence of BRCA1 and BRCA2 gene mutations in patients with early-onset breast cancer. *J Natl Cancer Inst* 91:943-949.

Petrij-Bosch A, Peelen T, van Vliet M, van Eijk R, Olmer R, Drusedau M, Hogervorst FB, Hageman S, Arts PJ, Ligtenberg MJ, Meijers-Heijboer H, Klijn JG, Vasen HF, Cornelisse CJ, van't Veer LJ, Bakker E, van Ommen GJ, Devilee P (1997) BRCA1 genomic deletions are major founder mutations in Dutch breast cancer patients. *Nat Genet* 17:341-345.

Piek JM, van Diest PJ, Zweemer RP, Jansen JW, Poort-Keesom RJ, Menko FH, Gille JJ, Jongsma AP, Pals G, Kenemans P, Verheijen RH (2001) Dysplastic changes in prophylactically removed Fallopian tubes of women predisposed to developing ovarian cancer. *J Pathol* 195:451-456.

Pike MC, Krailo MD, Henderson BE, Casagrande JT, Hoel DG (1983) 'Hormonal' risk factors, 'breast tissue age' and the age-incidence of breast cancer. *Nature* 303:767-770.

Piver MS, Jishi MF, Tsukada Y, Nava G (1993) Primary peritoneal carcinoma after prophylactic oophorectomy in women with a family history of ovarian cancer. A report of the Gilda Radner Familial Ovarian Cancer Registry. *Cancer* 71:2751-2755.

Plummer SJ, Anton-Culver H, Webster L, Noble B, Liao S, Kennedy A, Belinson J, Casey G (1995) Detection of BRCA1 mutations by the protein truncation test. *Hum Mol Genet* 4:1989-1991.

Puget N, Stoppa-Lyonnet D, Sinilnikova OM, Pages S, Lynch HT, Lenoir GM, Mazoyer S (1999) Screening for germ-line rearrangements and regulatory mutations in BRCA1 led to the identification of four new deletions. *Cancer Res* 59:455-461.

Quenneville LA, Phillips KA, Ozcelik H, Parkes RK, Knight JA, Goodwin PJ, Andrulis IL, O'Malley FP (2002) HER-2/neu status and tumor morphology of invasive breast carcinomas in Ashkenazi women with known BRCA1 mutation status in the Ontario Familial Breast Cancer Registry. *Cancer* 95:2068-2075.

Rebbeck TR, Friebel T, Lynch HT, Neuhausen SL, van't Veer L, Garber JE, Evans GR, Narod SA, Isaacs C, Matloff E, Daly MB, Olopade OI, Weber BL (2004) Bilateral prophylactic mastectomy reduces breast cancer risk in BRCA1 and BRCA2 mutation carriers: the PROSE Study Group. *J Clin Oncol* 22:1055-1062.

Rebbeck TR, Levin AM, Eisen A, Snyder C, Watson P, Cannon-Albright L, Isaacs C, Olopade O, Garber JE, Godwin AK, Daly MB, Narod SA, Neuhausen SL, Lynch HT, Weber BL (1999) Breast cancer risk after bilateral prophylactic oophorectomy in BRCA1 mutation carriers. *J Natl Cancer Inst* 91:1475-1479.

Rebbeck TR, Lynch HT, Neuhausen SL, Narod SA, van't Veer L, Garber JE, Evans G, Isaacs C, Daly MB, Matloff E, Olopade OI, Weber BL (2002) Prophylactic oophorectomy in carriers of BRCA1 or BRCA2 mutations. *N Engl J Med* 346:1616-1622.

Risch HA, McLaughlin JR, Cole DE, Rosen B, Bradley L, Kwan E, Jack E, Vesprini DJ, Kuperstein G, Abrahamson JL, Fan I, Wong B, Narod SA (2001) Prevalence and penetrance of germline BRCA1 and BRCA2 mutations in a population series of 649 women with ovarian cancer. *Am J Hum Genet* 68:700-710.

Rubin SC, Benjamin I, Behbakht K, Takahashi H, Morgan MA, LiVolsi VA, Berchuck A, Muto MG, Garber JE, Weber BL, Lynch HT, Boyd J (1996) Clinical and pathological features of ovarian cancer in women with germ-line mutations of BRCA1. *N Engl J Med* 335:1413-1416.

Rudkin TM and Foulkes WD (2005) BRCA2: breaks, mistakes and failed separations. *Trends Mol Med* 11:145-148.

Scott CI, Iorgulescu DG, Thorne HJ, Henderson MA, Phillips KA (2003) Clinical, pathological and genetic features of women at high familial risk of breast cancer undergoing prophylactic mastectomy. *Clin Genet* 64:111-121.

Shiloh Y (1995) Ataxia-telangiectasia: closer to unraveling the mystery. *Eur J Hum Genet* 3:116-138.

Smith RA, Saslow D, Sawyer KA, Burke W, Costanza ME, Evans WP, III, Foster RS, Jr., Hendrick E, Eyre HJ, Sener S (2003) American Cancer Society guidelines for breast cancer screening: update 2003. *CA Cancer J Clin* 53:141-169.

Spigelman AD, Murday V, Phillips RK (1989) Cancer and the Peutz-Jeghers syndrome. *Gut* 30:1588-1590.

Stoutjesdijk MJ, Boetes C, Jager GJ, Beex L, Bult P, Hendriks JH, Laheij RJ, Massuger L, van Die LE, Wobbes T, Barentsz JO (2001) Magnetic resonance imaging and mammography in women with a hereditary risk of breast cancer. *J Natl Cancer Inst* 93:1095-1102.

Stratton JF, Gayther SA, Russell P, Dearden J, Gore M, Blake P, Easton D, Ponder BA (1997) Contribution of BRCA1 mutations to ovarian cancer. *N Engl J Med* 336:1125-1130.

Swensen J, Hoffman M, Skolnick MH, Neuhausen SL (1997) Identification of a 14 kb deletion involving the promoter region of BRCA1 in a breast cancer family. *Hum Mol Genet* 6:1513-1517.

Swift M, Reitnauer PJ, Morrell D, Chase CL (1987) Breast and other cancers in families with ataxia-telangiectasia. *N Engl J Med* 316:1289-1294.

Tavtigian SV, Simard J, Rommens J, Couch F, Shattuck-Eidens D, Neuhausen S, Merajver S, Thorlacius S, Offit K, Stoppa-Lyonnet D, Belanger C, Bell R, Berry S, Bogden R, Chen Q, Davis T, Dumont M, Frye C, Hattier T, Jammulapati S, Janecki T, Jiang P, Kehrer R, Leblanc JF, Goldgar DE (1996) The complete BRCA2 gene and mutations in chromosome 13q-linked kindreds. *Nat Genet* 12:333-337.

The Breast Cancer Linkage Consortium (1999) Cancer risks in BRCA2 mutation carriers. *J Natl Cancer Inst* 91:1310-1316.

Thorlacius S, Olafsdottir G, Tryggvadottir L, Neuhausen S, Jonasson JG, Tavtigian SV, Tulinius H, Ogmundsdottir HM, Eyfjord JE (1996) A single BRCA2 mutation in male and female breast cancer families from Iceland with varied cancer phenotypes. *Nat Genet* 13:117-119.

Tobacman JK, Greene MH, Tucker MA, Costa J, Kase R, Fraumeni JF, Jr. (1982) Intra-abdominal carcinomatosis after prophylactic oophorectomy in ovarian-cancer-prone families. *Lancet* 2:795-797.

Tonin PN, Mes-Masson AM, Futreal PA, Morgan K, Mahon M, Foulkes WD, Cole DE, Provencher D, Ghadirian P, Narod SA (1998) Founder BRCA1 and BRCA2 mutations in French Canadian breast and ovarian cancer families. *Am J Hum Genet* 63:1341-1351.

Unger MA, Nathanson KL, Calzone K, Antin-Ozerkis D, Shih HA, Martin AM, Lenoir GM, Mazoyer S, Weber BL (2000) Screening for genomic rearrangements in families with breast and ovarian cancer identifies BRCA1 mutations previously missed by conformation-sensitive gel electrophoresis or sequencing. *Am J Hum Genet* 67:841-850.

Ursin G, Henderson BE, Haile RW, Pike MC, Zhou N, Diep A, Bernstein L (1997) Does oral contraceptive use increase the risk of breast cancer in women with BRCA1/BRCA2 mutations more than in other women? *Cancer Res* 57:3678-3681.

Vaughn JP, Cirisano FD, Huper G, Berchuck A, Futreal PA, Marks JR, Iglehart JD (1996) Cell cycle control of BRCA2. *Cancer Res* 56:4590-4594.

Venkitaraman AR (2002) Cancer susceptibility and the functions of BRCA1 and BRCA2. *Cell* 108:171-182.

Warner E, Plewes DB, Shumak RS, Catzavelos GC, Di Prospero LS, Yaffe MJ, Goel V, Ramsay E, Chart PL, Cole DE, Taylor GA, Cutrara M, Samuels TH, Murphy JP, Murphy JM, Narod SA (2001) Comparison of breast magnetic resonance imaging, mammography, and ultrasound for surveillance of women at high risk for hereditary breast cancer. *J Clin Oncol* 19:3524-3531.

Wooster R, Bignell G, Lancaster J, Swift S, Seal S, Mangion J, Collins N, Gregory S, Gumbs C, Micklem G (1995) Identification of the breast cancer susceptibility gene BRCA2. *Nature* 378:789-792.

Yoshida K and Miki Y (2004) Role of BRCA1 and BRCA2 as regulators of DNA repair, transcription, and cell cycle in response to DNA damage. *Cancer Sci* 95:866-871.

In: Leading Topics in Cancer Research
Editor: Lee P. Jeffries, pp. 95-123

ISBN 1-60021-332-4
© 2007 Nova Science Publishers, Inc.

Chapter 4

SCREENING FOR OVARIAN CANCER IN WOMEN AT HIGH RISK FOR DISEASE

Laurie Elit
McMaster University, Hamilton, Canada

ABSTRACT

Background

Ovarian cancer is the sixth most common malignancy in women and the leading cause of death from gynecologic malignancies. Seventy percent of ovarian cancers present as advanced disease, which is associated with an overall five-year survival of 30%. The earlier the stage of disease, the better the survival (Stage 1 - 85% 5-year). Risk factors associated with ovarian cancer include: advancing age and family history of breast and/or ovarian cancer or Hereditary Non-Polyposis Colon Cancer or known BRCA 1 or 2 mutation. There is no known precursor status for ovarian cancer; however, if earlier stage disease could be identified then survival could be enhanced. Much work has been done addressing the role of various imaging modalities (ie., ultrasound) with or without tumor markers (ie., CA125) to identify women with early stage disease.

Methods

This chapter will address the role of screening for ovarian cancer in higher risk women such as postmenopausal women or those with a family history of disease or premenopausal breast cancer or known BRCA1 or 2 mutations. Several databases were searched including MEDLINE, CANCERLIT, Physician Data Query, Canadian Medical Associate Infobase and the National Guidelines Clearinghouse. To be included in this review were: clinical trials or systematic reviews of clinical trials; evaluated tests to detect ovarian cancer; included asymptomatic women from the populations of interest; and reported rates of confirmed ovarian cancer.

Results

In postmenopausal women, who were screened with either ultrasound or CA125 or both, approximately 10% of women all called back for further testing and the false positive rate is 0.6% for CA125 to 2.5% for ultrasound and diagnosis of ovarian cancer of 0.1% over eight years. Currently there is no screening strategy available for ovarian cancer in the general population. In women with a family history for disease, no screening intervention was found superior to another and the detection rate was 0.2%. Women who are interested in screening should participate in clinical trials addressing novel screening modalities. Women with a known BRCA1 or 2 mutations are at a substantial lifetime risk for developing ovarian cancer (BRCA1-60% and BRCA2 25%) and should consider prophylactic oophorectomy at the culmination of reproductive activity to decrease the risk of de novo ovarian cancer (1.8%-4%) or breast cancer (decreased by 53%) or recurrent breast cancer.

Conclusion

Screening for ovarian cancer is not advocated for the general population, postmenopausal women or women with a hereditary predisposition to ovarian cancer at this time. Women interested in pursuing screening should participate in research studies to help identify beneficial novel screening modalities.

BACKGROUND

Epithelial ovarian cancer affects 1000 women in Ontario, Canada annually with 620 deaths in 2005[1]. Ovarian cancer is the sixth leading cause of cancer after breast, lung, colon, uterus and non-Hodgkin's lymphoma. It is the leading cause of gynecologic cancer death. The lifetime risk for developing ovarian cancer is 1 in 70 women. Seventy percent of ovarian cancers present as advanced disease (stage 3 and 4) which is associated with a poor five year survival of 30%. Although early disease (stage 1) has a 80-90% survival there is a lack of specific symptoms for early stage disease. Ovarian cancer can arise from the surface epithelial cells, the germ cells or the stromal cells. The most common type of ovarian cancer arises from the surface epithelial. For the purposes of this chapter we will confine are remarks to this group.

The objectives of this chapter are to:

1. Outline the risk factors for ovarian cancer
2. Review the important methodologic factors to consider when evaluating screening tests.
3. Discuss potential screening strategies for those in higher risk groups such as postmenopausal age and those with a hereditary predisposition to ovarian cancer.
4. Assess the adverse effects of screening.
5. Outline potential novel strategies for screening that are currently under investigation.

Risk Factors for Epithelial Ovarian Cancer

There are several risk factors associated with the development of ovarian cancer. It is well known that the risk for epithelial ovarian cancer rises with advancing age. The incidence of ovarian cancer increases markedly over the age of 40 years; 94% of cases occur in women over 40 years and 48% in women between 50-69 years [2] The mortality rate for ovarian cancer was 14.7 per 100,000 women in 1994. Mortality rises with age such that between the ages of 50 – 69 years, the mortality rate was 30 per 100,000 in 1994 [2]. A second risk factor is hereditary ovarian cancer which was first described by Lynch more than 20 years ago. About 30% of epithelial ovarian cancer cases have a family history of ovarian or premenopausal breast cancer. With one first or second degree relative with ovarian cancer the relative risk is 3.1 (2.2-4.4) compared to 4.6 (1.1-18.4) with two or three relatives with ovarian cancer [2]. The BRCA1 gene was cloned in 1993 and the BRCA2 gene was cloned in 1995. Both genes have been linked to ovarian and breast cancer. In 15% of these cases a BRCA 1 or 2 mutation can be documents [3,4]. The most common histology in these women with ovarian tumors is serous. These BRCA 1 or 2 mutations appear to be clustered in certain cultural groups such as Ashekanzi Jewish women, and French Canadian women. The risk of developing ovarian cancer by age 70 with BRCA1 mutation is 39%, BRCA2 mutation 11% and with no mutation it is 1.4% [5]. Since ovarian cancer has a low prevalence (1 in 70 women) in the general population, many screening modalities have been assessed in higher risk populations. We will review the role of screening in both the postmenopausal women and those with a hereditary predisposition for cancer.

METHODS

Several databases were searched using the search terms of ovarian cancer, screening, systemic reviews, practice guidelines, and reports. The sources included: MEDLINE (1966-Mar 2005), CANCERLIT (1983 through Mar 2005), Cochrane Library (2004) reference lists of papers and review articles, abstracts 1997-2002 of the American Society of Clinical Oncology (ASCO), Physician Data Query (PDQ), Canadian Medical Association (CMA) Infobase (http://mdm.ca/cpgsnew/cpgs/index.asp) and The National Guidelines Clearinghourse (http://www.guideline.gov/).

SCREENING

Principles of Screening

The role of screening is to identify women at a preinvasive point in disease when the disease is amenable to treatment at low cost and low morbidity. The criteria for an effective screening test as proposed by the World Health Organization are [6,7]:

1. The condition should be an important health problem (significant prevalence and cause of mortality)

2. The natural history of the condition including development from latent to declared disease, should be adequately understood
3. There should be a recognizable latent or early symptomatic stage in which treatment improves outcome
4. There should be a suitable test or examination that is acceptable to the population
5. There should be efficacious treatment for patients with recognized disease
6. Facilities for diagnosis and treatment should be available.
7. There should be an agreed policy on whom to treat
8. The screening program must be cost effective
9. The screening test should have a high sensitivity, to detect disease (low false negative rate), a high specificity (low false positive rate) and high positive and negative predictive values.

These requirements along with six factors are used for evaluating screening programs: validity (how well a screening test detects ovarian cancer), reliability, yield (the number of cases of ovarian cancer detected), cost, acceptance and follow-up services.

Ovarian cancer occurs at a low prevalence in the general population (1 in 70 women). Thus, many screening studies are conducted in high-risk groups where the prevalence of disease is increased. In ovarian cancer there is no known preinvasive form of the disease. Thus the aim of screening is to detect the ovarian cancer at an earlier stage when treatment is more effective. A screening test will increase the probability of the disease. However, to confirm the disease, harm may occur. The balance of benefits and harms is expressed in terms as:

*   True positive: women with a positive screening test have confirmed ovarian cancer (A)
*   False positive: women with a positive screening test but who do not have ovarian cancer (B)
*   True negative: women with a negative screening test and who do not have ovarian cancer (D)
*   False negative: women with a negative screening test but who have ovarian cancer (C)
*   Positive predictive value: the proportion of women with a positive screening test who have confirmed ovarian cancer (true positives/true + false positives or a/a+b)
*   Sensitivity: Proportion of women with ovarian cancer found by screening (true positives/true positives + false negatives or a/a+c) ie., the chance that a person with cancer has a positive test
*   Specificity: proportion of women who do not have ovarian cancer who test negative (true negative/(true negative+false positive or d/d+b) ie., the chance that a person without cancer has a negative test.
*   Prevalence: True cases of disease (a+c) in the population (a+b+c+d).

A test that discriminates well between those with ovarian cancer and healthy women will have a high sensitivity and specificity. Different factors affect sensitivity and specificity. These include the threshold at which a test is considered abnormal and the interval between screens. For example a fast growing cancer may be missed by too long a screening interval.

Harm will depend on the test's specificity. The more specific the test, the lower the proportion of false-positive women who are exposed to invasive procedures. These harms can involve invasive procedures (i.e., surgery) or the anxiety of being recalled for further tests.

In assessing the role of screening in ovarian cancer, the first question to answer is whether a case of ovarian cancer detected by screening can have improved outcomes. If this is proven, then the benefits versus harms must be determined. Lastly the costs for screening, follow-up test and such must be quantified.

Table 1. Screening Test Parameters

	Confirmed Ovarian Cancer	No confirmed ovarian cancer	Total
Positive test for ovarian cancer	A	B	A+B
Negative test for ovarian cancer	C	D	C+D
Total	A+C	B+D	A+B+C+D

Screening Tests that Have Been Evaluated in Ovarian Cancer

The screening tests that have been evaluated in ovarian cancer assess morphology (endovaginal ultrasound with or without color Doppler) or biology (Cancer Antigen 125 (CA125)). Ultrasound assesses the change in size and shape and consistency of the ovary. Criteria exist defining abnormal ovaries and these vary depending on age and menopausal status. CA125 is a glycoprotein produced by some ovarian cancers. CA125 levels have been elevated in 25-75% of stage 1 ovarian cancers [2]. However, elevated values are also seen in other malignancies (pancreatic, endometrial), benign gynecologic disorders (ie., endometriosis), other benign conditions (ie., diverticulitis).

Given that none of these tests have high enough sensitivity and specificity alone, most screening protocols have combined tests to improve sensitivity and specificity. Thus, the approaches for screening have included:

1. Ultrasound as the primary screening test with CA125 used for further testing of women with abnormal ultrasound results or;
2. CA125 as the primary screening test and secondary ultrasound for those with high CA125 values.

Table 2. Recommendations for screening postmenopausal women

Year and Organization	Recommendation
1994 Canadian Task Force on Preventive Health Care [8]	Screening for ovarian cancer either by abdominal examination, pelvic or transvaginal sonography or CA125 levels should not be a part of the periodic health examination of asymptomatic postmenopausal women
1994 American College of Physicians [9,10]	Screening with ultrasound or CA125 for women without a family history is not recommended.

Table 2. Recommendations for screening postmenopausal women (Continued)

Year and Organization	Recommendation
1995 National Institute of Health Consensus conference [11]	There is no evidence available yet that the current screening modalities of CA125 and transvaginal ultrasonography can be effectively used for widespread screening to reduce mortality from ovarian cancer nor that their use will result in decreased rather than increased morbidity and mortality
1996 United States Preventive Task Force [12]	Screening asymptomatic women for ovarian cancer with ultrasound, the measurement of serum tumor markers or pelvic examination is not recommended
1997 American College of Preventive Medicine [13]	The evidence is insufficient at this time to recommend physical examination, ultrasonography, biochemical markers or genetic screening for asymptomatic women for early detection of ovarian malignancy. The research has not convincingly detected that screening will reduce morbidity of mortality from ovarian cancer or improve the health status of women.
2003 Program in Evidence-based care, Cancer Care Ontario -Screening Postmenopausal Women for Ovarian cancer 4-6a [7]	There is insufficient evidence currently to support the introduction of screening in the asymptomatic, general risk postmenopausal population. Screening is associated with increased rates of surgery and patient anxiety. The benefits of screening in terms of lives saved, pain and suffering do not appear to be outweighed by the social costs of unnecessary investigations and treatments, Detection of early stage cancers may not lead to increased survival rates. No optimal interval for screening can be defined. The positive predictive value of the screening tests needs to be improved. Any further recommendations regarding screening for ovarian cancer in this group of women must await the conclusions of the three major ongoing trials. Efforts to impact ovarian cancer-related mortality rates should focus on prevention including --identifying women at high risk followed by genetic counseling and BRCA 1 and BRCA2 identification. --make available information about the benefits of oral contraception, tubal ligation and prophylactic oophorectomy to this population.
2003 Scottish Intercollegiate Guidelines Network (SIGN) [14]	Value of general population screening remains uncertain and cannot be recommended.
2004 Institute for Clinical Systems Improvement (ICSI) [15]	CA125 and pelvic ultrasound screening for ovarian cancer in asymptomatic women should not be done due to physical, psychological and financial harm from false positives resulting in unnecessary surgery.
2004 US Preventive Services Task Force [16]	The routine screening of well women for ovarian cancer results in more harm than benefit

Screening for the Postmenopausal Woman

Practice Guidelines, Task Force and Consensus Recommendations
In the last decade, there have been several practice guidelines, task force, and consensus recommendations regarding screening for postmenopausal women [7-13]. No group recommends screening for women where age is the only risk factor.

Systematic Review [2]
In 1998, the National Health Service Center for Reviews and Dissemination at University of York (United Kingdom) published a comprehensive review on Ovarian Cancer Screening [2]. The goals of the report were:

- to evaluate the performance of current screening tests for ovarian cancer;
- assess the adverse effects of screening, including morbidity associated with surgical intervention and psychological morbidity associated with false positive diagnosis;
- report on the stage of diagnosis of newer methods of screening

The key evidence was that:

- In the absence of evidence of effectiveness, it is premature to establish any kind of screening program
- The evidence suggests that both CA125 based screening (50%, 95% CI 23-77) and U/S screening (75%, 95%CI 35-97) can detect higher proportions of ovarian cancers at Stage 1 than that currently observed with no screening (22-28%). These numbers should be interpreted with caution given they are based on a small number of studies on mainly self-selected women.
- Annual ultrasound screening for the general population detects 100% of ovarian cancer (sensitivity) and Ca 125 screening detects 80% of cases. Due to varying sizes of the study population the confidence intervals are wide. With ultrasound (alone or with other tests) 8 ovarian cancers were detected among 15,824 women. With CA125 followed by ultrasound there were 14 ovarian cancers detected among 27,560 women screened.
- False positive rates ranged from 1.2% to 2.5% by U/S and 0.1%-0.6% for Ca125 screening.
- About 0.5-1% of women suffer a significant complication due to surgery and most of those who do not have ovarian cancer will have a benign gynecologic condition. There is a risk that detection of benign and borderline tumors may become the target of ovarian screening even though they would not have been associated with any morbidity during a patient's lifetime.
- Intervals of 1-3 years for U/S and annual for CA125 are underway.
- About 3-12% of screened women are recalled for further testing and assessment resulting in potential distress and anxiety to otherwise healthy women.
- The low positive predictive value of ovarian screening (3% surgery, 0.6% for initial recall for annual ultrasound screening, 15% for surgery and 1% for initial recall for

annual CA125 screening) is due to the low prevalence of ovarian cancer and this limits the cost-effective of general population screening.

- Although ultrasound screening is more sensitive than CA125 screening, CA125 has fewer false positives and so a high positive predictive value.

In conclusion: the most effective screening method and interval is not known and the effectiveness of screening programs for the general populations can not be determined.

Table 3. Studies of ultrasonography alone (Reprinted with permission from the Program in Evidence-Based Care, Cancer Care Ontario (CCOPEBC, 2003, 4-6a)[7]

Study	Van Nagell 2000 [17]	Hayashi 1999 [18]	Tabor 1994 [22]	Campbell 1989 [20]	Millo 1989 21]
Type	Cohort	cohort	pilot	cohort	cohort
Population	>50 yo or >25 yo with FHOC	> 50 yr	46-65 yr	> 45 yr	> 45 yo
Type of U/S	vaginal	vaginal	Vaginal	vaginal	vaginal
# screens	Annual 1987-1999	1 screen	1 screen	3 annual screens	1 screen
# participants	14,469	23,451	435[a]	5,479	500
# of abnormal U/S tests	180 persistent	258	54	326	12
# undergoing surgery	180 (1.2%)	95 (0.04%)	9 (2.1%)	326 (5.9%)	6 (1.2%)
# ovarian cancers detected	17 11 stg 1 3 stg 2 3 stg 3	7	0	9 5 stg 1 4 mets 5 @ 1st 4 @ 2nd	0
# false positives	163	88	9	317	6
PPV	9.4%	7.4%	0	1.5%	0
# of cancers developing amoung women with negative screening tests	4 within 12 mos 2 stg 2 2 stg 3	NR	NR	NR	NR

NR – not reported U/S – ultrasound;
a-There were 950 women in the study but only 435 women were randomized to the screening group.

The Program in Evidence Based Care through Cancer Care Ontario published their report in 2003 with an update in 2004 [7]. We will review the specific screening strategies as described in their report with literature updates as were identified in the intervening year.

Ultrasound Alone

There are 4 cohort and 1 pilot randomized trial on ultrasonography alone [17-21]. Between 0.04-5.9% of women underwent surgery because of a persistent abnormal screening ultrasound. Between 3-9.4% of those receiving surgery had cancer with half of the cases being early stage. There was no difference in ovarian cancer mortality between those women screened and the general population in Crayford's followup study to Campbell's screening study [20]. Ultrasound alone has a low positive predictive value for the high rate of harm (surgery) to deal with the false positive screens.

Color Doppler Imaging

There have been 2 prospective cohort studies and one pilot randomized trial assessing color Doppler imaging in postmenopausal women [23-25]. The rate of persistent positive screens was 0.2-0.8% which is improved over ultrasound alone. The rate of ovarian cancer for those who underwent surgery was 10%. All the cases were early stage disease. Unfortunately 3 patients with a negative screen developed ovarian cancer within 2 years of the test.

Table 4. Studies of ultrasonography followed by CA125
(Reprinted with permission from the Program in Evidence-Based Care,
Cancer Care Ontario (CCOPEBC, 2003, 4-6a)[7]

Study	Sato 2000 [19]	Vuento 1997 [23]	Holbert 1994 [26]
Type of study	Cohort	cohort	Cohort
Population	>35 yr, 52% postmenopausal	postmenopausal	Postmenopausal
CA125	NR	>30U/ml	>35U/ml
#screenings	51,550	1291	478
# participants	Annually 10 yr	1 screening	1 screening
# positive screening U/S	4452	NR	33
# elevated CA125	2554	14	29
# undergoing surgery (%)	320 (0.6%)	NR	11 (2.3%)
# ovarian cancers detected	22 (4-LMP, 13 Stg ½, 3 stg ¾)	1 (LMP)	1 (stg 1)
# False positive	298	NR	10
PPV	6.9%	NR	9.1%
# cancers found in women with negative tests	4 stg 1	4 1 stg 1 2 stg 1 uterine 1 abdominal carcinomatosis	NR

LMP   – Low malignant potential
NR   – not reported; U/S – ultrasound

Table 5. Studies of CA125 followed by ultrasound (Reprinted with permission from the Program in Evidence-Based Care, Cancer Care Ontario (CCOPEBC, 2003, 4-6a) [7]

Study	Jacobs 1999 [27]	Adonakis 1996 [28]	Grover 1995 [29]	Jacobs 1993 [30]	Einhorn 1992 [31]
Type of study	Pilot RCT	Cohort	Cohort	Cohort	Cohort
Population	Age > 45	Age >45	Age >40 or family history	Age >45	Age >40
CA125	>30U/ml	>35U/ml	>35U/ml	>30U/ml	>30U/ml
#screenings	3 annual	1 screen	1 screen	1 screen	2 screens
# participants	10958 screened 10977 control	2000	2550	22,000	5,550
# elevated CA125	468	18	101	339	175
# positive screening U/S	29	18	16	41	NR
# undergoing surgery (%)	29 (0.3%)	14 (0.7%)	16 (0.6%)	41 (0.2%)	39 (0.7%)
# ovarian cancers detected	6 (ov or tube) 3 @ 1st 3 @ 3rd	3 (1 invasive, 1 borderline, 1 metastatic)	0	11 (3 stage 1, 1 stage 2, 7 stage 3,4)	7 (2 stg 1, 2 stg 2, 2 stg 3, 1 NR)
# False positive	23	12	8	30	32
PPV	20.7%	14.3%	0	26.8%	15.4%
# cancers found in women with negative tests	NR	NR	NR	8 ovarian (5 stg 1, 3 stg 3) within 6-22 mos of screening	6 ovarian cancer within 3 years of screening
Cancer arising after 1 yr	NR	0	1	3	1
Sensitivity after 1 yr	NR	100%	NR	79%	NR
# of patients followed	19,960 (91%)			19,464 (88%)	NR
Duration of Followup	7 yr			6.76 yr	10 year
# ovarian cancers detected since the original study	16 screened 20 non-screened			49	20

NR – not reported

Patients in both Jacobs et al studies[27,30] are from the same patient population.

PPV – positive Predictive Value

RCT-Randomized controlled trial

U/S – ultrasound

Ultrasound Followed by CA125

Three cohort studies [19,23,26] assessed the combined approach of ultrasound followed by CA125 evaluation for those with an abnormal scan. When both tests were positive, surgery was completed for 0.6-2.3%. The rate of ovarian cancer for those with both tests positive (PPV) was low 6.9-9.1%. Twenty percent of those cases being low malignant potential and 60% being early stage disease.

CA125 Followed by Ultrasound

Four cohort and one pilot randomized study described screening using CA125 followed by ultrasound for those with abnormal results. When both tests were abnormal, between 0.2-0.7% underwent surgery. For those who had surgery, the rates of ovarian cancer (PPV) were 14.3-26.8%. About 30% of the cases were early stage disease. In the two years following a negative screening test, approximately an equal number of cancer cases were found. The authors felt CA125 followed by ultrasonography was effective but further work was required.

Ongoing Work

The York document [2] outlined three ongoing prospective trials [32-34] assessing various combinations of ultrasound with or without CA125 testing.

Future Research

Research is currently evaluating other markers or proteomic patterns that may be useful for the detection of early stage ovarian cancer. Lysophosphatidic acid (LPA) is associated with an invasion of the extracellular matrix in ovarian cancer. Serum LPA concentrations are elevated in 96% of women with ovarian cancer including 90% of those with stage 1 disease [35-37]. Multiple markers or panels of tumor markers may be more sensitive than single markers for detection of early stage ovarian cancer. OVX1, CA-125 and macrophage-colony stimulating factor were measured in 281 women with ovarian tumors (175 malignant, 29 borderline and 77 benign) and 117 normals [38]. The panel was significantly more sensitive than CA125 alone for presence of any ovarian malignancy (sensitivity 85% vs 80% for stage 1 ovarian cancer (76 vs 66%) but no single marker performed better than CA125. Proteomic patterns measured in serum may allow for detection of early stage ovarian cancer. One study using mass spectroscopy proteomic analysis of serum found that the 50 samples of women with ovarian cancer were correctly classified including 18 women with stage 1 cancer. In the samples of 63 of 66 women without ovarian cancer, were correctly classified [39]. Further work is required to assess these tests in prospective screening studies.

Defining Families with a History of Breast or Ovarian Cancer

There are several situations in which a cancer can appear in families:

Hereditary cancer (at risk families): Any pedigree that demonstrates autosomal dominant transmission of a cancer suggests an inherited cancer predisposition. Most hereditary cancer syndromes are characterized by incomplete penetrance (a probability that cancer will develop but not a certainty) and variable expressivity (age of onset, number of primary tumors and tumor site can vary within and among families). Hereditary breast ovarian cancer syndrome is an example of hereditary cancer. Models for determining the probability that genetic testing will reveal a mutation in BRCA1 or BRCA2 are available. These models include age of onset of cancer, number of affected relatives, presence/absence of associated malignancies, ancestry.

Table 6. Ongoing Randomized Controlled Trials [2]

	Randomized trial of screening for ovarian cancer (Bart's study)[32]	European randomized trial of ovarian cancer screening [33]	National Cancer Institute sponsored screening trial for prostate, lung, colorectal and ovarian carcinomas. [34]
Control group	Yes	Yes	Standard medical care
Screening method	Ca125 followed by ultrasound for test positive Annual screen for 6 years	Transvaginal ultrasound every 18 or 36 mos	Transvaginal ultrasound and CA125 every year for 4 years
Reason for recall	Based on woman's risk for ovarian cancer, age and rate of CA125 change	Ovarian abnormality	
Study population	Postmenopausal	50-64 year	60-74 years
Target number	60,000 in each arm	30,000 in each intervention and 60,000 in control group Total 120,000	37,000 in each arm Total 74,000
Sub studies	Economic Psychological impact Serum Bank	Economic Serum Bank	Serum Bank
Completion	7 year follow-up	10 year follow-up	10 year follow-up
Follow-up	Questionnaire		Annual Periodic Survey of Health questionnaire
Results expected	2011		

Familial cancer: Here more cases of a specific type of cancer occur than are expected on the basis of chance alone but not exhibiting classic features of hereditary cancer such as early age of onset, multifocal tumors or dominant inheritance. Genetic testing is often less likely to provide information about cancer risk in these cases. Models are available to estimate cancer risk in familial cases of ovarian cancer and they take into account factors such as age of onset, number of affected relatives, and the degree of relationship between the patient and the affected relative in estimating lifetime cancer risks. Empiric risks are useful because they can demonstrate that not everyone with a family history of cancer is at significantly increased risk of developing the disease.

Table 7. Criteria for Referral to the Genetics Assessment Program or Testing

---

The Ministry of Health and Long Term Care Criteria for Referral to the Genetics Assessment Program or Testing

Referral to the Genetics Assessment Program
Referral for Hereditary Breast Ovarian Cancer
- Multiple cases of breast cancer (particularly where diagnosis occurred at less than 50 years) and/or ovarian cancer (any age) in the family
- Age at diagnosis of breast cancer less than 35 years
- A family member diagnosed with both breast and ovarian cancer
- Breast and/or ovarian cancer in Jewish families
- Family member(s) with primary cancer occurring in both breasts-especially if one or both cancers were diagnosed before age 50
- A family member diagnosed with invasive serous ovarian cancer
- Presence of male breast cancer in the family
- Family member with an idenfitied BRCA1 or BRCA2 mutation
- Presence of other associated cancers or conditions suggestive of an inherited cancer syndrome.

Referral for Colorectal Cancer
- Multiple cases in the family of the following cancers related to the hereditary non-polyposis colorectal cancer (HNPCC) spectrum, with at least one relative affected with colorectal or endometrial cancer. Age of onset less than 50 years, in closely related relatives and in more than one generation, would raise the index of suspicion.
- Age at diagnosis of colorectal cancer < 35 year
- Multiple primary cancers in one family member
- Family member with familial adenomatous polyposis or 10 or more adenomatous polyps
- Family member with a colonic adenoma or cancer with high microsatellite instability
- Family member with a known mutation causing either HNPCC or FAP

Testing for Hereditary Breast or Ovarian Cancer
Testing for affected individuals with breast or ovarian cancer
At least one case of cancer
- Jewish and breast cancer < 50 years, or ovarian cancer at any age
- Breast cancer <35 years of age
- Male breast cancer (only BRCA2 testing)
- Invasive serous ovarian cancer at any age
At least two cases of cancer on the same side of the family
- Breast cancer <60 years and a 1st or 2nd degree relative with ovarian cancer or male breast cancer.
- -Breast and ovarian cancer in the same individual, or bilateral breast cancer with first cancer < 50 years
- Two cases of breast cancer, both < 50 years, in first or second-degree relatives
- Two cases of ovarian cancer, any age, in first or second-degree relatives
- Jewish and breast cancer at any age, and any family history of breast or ovarian cancer
At least three cases of cancer on the same side of the family
- Three or more cases of breast or ovarian cancer at any age, in a suggestive pattern

Table 7. Criteria for Referral to the Genetics Assessment Program or Testing (Continued)

The Ministry of Health and Long Term Care Criteria for Referral to the Genetics Assessment Program or Testing (Continued)

Testing for Hereditary Breast or Ovarian Cancer (Continued)

Testing for unaffected individuals (This should only be done if affected individuals are unavailable (i.e., deceased)
- Relative of individual with known BRCA1 or BRCA2 mutation (specific family mutation only tested)
- Jewish and first or second-degree relative of individual with:
  - breast cancer < 50 years or
  - ovarian cancer at any age or
  - male breast cancer or
  - breast cancer any age with positive family history of breast or ovarian cancer
- In exceptional cases, testing may be offered to a first-degree relative of an affected individual who has breast or ovarian cancer, and who also has a pedigree strongly suggestive of hereditary breast/ovarian cancer, i.e., risk of carrying a mutation for the individual being tested is >10%. Every attempt must be made to contact and offer testing to the highest-risk member first.

Testing for Hereditary NonPolyposis Colon Cancer

- Affected and unaffected individuals from families with a known HNPCC mutation
- Affected individual from Modified Amsterdam families. Family must meet all of the following criteria:
  - Three affected relatives, one with colorectal cancer, and the other two with any combination of colorectal, endometrial, small bowel, ureter, transitional cell kidney cancer, and/or sebaceous adenoma/carcinoma
  - One should be a first-degree relative of the other two
  - At least one diagnosis of colorectal cancer must be made before age 50
  - Tumor type should be confirmed by review of pathology or other medical records.
- Affected individuals from families with:
  - Three affected individuals, one with colorectal cancer, and the other two with any combination of: colorectal, endometrial, small bowel, ureter, sebaceous adenoma/carcinoma, ovarian, pancreatic, kidney (transitional cell cancer only), gastric, primary brain or primary hepatobiliary cancer.
  - Two of the three family members must be in a first-degree relationship
  - At least one diagnosis under the age of 50
  - Tumors should be verified by pathological examination
- Individual affected with colorectal cancer and a second primary HNPCC-associated cancer. This includes synchronous and metachronous colorectal cancers. At least one primary cancer must be diagnosed under age 55. Families are eligible with or without family history of HNPCC-associated cancer, and tumors should be verified by pathological examination.
- Individual diagnosed with colorectal cancer under the age or 35. Families are eligible with or without family history of HNPCC-associated cancer, and tumors should be verified by pathological examination.

Table 7. Criteria for Referral to the Genetics Assessment Program
or Testing (Continued)

The Ministry of Health and Long Term Care Criteria for Referral to the Genetics Assessment Program or Testing (Continued)

Women at High Risk for Ovarian cancer as per the American Society of Clinical Oncology [40]

The definition of **high risk** for ovarian cancer as a woman having one of the following:
- first degree relative diagnosed with ovarian cancer before age 40
- first-degree relative diagnosed with breast and ovarian cancer (one cancer diagnosis before age 50)
- two or more first- and second-degree relatives (of same lineage) with ovarian cancer
- two or more first- and second-degree relatives (of same lineage) with breast cancer and one relative with ovarian cancer
- One first- or second-degree relative with breast cancer before age 40 and one first- or second-degree relative with ovarian cancer before age 50 (of same lineage)
- Two or more first-and second-degree relatives (of same lineage) diagnosed with breast cancer before age 50
- Two or more first- and second-degree relatives (of same lineage) diagnosed with breast cancer, one before age 40.

Women at High Risk for Ovarian Cancer as per Scottish Intercollegiate Guidelines Network [14]

High risk individuals meet one of the following criteria:
- two or more individuals with ovarian cancer, who are first degree relatives of each other
- one individual with ovarian cancer at any age, and one with breast cancer diagnosed under age 50 years, who are first degree relatives of each other *
- one relative with ovarian cancer at any age, and two with breast cancer diagnosed under 60 years, who are connected by first degree relationships*
- know carrier of relevant cancer gene mutations (eg BRCA1 and 2)
- untested first degree relative of a predisposing gene carrier
- three or more family members with colon cancer, or two with colon cancer and one with stomach, ovarian endometrial, urinary tract or small bowel cancer in two generations. One of these cancers must be diagnosed under age 50 years.
- an individual with both breast and ovarian cancer.

* In these categories a second degree relative may be counted if the transmission is via the paternal line (eg, a sister and a paternal aunt or a sister and two paternal aunts.

Sporadic cancer means that the cancer in the family is mainly due to nonhereditary causes.

Uncertain significance means that the reasons for difficulty in pedigree assessment can include small family size, reduced penetrance, paucity of susceptible gender for sex-influenced or sex-limited cancers, prophylactic surgeries in at-risk members, lack of information regarding key relatives in the pedigree (ie., adoption).

Family history can be used to define women who are at high risk for developing ovarian cancer. Different organizations use different criteria to inform those women and/or families who will be invited for more intense counseling (Table 7). During this process a detailed personal and family medical history will be obtained as outlined in table 8. A psychological assessment will inform those factors that affect the woman's risk perception and the way she will utilize the genetic information. Risk assessment and information about the patient's candidacy for testing are discussed. This includes a discussion of possible risks and benefits of genetic testing. Testing is not recommended in situations where there is a low probability of carrying a mutation given the financial cost of cancer genetic testing as well as the potential psychological ramifications. To offer genetic testing means to take responsibility for the adequate pretest education, the process of informed consent and posttest counseling. If the patient carries a gene mutation then the benefits and harms of cancer early detection and prevention modalities must be reviewed.

Table 8. Information exchange during Genetic Counseling

Purpose	Domain	Details
Information gathering and risk assessment	Medical information	Age, personal history of benign or malignant tumors, major illnesses, hospitalizations, surgeries, biopsy history, reproductive history, cancer surveillance, environmental exposures (occupation, alcohol consumption, tobacco use and diet). If the patient has had cancer then the following needs to be defined: organ in which the tumor developed, age at diagnosis, number of tumors, pathology, stage and grade of malignant tumor, pathology of benign tumors, treatment (surgery, chemotherapy, radiotherapy).
	Family pedigree	To the 3rd to 4th generation pedigree. Information on ethnicity and consanguinity is necessary. If a relative had cancer the date of diagnosis, the diagnosis, the date of death and reason for death is important.
Information gathering and risk assessment	Psychosocial assessment	The optimal method to appreciate all of the factors that affect risk perception and utilization of cancer genetic information. This will also provide insight into the potential impact of cancer genetic information on the client's quality of life, educational and career goals, reproductive options and other life choices. The areas to be probed include: motivations for seeking a cancer risk consultation, beliefs about cancer etiology and perception of risk, ethnocultural information, socioeconomic and demographic information, psychosocial factors such as emotional reactions to cancer risk, current screening practice, health behaviors and coping strategies.
Information delivery	Genetic Testing	purpose of the test and who to test, general information about the gene(s), possible test results, likelihood of positive result, technical aspects and accuracy of the test, economic considerations, risk of genetic discrimination, psychosocial aspects, confidentiality, utilization of test results, alternatives to genetic testing, storage and potential reuse of genetic material.
Information exchange	Genetic test results	Disclosure and post-test counseling include: results disclosure, significance of the test results, impact of test results, medical management, informing other relatives, future contact, resources.
Information exchange	On going surveillance	Discussion of cancer screening guidelines, reviewing limitations if relevant, methods for reducing cancer risk if known and referral to appropriate professionals if needed.

Table 9. Practice Guideline, Task Force and Consensus Recommendations

Agency	Screening Recommendations
1994 American College of Physicians [9]	In women with a family history of ovarian cancer in one or more relatives (without evidence of a hereditary cancer syndrome), routine screening with CA125 or ultrasound in general is not recommended. Women requesting screening should be counseled about their individual risk (considering age, parity, and a history of oral contraceptive pill use), abour the potential adverse effects of screening and about the lack of scientific evidence that deaths from ovarian cancer are decreased by screening. Women and their physicians should consider this information in making individual decisions about screening. For women from a family with the rare hereditary ovarian cancer syndrome, referral for specialist care is recommended.
1997 National Health Service (NHS) centre for reviews and dissemination at the University of York [2]	In the absence of evidence from randomized controlled trials, no assumptions about the effectiveness of screening programs for women with a family history of ovarian cancer can be made.
2003 Scottish Intercollegiate Guidelines Network [14]	Screening for ovarian cancer in high risk groups should only be offered in the context of a research study designed to gather data on – sensitivity and specificity of a screening tool, stage of cancer detected through screening and residual risk of primary peritoneal cancer following prophylactice oophorectomy. D* Screening programmes for women at increased risk of ovarian cancer should include mechanisms for providing emotional and psychological support. D* women with genetic mutations of BRCA1 or BRCA2 genes should be counseled regarding prophylactic oophorectomy and removal of fallopian rubes at a relevant time of their life. C* Screening programmes for women at increased risk of ovarian cancer should include mechanisms for providing emotional and psychological support. D*
2004 Program in Evidence-based Care. Screening High Risk Women for Ovarian Cancer 4-6b [41]	The lack of sufficient high quality evidence precludes definitive recommendations being made. The Gynecology Cancer Disease Site Group offers the following opinions based on the evidence reviewed: − Studies are inadequate to establish benefits from screening the population of women who are at risk for developing ovarian cancer. − The population of women who are at high risk for developing ovarian cancer has not been studied adequately enough to establish that screening is beneficial. − More long-term studies of women who are at high risk for developing ovarian cancer need to be conducted in order to determine if there is any benefit from screening. − Women may experience distress about their perceived risk of ovarian cancer regardless of their familial ovarian cancer risk. Practitioners should acknowledge this distress and educate women about their risk of developing ovarian cancer and the effectiveness of available screening tests. − There are no high-quality randomized controlled trials examining the role of screening women at high risk for developing ovarian cancer. Such trial would be of benefit to health care providers and the patients they serve. Patients and practitioners should be encouraged to take part in such trials.

- See Appendix for Level of Recommendations and Strength of Evidence

Screening in Families with a History of Ovarian Cancer

Practice Guideline, Task Force and Consensus Recommendations

Recommendations have been published regarding the role of screening for women at high risk for ovarian cancer based on family history.

The Program in Evidence based Care through Cancer Care Ontario published their report in 2004 [42]. We will review the specific screening strategies as described in their report with updates as they were identified in the intervening year.

Ultrasound

Two prospective cohort studies addressed the role of transabdominal and transvaginal ultrasound in women with a family history of ovarian cancer. Between 2.7-4.8% of women underwent surgery and there were 7.7-9.4% cancers identified (PPV). In the van Nagel study [17], 64% of these were early stage disease. Unfortunately in the van Nagel study [43], 4.9% of women (8) developed ovarian cancer in the 24 months following surgery.

Table 10. Studies on ultrasound alone (Reprinted with permission from the Program in Evidence-Based Care, Cancer Care Ontario (CCOPEBC, 2004, 4-6b) [2,41]

Study	Andolf 1986 [43]	Van Nagell 2000 [17]
Population	40-70 yr	Women > 25 yo with FHOC or women >50
# participants	805	14,469
Type of ultrasound	Transabdominal	Transvaginal
# undergoing surgery (%)	39 (4.8%)	395 (2.7%)
# undergoing surgery due to abnormal results (%)	39 (4.8%)	180 (1.2%)
# ovarian cancers detected	3 (2 LMP)	17 (11 stg 1, 3 stg 3, 3 stg 3)
# false positives	36	163
PPV	7.7%	9.4%
Cancers arising during follow-up	NR	4 within 12 months 4 after 12 months

PPV – Positive predictive value
FHOC – Family history of ovarian cancer
NR   – not reported

Ultrasound and Color Flow Doppler

Weiner [44] screened 600 women with prior breast cancer using ultrasound and color flow Doppler. There were 64 were abnormal cases and 12 women (2%) subsequently underwent surgery. Four women had ovarian cancer: 3 non-metastatic and 1 metastatic for a PPV 33%.

Table 11. Studies of concurrent CA125 and ultrasonography (Reprinted with permission from the Program in Evidence-Based Care, Cancer Care Ontario (CCOPEBC, 2004, 4-6b) [2,41]

Study	Karlan 1993 [6]	Muto 1993 [45]	Schwartz 1995 [46]	Belinson 1995 [47][a]	Dorum 1996 [48]	Laframboise 2002 [52]	Taylor 2003 [51]	Vasen 2005 [53]
Population	>35yo FHOB	>25yo FHOC	>30yo FHOC	>25yo FHOC	>18yo 2 FDR B+OC or 1 FDR B+OC	2FRD OC 2FDC B+1OC 1FDR OC and Ash jew, French Canadian, Dutch 1 FDR OC + 1 male FDR B 1FDR OC + 2 FDR early onset Br, pancreatic or prostate know mutation in family	1FDR OC[b]	BRCA1 (77) BRCA2 (18) others from known BRCA1/2 families
C125 u/ml	>35	>35	>35	>35	>35	>35	?	?
No. screened	597	384	247	137	180	311	2,500	138
No. Surgery	19 (3.2%)	38 (9.9%)	1 (0.4%)	2 (1.5%)	27 (15.0%)	57 (18.3%)	?	132
No. with abnormal test and surgery	10 (1.7%)	15 (3.9%)	1 (0.4%)	2 (1.5%)	14 (7.8%)	9 (2.9%)	?	?
Ov Ca[c]	1 (LMP)	0	0	1	7 (3LMP)	1 (LMP)	11 (4LMP)	6
False-positive	9	15	1	1	7	8	93[d]	30
PPV	10%	0%	0%	50%	50%	11%	10.5%	17%

FDR – first degree relative; FHBO – family history of breast and ovarian cancer.

OC – ovarian cancer; LMP – low malignant potential.

[a] Colour Doppler imaging used in addition to transvaginal ultrasound and CA125.

[b] Inclusion criteria changed over time, eventually women included in the study had to have one first degree relative with ovarian cancer, and at least one other relative with first or second degree with any cancer.

[c] Number of ovarian cancers detected among women who underwent surgery for abnormal test results.

[d] False positive value is based on the number of abnormal screening tests as opposed to the number of surgery performed that did not identify malignant disease.

Concurrent CA125 and Ultrasonography

Eleven prospective cohort studies [6,17,43-51] and one retrospective study [52] met the inclusion criteria: reported clinical trials (RCT, comparative cohort study or single cohort study) or systematic review of clinical trials; 2. evaluated tests to detect ovarian cancer; 3. included asymptomatic women at high risk for developing ovarian cancer by ASCO definition; 4. reported rates of confirmed ovarian cancer.

Several studies have involved screening women with a family history of ovarian/breast cancer or known BRCA 1 or 2 mutation status using concurrent ultrasound and CA125. Between 0.4%-7.8% of women underwent surgery for abnormal tests while 0.4%-18.3% underwent surgery for reasons including prophylaxis. The positive predictive value of both tests had a wide range of 0-50%. The number of false positives (harm) was also high at 50-100%. There were a significant number of low malignant potential tumors identified in the group.

Sequential CA125 and Ultrasonography

There were two prospective cohort studies [50,51] assessing sequential CA125 and ultrasonography. Between 1.2-4.1% of women underwent surgery for an abnormal results and the PPV ranged from 0-11.2%. Further work would be required to determine whether there is a benefit between concurrent versus sequential testing.

Table 12. Studies of sequential CA125 and ultrasonography (Reprinted with permission from the Program in Evidence-Based Care, Cancer Care Ontario (CCOPEBC, 2004, 4-6b) [2,41]

Study	Bourne 1994 [50]	Taylor 2001 [51]
Population	>25 yr family history of ov ca	>25 yr family history of ov ca
CA125 cut off for repeat screening	Varied (10-35 U/ml)	>20 U/ml (premenopausal) >6U/ml (postmenopausal)
# participants	1601	252
#undergoing surgery	62 (4.1%)	24 (9.5%)
#undergoing surgery because of abnormal test result	62 (4.1%)	3 (1.2%) [a]
# ovarian cancers detected	7 3 were LMP	0
# false positives	55	3
PPV	11.2%	0%

PPV – positive predictive value

LMP – low malignant potential

Ov ca – ovarian cancer

A – Taylor et al reported that 3 surgeries were 'initiated' by the study. It is not clear whether the other women undergoing surgery chose prophylactic surgery or not.

Psychological Consequences of Screening

Women with a family history of ovarian cancer who seek advice and screening may have higher levels of anxiety and depression than are found in the general population.

Pernet [54] conducted a small case series study evaluating the psychological effects of a false positive diagnosis of ovarian cancer in women undergoing screening for a family history of ovarian cancer. Questionnaires were used to measure psychological distress, anxiety and depression in 15 women before and 3 months after surgery for abnormal screen. There were no cases of ovarian cancer identified. Ten women were interviewed at 12-21 months after surgery. Anxiety was highest in the time between surgery and biopsy results being available.

Table 13. Practice Guidelines for decreasing ovarian cancer in women with known BRCA1 or 2 mutations

Guideline	Recommendation
2003 SIGN [14]	Women with genetic mutation of BRCA1 or BRCA 2 genes should be counseled regarding prophylactic oophorectomy and removal of fallopian tubes at a relevant time of their life. C (2++,3)* High risk women in whom mutations have not been identified should be counseled at around the age 40 years regarding prophylactic oophorectomy. X* Women who decide to have prophylactic oophorectomy should be offered counseling support and information before and after surgery. X (3,4)*
2003 PEBC [42]	The lack of sufficient high quality evidence precludes definitive recommendations from being made. Instead, the Gynecology Cancer Disease Site Group offers the following opinions based on the evidence reviewed: − Women with a personal or family history of ovarian cancer should be referred for genetic counseling and testing to identify BRCA1 and 2 mutations. Other women who are concerned about their risk of ovarian cancer may also be referred for genetic counseling. − For women choosing prophylactic oophorectomy, peritoneal washings take at the time of surgery may assist in identification of occult cancers. − When deciding on whether or not to include hysterectomy as part of the surgical procedure, the surgeon needs to inform the patients about the risk of fallopian tube cancer. − Hormone replacement therapy remains the best treatment for distressing menopausal symptoms, and therefore a short term trial of HRT may be indicated to relieve these symptoms. − It is crucial that the entire ovary is removed during prophylactic surgery. Any remnant of ovarian tissue is at risk for developing cancer. − For BRCA1 mutation carriers who may be reluctant to have definitive prophylactic surgery, oral contraceptives and/or tubal ligation may reduce their risk of developing ovarian cancer.

* See Appendix 1 for strength of Recommendation and Levels of Evidence

Ongoing Studies

UK Committee for Coordinating Cancer Research (UKCCCR) [2,55] are conducting a prospective uncontrolled screening study for women with a family history of ovarian cancer. Eligible patients have a history of more than one affected close relative such that the average lifetime risk is at least 15%. There is no planned comparison group. Screening will involve annual CA125 and ultrasound.

Future Research

There are a number of markers being evaluated to increase the specificity (decrease the false positive rate) of screening tests. These include Herceptin [56], urinary gonadotropin peptide [56], lipid-associated sialic acid (LASA) [56], Dianon marker 70/K (DM/70K) [56], prostasin [57], human kallikrein 6 (hK6) and 10 (hK10) [58,59]. Petricoin [39] is using proteomic pattern technology to define an algorithm to identify ovarian cancer. They identify a cluster pattern that was able to distinguish all ovarian cancer cases from non-ovarian cancer cases

Table 14. Benefits of Prophylactic Surgery for Those with a BRCA 1 and 2 mutation. (Reprinted with permission from the Program in Evidence-Based Care, Cancer Care Ontario (CCOPEBC, 2003, 4-4) [42]

Study	Kauff 2002 [59]	Rebbeck 2002 [61]	Struewing 1995 [60]
Type of study	Prospective followup	Retrospective	Prospective follow-up
Age of patients	> 35 yr	No specific age	NR
# patients with BRCA1 or 2 mutations	170	551	390
# patients undergoing PO	98	259	44
# patients in control group	72 known BRCA 1 or 2	292 known BRCA 1or 2	346 first degree relative
Incidence of cancer among PO group	1 peritoneal 3 breast	6 ovarian 2 peritoneal	2 peritoneal
Incidence of cancer among control group	4 ovarian 1 peritoneal 8 breast	58 ovarian/peritoneal	8 ovarian
Mean FUP	24.2 mos	8.2 yr in PO 8.8 yr in FUP	NR
Outcome measures	DFS 98% for PO and 83% in control p=0.04	Incidence of cancer: 0.8% in PO 19.9% in control p<0.001	PO – 13 times increased risk of ovarian cancer compared to general population Control – 24 times increased risk of general population

DFS – Disease free survival
PO   – prophylactic oophorectomy

Definitive Treatment for Women with BRCA1 or 2 Mutations

Women identified as being at high risk of ovarian cancer can be offered oral contraceptives, tubal ligation or prophylactic oophorectomy as methods for decreasing their risk for developing invasive disease. Prophylactic oophorectomy is the superior strategy for decreases the risk of ovarian cancer and breast cancer.

Practice Guideline, Task Force and Consensus Recommendations

All the guidelines clearly advocate for prophylactic oophorectomy for those women interested in decreasing their risk for invasive disease.

The Program in Evidence based Care through Cancer Care Ontario published their report on Management Options for women with a Hereditary Predisposition to Ovarian Cancer in 2003 [42]. We will review the specific screening strategies as described.

Two prospective follow-up [59,60] and one retrospective [61] reports show that prophylactic oophorectomy for BRCA1 and 2 carriers decreases the risk of primary peritoneal cancer to 0.1% to 0.5%. The rate of new onset breast cancer is decreased by 50%. The risk of recurrent breast cancer is also decreased.

CONCLUSION

Ovarian cancer affects 1 in 70 women in their lifetime. The women at higher risk for disease are postmenopausal women, those with a family history for ovarian cancer or a known BRCA1 or 2 mutation. When assessing the benefits of a screening test, the important factors to consider include whether the test has high sensitivity (identifies accurately those with the disease) especially at point in the disease where treatment is more beneficial with a low chance of causing harm to those false test positive cases. We have reviewed the role of ultrasound alone, with the addition of colour flow Doppler, with the addition of concurrent or sequential CA125 use in these high risk populations. At this point in time, effectiveness of any strategy for decreasing ovarian cancer is not known. The strategies do detect a high proportion of women with stage 1 disease. Because the false positive rate of any strategy is as high as 12%, many women need subsequent testing. This may increase anxiety. Even with multiple tests, up to 2%, women receive surgery for findings that are not ovarian cancer (FP). Three large prospective studies will address whether ovarian cancer screening can decrease ovarian cancer rate. Potential strategies for the future include novel biomarkers or proteonomic assessment.

APPENDIX 1. GRADES OF RECOMMENDATIONS AND LEVELS OF EVIDENCE FOR THE SCOTTISH INTERCOLLEGIATE GUIDELINE NETWORK (SIGN)

		Grades of Recommendation
A		At least one meta-analysis, systematic review of randomized controlled trials or RCT rated as 1++ and directly applicable to the target population or a body of evidence consisting principally of studies rates as 1+ directly applicable to the target population and demonstrating overall consistency of results
B		A body of evidence including studies rated as 2++ directly applicable to the target population and demonstrating overall consistency of results or extrapolated evidence from studies rated as 1++ or 1+
C		A body of evidence including studies rated as 2+ directly applicable to the target population and demonstrating overall consistency of results or extrapolated evidence from studies rated as 2++
D		Evidence level 3 or 4 or extrapolated evidence from studies rated as 2+
		Levels of Evidence
1++		high quality meta-analysis, systematic reviews or RCTs, or RCTs with a very low risk of bias
1+		well conducted meta-analyses, systematic reviews of RCTs or RCTs with a low risk of bias
1		meta-analyses, systematic reviews of RCTs or RCTs with a high risk of bias
2++		High quality systematic reviews of case control or cohort studies, high quality case control or cohort studies with a very low risk of confounding or bias and a high probability that the relationship is causal
2+		Case control or cohort studies with a high risk of confounding or bias and a significant risk that the relationship is not causal
3		Non-analytic studies ie., case reports, case series
4		Expert opinion

APPENDIX 2. ACRONYMS

Acronyms	Meaning
DFS	Disease Free Survival
FDR	First degree relative
FHBO	Family history of breast and ovarian cancer
FHOC	Family history of ovarian cancer
FP	False positive
HNPCC	Hereditary Non-polyposis Colon Cancer
HK6	Human kallikrein 6
Hk10	Human kallikrein 10
ICSI	Institute for Clinical Systems Improvement
LMP	Low Malignant Potential
NR	Not reported
Ov Ca	Ovarian Cancer
PEBC	Program in Evidence Based Care
PPV	Positive Predictive Value
RCT	Randomized Controlled trial
SIGN	Scottish Intercollegiate Guidelines Network
U/S	ultrasound

REFERENCES

[1]   Canadian Cancer Society/National Cancer Institute of Canada. Canadian Cancer Society/National Cancer Institute of Canada, editors.Canadian Cancer Statistics. 2005th ed. Toronto, Canada: 2005;Canadian Cancer Statistics 2005. p. 1-107.

[2]   Bell, R., Petticrew, M., Luengo, S., and Sheldon, T.A. Screening for ovarian cancer: a systematic review. *Health Technol Assess 1998,* 2,1-83.

[3]   Ford, D., Easton, D.F., Stratton, M., Narod, S., Goldgar, D., Devilee, P., Bishop, D.T., Weber, B., Lenoir, G., and Chang-Claude, J. Genetic heterogeneity and penetrance analysis of the BRCA1 and BRCA2 gene in breast cancer families. The Breast Cancer Linkage Consortium. *Am J Hum Genet 1998,* 62,676-689.

[4]   Berchuck, A., Schildkraut, J.M., Marks, J.R., and Futreal, P.A. Managing hereditary ovarian cancer risk. *Cancer 1999,* 86,2517-2524.

[5]   Risch, H.A., McLaughlin, J.R., Cole, D.E., Rosen, B., Bradley, L., and Kwan, E. Prevalence and penetrance of germline BRCA1 and BRCA2 mutations in a population series of 649 women with ovarian cancer. *Am J Hum Genet 2001,* 68,700-710.

[6]   Karlan, B.Y., Raffel, L.J., Crvenkovic, G., Smrt, D., Chen, M.D., and Lopez, E. A multidisciplinary approach to the early detection of ovarian carcinoma: rationale, protocol design, and early results. *Am J Obstet Gynecol 1993,* 169,494-501.

[7]   Fung, M.F.K., Bryson, P., Johnston, M. et al. Screening Postmenopausal Women for Ovarian Cancer. Toronto. Program in Evidence-Based Care. 2004; 4-6a. p.1

[8]   Gladstone CQ. ; Canadian Task Force on the Periodic Health Examination. editors.Canadian Guide to Clinical Preventive Health Care. Ottawa: Health Canada, 1994;Screening for ovarian cancer. p. 870-81.

[9]   American College of Physicians. Screening for ovarian cancer: recommendations and rationale. *Ann Int Med 1994*, 121,141-142.

[10] Carlson, K.J., Skates, S.J., and Singer, D.E. Screening for ovarian cancer. *Ann Int Med 1994*, 121,124-132.

[11] NIH Consensus Conference. Ovarian Cancer: Screening, treatment and follow-up. *J Am Med Asso 1995*, 273,491-497.

[12] U.S.Preventive Services Task Force. ; U.S.Preventive Services Task Force. editors.Guide to clinical preventive services. 2nd ed. Baltimore: Williams and Wilkins, 1996;Guide to clinical preventive services. p. 159

[13] Ferrini, R. Screening asymptomatic women for ovarian cancer: American College of Preventive Medicine practice policy. *Am J Prev Med 1997*, 13,444-446.

[14] Scottish Intercollegiate Guidelines Network (SIGN). Epithelial ovarian cancer. A national clinical guideline. Edinburgh, Scotland. SIGN. 2003; 75. p.1

[15] Institute for Clinical Systems Improvement (ICSI). Preventive services for adults. Bloomington (MN). Institute for Clinical Systems Improvement (ICSI). 2005; 51. p.1

[16] U.S.Preventive Services Task Force. Screening for ovarian cancer: recommendation statement. *Am Fam Physicia 2005*, 71,759-762.

[17] van Nagell, J.R., DePriest, P.D., Reedy, M.B., Gallion, H.H., Ueland, F.R., and Pavlik, E.J. The efficacy of transvaginal sonographic screening in asymptomatic women at risk for ovarian cancer. *Gynecol Oncol 2000*, 77,350-356.

[18] Hayashi, H., Yaginuma, Y., Kitamura, S., Saitou, Y., Miyamoto, Y., and Komori, H. Bilateral oophorectomy in asumptomatic women over 50 years old selected by ovarian cancer screening. *Gynecol Obstet Invest 1999*, 47,58-64.

[19] Sato, S., Yokoyama, Y., Sakamoto, T., Futagami, M., and Saito, Y. Usefulness of mass screening for ovarian cancinoma using transvaginal ultrasonography. *Cance r2000*, 89,582-588.

[20] Campbell, S., Bhan, V., and Royston, P. Transabdominal ultrasound screening for ovarian cancer. *BMJ 1989*, 299,1363-1367.

[21] Millo, R., Facca, M.C., and Alberico, S. Sonographic evaluation of ovarian volume in postmenopausal women: a screening test for ovarian cancer? *Clin Exp Obstet Gynecol 1989*, 16,72-78.

[22] Tabor, A. Feasibility study of a randomized trial of ovarian cancer screening. *J Med Screen 1994* 4,215-219.

[23] Vuento, M.H., Stenman, U.H., Pirhonen, J.P., Makinen, J.I., Laippala, P.J., and Salmi, T.A. Significance of a single CA125 assay combined with ultrasound in the early detection of ovarian and endometrial cancer. *Gynecol Oncol 1997*, 64,141-146.

[24] Parkes, C.A., Smith, D., Wald, N.J., and Bourne, T.H. Feasibility study of a randomized trial of ovarian cancer screening among the general population. *J Med Screen 1994*,4,209-214.

[25] Kurjak, A., Shalan, H., Kupesic, S., Kosuta, D., Sosic, A., and Benic, S. An attempt to screen asymptomatic women for ovarian and endometrial cancer with transvaginal color and pulsed Doppler sonography. *J Ultrasound Med 1994*, 13,295-301.

[26] Holbert, T.R. Transvaginal ultrasonographic measurement of endometrial thickness in postmenopausal women receiving estrogen replacement therapy. *Am J Obstet Gynecol 1997,* 176,1334-1338.

[27] Jacobs, I.J., Skates, S.J., MacDonald, N.D., Menon, U., Rosenthal, A.N., and Davies, A.P. Screening for ovarian cancer: a pilot randomised controlled trial. *Lancet 1999,* 353,1207-1210.

[28] Adonakis, G.L., Parraskevaidis, E., Tsiga, S., Seferiadis, K., and Lolis, D.E. A combined approach for the early detection ovarian cancer in asymptomatic women. *Europ J Obstet Gynec Reprod Biol 1996,* 65,221-225.

[29] Grover, S., Quinn, M.A., Weideman, P., Koh, H., Robinson, H.P., and Rome, R. Screening for ovarian cancer using serum CA125 and vaginal examination: report on 2550 females. *Int J Gynecol Cancer 1995,* 5,291-295.

[30] Jacobs, I., Davies, A.P., and Bridges, J. Prevalence screening for ovarian cancer in postmenopausal women by CA125 measurement and ultrasonography. *BMJ 1993,* 306,1030-1034.

[31] Einhorn, N., Sjovall, K., Knapp, R., Hall, P., Scully, R., Bast, R., and Zurawski, V. Prospective evaluation of serum CA 125 levels for early detection of ovarian cancer. *Obstet Gynecol 1992,* 80,14-18

[32] The Royal Hospitals Trust. Ovarian Cancer Screening Unit, editor. Randomized trial of screening for ovarian cancer (protocol). England. 1995; p.1

[33] Wolfson Institute of Preventive Medicine. Department of Environmental and Preventive Medicine, editor. European randomized trial of ovarian cancer screening (protocol). London. 1995; p.1

[34] Kramer, B.S., Gohangan, J., Prorok, P.C., and Smart, C.A. National Cancer Institute-sponsored screening trial for prostatic, lung, colorectal, and ovarian cancer. *Cancer1993,*89-593.

[35] Xu, Y., Shen, Z., and Wiper, D.W. Lysophosphatidic acid as a potential biomarker for ovarian and other gynecologic cancers. *JAMA1 1998,* 80,719.

[36] Fishman, D.A., Liu, Y., Ellerbroek, S.M., and Stack, M.S. Lysophosphatidic acid promotes matrix metalloproteinase (MMP) activation and MMP-dependent invasion in ovarian cancer cells. *Cancer Res2001,* 61,3194.

[37] Sansom, C. Biochemical marker allows early detection of ovarian cancer. *Oncology 2001,* 2,494.

[38] van Haaften-Day, C., Shen, Y., and Xu, F. OVX1, macrophage-colony stimulating factor and CA125-II as tumor markers for epithelial ovarian carcinoma: a critical appraisal. *Cancer 2001,* 92,2837.

[39] Petricoin, E.F., Ardekani, A.M., Hitt, B.A., Levine, P.J., Fusaro, V.A., and Steingerg, S.M. Use of proteomic patterns in serum to identify ovarian cancer. *Lancet 2002,* 359,572-577.

[40] American Society of Clinical Oncology. American Society of Clinical Oncology Policy Statement Update: Genetic Testing for Cancer Susceptibility. *JCO 2003,* 21,2397-2406.

[41] Rosen, B., Elit, L., Fung, M.F.K. et al. Screening High-risk Women for Ovarian Cancer. Practice Guideline. Toronto. Program in Evidence-based Care. 2004; 4-6b. p.1

[42] Rosen, B., Kwon, J., Fung, M.F.K. et al. Management options for women with a hereditary predisposition to ovarian cancer. Toronto. Program in Evidence-Based Care. 2003; 4-4. p.1

[43] Adolf, E., Svalenius, E., and Astedt, B. Ultrasonography for early detection of ovarian carcinoma. *Br J Obstet Gynecol 1986*, 93,1286-1289.

[44] Weiner, Z., Beck, D., Shteiner, M., Borovik, R., Ben-Shachar, M., and Robinson, E. Screening for ovarian cancer in women with breast cancer with transvaginal sonography and color flow imaging. *J Ultrasound Med 1993*, 12,387-393.

[45] Muto, M.G., Cramer, D.W., Brown, D.L., Welch, W.R., Harlow, B.L., Xu, H., Brucks, J.P., Tsao, S.W., and Berkowitz, R. Screening forovarian cancer: the preliminary experience of a familial ovarian cancer center. *Gynecol Oncol 1993*, 51,12-20.

[46] Schwartz, P.E., Chambers, J.T., and Taylor, K.J. Early detection and screening for ovarian cancer. *J Cell Biochem 1995* 23,233-237.

[47] Belinson, J.L., Okin, C., Casey, G., Ayoub, A., Klein, R., and Hart, W.R. The familial ovarian cancer registry: Progress Report. *Cleveland Clinic Journal of Medicine.1995*, 62,129-134.

[48] Dorum, A., Kristensen, G.B., Abeler, V., Trope, C., and Moller, P. Early detection of familial ovarian cancer. *Eur J Cancer 1996*, 32A,1645-1651.

[49] Tailor, A., Bourne, T.H., Campbell, S., Okokon, E., Dew, T., and Collins, W.P. Results from an ultrasound-based familial ovarian cancer screening clinic: a 10-year observational study. *Obstet Gynecol 2003*, 21,378-385.

[50] Bourne, T.H., Campbell, S., Reynolds, K., Hampson, J., Bhatt, L., and Crayford, T.J.B. The potential role of serum CA125 in an ultrasound-based screening program for familial ovarian cancer. *Gynecol Oncol 1994*, 52,379-385.

[51] Baylor, K.J., Schwartz, P.E. Cancer screening in a high risk population: a clinical trial. *Ultrasound in Med and Biol 2001*, 27,461-466.

[52] Laframboise, S., Nedulcu, R., Murphy, J., Cole, D.E.C., and Rosen, B. Use of CA-125 and ultrasound in high-risk women. *Int J Gynecol Cancer 2002*, 12,86-91.

[53] Vasen, H.F.A., Tesfay, E., Boonstra, H., Mourits, M.J.E., Rutgers, E., Verheyen, R., Oosterwijk, J., and Beex, L. Early detection of breast and ovarian cancer in families with BRCA mutations. *Eur J Cancer 2004*, 41,549-554.

[54] Pernet, A.L., Wardle, J., Bourne, T.H., Whitehead, M.I., Campbell, S., and Collins, W.P. A qualitative evaluation of the experience of surgery after false positive results in screening for familial ovarian cancer. *Psycho-Oncology 1992*, 1,217-233.

[55] Jacobs, I., Mackay, J., and Skates, S. UKCCCR Gynecological Subcommittee, editor. UKCCCR national familial ovarian cancer screening study (protocol). London. 1997; p.1

[56] Crump, C., McIntosh, M.W., Urban, N., Anderson, G., and Karlan, B.Y. Ovarian cancer tumor marker behavior in asymptomatic healthy women: Implications for screening. *Cancer Epidemiol Biomarkers Prev 2000*, 9,1107-1111.

[57] Mok, S.C., Chao, J., Skates, S., Womg, K., Yiu, G.K., and Muto, M.G. Prostasin, a potential serum marker for ovarian cancer: identification through microarray technology. *J Natl Cancer Inst 2001*, 93,1458-1464.

[58] Katasaros, D., Fracchioli, S., Yousef, G.M., Luo, L.Y., Scorilas, A., and Puopolo, M. Human kallikrein 6 (hK6) and 10 (hK10): New potential serum biomarkers for diagnosis and prognosis of epithelial ovarian cancer [abstract]. *Proceedings of ASCO* 20(2002).

[59] Kauff, N.D., Satagopan, J.M., Robson, M.E., Scheuer, L., Hensley, M., and Hudis, C.A. Risk-reducing salpingo-oophorectomy in women with a BRCA1 or BRCA2 mutation. *NEJM 2002,* 346,1609-1615.

[60] Struewing, J.P., Watson, P., Easton, D.F., Ponder, B.A.J., Lynch, H.T., and Tucker, M.A. Prophylactic oophorectomy in inherited breast/ovarian cancer families. *Monogr Natl Cancer Inst 1995,* 17,33-35.

[61] Rebbeck, T., Lynch, H., Neuhausen, S., Narod, S., Van't Veer, L., and Garber, J.E. Prophylactic oophorectomy in carriers of BRCA1 and BRCA2 mutations. *NEJM 2003,* 326,1616-1622.

In: Leading Topics in Cancer Research
Editor: Lee P. Jeffries, pp. 125-142

ISBN 1-60021-332-4
© 2007 Nova Science Publishers, Inc.

Chapter 5

DETERMINING ELIGIBILITY CRITERIA FOR CANCER SUSCEPTIBILITY GENETIC TESTING

Chris D. Bajdik, Steve Sung and Richard P. Gallagher
BC Cancer Agency, Vancouver BC, Canada

ABSTRACT

A genetic testing service can determine which members of a population might benefit most from prevention measures. The eligibility criteria for a service will affect the number of people who use it and the portion that test positive, and this affects both the service's costs and benefits. In this chapter, a computer simulation model is used to estimate the effects of eligibility restrictions on the performance of a genetic testing service. In particular, restrictions might apply to someone's age, gender and family history of disease. The effects are considered in terms of the eligibility criteria's sensitivity, specificity and "post-test likelihoods" for a genetic test result. All of these measures are affected differently by eligibility restrictions, and criteria should be chosen according to outcomes that are considered most important. We focus on a testing service for cancer susceptibility, but the extension to other diseases is straightforward.

INTRODUCTION

British Columbia (BC) is the western-most province of Canada. There were about 4.2 million people and 19,300 new diagnoses of cancer in BC during 2005 (NCIC 2005). Previous studies suggest that about 10% of these cancer patients have a family history of the disease (Yang et al 1992, Gallagher et al 1995, Ghadirian et al 1997, McBride et al 1999, McDuffie et al 2001, Begg et al 2004). Someone might have a family history because of genetic susceptibility that was inherited from his or her parents, or because of non-genetic factors that are shared between family members. The latter include lifestyle characteristics such as diet, and environmental exposures such as pesticide exposure. A family history can also arise by chance, with probability affected by the size and structure of someone's family. Most family histories are likely the result of genetic factors, environmental exposures and chance combined.

Genetic testing allows for disease surveillance of susceptibility carriers and avoids unnecessary surveillance of non-carriers. A population-based service can be introduced to provide genetic testing, but this is a *service* -- not mandatory screening of the population. The cost of a service includes that of identifying high-risk families, and there are non-financial costs such as the anxiety that a service might create. The service's benefits depend on the improvement that is achieved in the population's health, including changes in psychological and emotional outcomes, and reductions in cancer morbidity and mortality. People who are found not to carry genetic susceptibility are assured that they do not have a higher cancer risk than people in the general population. This is expected to reduce anxiety and the demand for disease surveillance. To assess the service's impact, we need to know how many people will be eligible for the service and how many people with genetic susceptibility will be identified. Both numbers are determined by the population's characteristics relative to the service's eligibility criteria.

This chapter will present a computer model for simulating a family history of cancer. In examples, we will use the model to generate millions of family histories and determine how various eligibility criteria might identify people with genetic susceptibility. We restrict the chapter to genetic susceptibility that is determined by a genetic mutation with autosomal dominant inheritance.

ELIGIBILITY CRITERIA

The eligibility criteria used in this chapter are binary: someone is either eligible or ineligible for the service. Other criteria could be used, but binary criteria imply a decision rule, and are more applicable to the circumstance under consideration. Ideal criteria should

- account for someone's cancer history
- account for someone's cancer family history
- account for family size and structure
- account for biologic relationships between affected family members
- account for the rate of disease incidence in the population
- be simple to determine

Someone's cancer history includes any diagnoses they have received in the past and the age at which they were diagnosed. Someone's cancer family history includes the same information for his or her blood relatives. Accounting for biologic relationships and ages in a family is important because first-degree relatives share twice as much genetic material on average as second-degree relatives, and relatives from the same generation are likely to share more environmental exposures than relatives one or more generations apart. However, most people have more distant relatives than close relatives (e.g., more cousins than siblings), so the inclusion of distant relatives might substantially improve the predictive ability of family history. Many sets of eligibility criteria require a minimal number of affected family members, but some criteria also restrict the relationship between them. For example, the Amsterdam criteria that define Hereditary Non-Polyposis Colorectal Cancer (HNPCC) (The International Collaborative Group on Hereditary Nonpolyposis Colorectal Cancer (ICG-HNPCC) 1991) require someone's cancer family history include three affected people, one of whom is a first-degree relative of the other two, and that at least two successive generations are affected. The disease incidence in a population is important because the interpretation of someone's disease history, and family history, will depend on whether the disease is common. Finally, some measures are simpler to determine. This affects the resources that are necessary and level of knowledge that is required to assess the criteria. Eligibility criteria should be easier to assess than performing a genetic test, and not require sophisticated laboratory resources or expertise.

Eligibility criteria might be restricted to information about family members from the same or previous generations because relatives from subsequent generations will often be young and only early-life events will be observed in them. As a result, the inclusion of someone's relatives in subsequent generations may sensitize a family history measure to early-onset cases of disease. All disease information should be verified by medical records, and the ease of doing so depends on what information is involved. First-degree relatives usually live nearer than second-degree relatives, and so medical records might be easier to obtain. Medical records are often destroyed after a person's death, so information might be more difficult to obtain for deceased relatives. Finally, people are more likely to provide accurate information about close family members than distant ones.

The eligibility criteria we consider are generally restricted to the first person in a family who uses the genetic testing service (hereafter called the proband) and his or her first-degree and second-degree relatives. We do not consider eligibility criteria that incorporate information about multi-focal cancers because it is sometimes difficult to distinguish between multi-focal and metastatic disease.

MEASURING THE EFFECTS OF ELIGIBILITY CRITERIA

A genetic testing service can be evaluated in the same way as a diagnostic test, except the goal is to assess the ability of eligibility criteria to predict whether someone carries genetic susceptibility. For the remainder of this chapter, we assume that genetic cancer susceptibility is the result of a germline mutation in a gene with autosomal inheritance. Accordingly, people with genetic cancer susceptibility are sometimes referred to as "mutation carriers" or just "carriers". Data from a population can be classified in a simple 2x2 table according to the people's eligibility for the service and whether they test positive for genetic susceptibility.

		Genetic Test for Susceptibility	
		+	−
Eligible	Yes	a	b
	No	c	d

The ability of eligibility criteria to identify carriers is measured by four parameters:

$sensitivity = a / (a + c)$
$specificity = d / (b + d)$
$PTL+ = a / (a + b)$
$PTL- = c / (c + d)$

Sensitivity is the proportion of carriers who fulfill the eligibility criteria. Specificity is the proportion of non-carriers who are ineligible. The positive post-test likelihood ($PTL+$) is the proportion of eligible people who are mutation carriers, and the negative post-test likelihood ($PTL-$) is the proportion of ineligible people who are carriers. The name "post-test likelihood" comes from the historical use of a 2x2 table to measure the performance of a diagnostic test, and "post-test" referred to the likelihood of having the disease given the test result. Our use of a similar 2x2 table to measure the performance of eligibility criteria is more recent, but we will retain the name "post-test likelihood" to describe the measures that the table provides. Finally, again based on the original 2x2 tables use for evaluating diagnostic tests, $PTL+$ is sometimes called the positive predictive value, or PPV, and the $PTL-$ is sometimes called ($1-NPV$) where NPV is the negative predictive value.

The prevalence of genetic susceptibility (p_c) in the 2x2 table can be measured as:

$p_c = (a + b) / (a + b + c + d)$

The sensitivity and specificity of eligibility criteria do not depend on the prevalence of genetic susceptibility in the 2x2 table, and can be measured in a study with an arbitrary number of carriers and non-carriers. This is important because carriers might be rare in a population and researchers will conduct a study that includes a disproportionately high number of carriers. Unlike sensitivity and specificity, the prevalence of carriers has a direct effect upon the post-test-likelihoods.

A genetic testing service typically offers both genetic counseling and genetic testing. This is always true in Canada, but not so for other parts of the world. The eligibility criteria for the service might only refer to eligibility for genetic counseling (which usually precedes genetic testing) and genetic testing might involve further restrictions. These added restrictions are often based on information gathered during genetic counselling. For example, genetic counseling may be offered to unaffected members of a family, but genetic testing might only be pursued in a family member with cancer. (The testing of family members usually happens regardless of the service's usual eligibility criteria.) This is done because testing relatives is less costly if a positive test result has been obtained in some other family member. If a family member is tested and the result is negative, the likelihood of anyone in the family carrying a mutation may be substantially lessened, and so no one else in the family will be offered testing. For HNPCC, probands who are eligible for genetic testing are often pre-tested for DNA mismatch repair (MMR) defects, and receive MSH2/MLH1 mutation testing only when the results of the preliminary test are positive. This increases the prevalence of gene mutations in the population subset who proceed to direct MSH2/MLH1 gene testing.

The post-test likelihoods can also be calculated as

$$PTL+ = \frac{1}{2} * \frac{p_c LR+}{(1-p_c) + p_c LR+}$$

and

$$PTL- = \frac{1}{2} * \frac{p_c LR-}{(1-p_c) + p_c LR-}$$

where p_c is the probability that a parent who is randomly selected from the population is a mutation carrier and LR+ is the positive likelihood ratio:

$LR+ = sensitivity / (1-specificity)$

and

$LR- = (1- sensitivity) / specificity$

If someone is a mutation carrier, then only half of his or her children will inherit the mutation on average. If mutations are rare in the study population, p_c is twice the probability that anyone in the study population is a carrier. $LR+$ is the probability of eligibility in someone with a mutation, divided by the probability of eligibility in someone without a mutation. $LR-$ is the probability of ineligibility in someone with a mutation, divided by the probability of ineligibility in someone without a mutation. These definitions should not be confused with the sensitivity (etc.) of a genetic test to detect mutations in a biological sample.

We do not use these formulae to calculate the post-test likelihoods, but present them to show how PTL+ and PTL- depend on the prevalence of genetic susceptibility.

We should not confuse the service's sensitivity with the carrier detection rate. The latter is the proportion of mutation carriers in the population who are identified by the program. This is distinct from sensitivity in that the carrier detection rate refers to a whole population and not just the subset that are screened. Each measure assumes that the genetic tests are completely accurate in their ability to detect mutations, and that all eligible people will come forward and request genetic testing. The latter assumption is a big one. If only 50% of eligible people in a population use the genetic testing service, then only half of the carriers predicted by the carrier detection rate will be identified. In the end, each measure must be interpreted relevant to the number of false positive and false negative results they entail.

False positive results occur when someone satisfies the service's eligibility criteria but is subsequently found to not carry increased genetic susceptibility. Note that "false" refers to the eligibility criteria as an indication of genetic susceptibility, and only the type of genetic susceptibility under study. Only half of the people with a parent who is carrier will inherit the mutation, and therefore many false positives are unavoidable. There are emotional and psychological effects that result if someone is false positive in this sense, and economic consequences for the genetic testing service, but other effects are beneficial. In particular, receiving a negative genetic test result might reduce someone's anxiety about disease risk that arose because of his or her family history. (Recall that the genetic test is assumed to be accurate.) In addition, the determination of non-carrier status is expected to reduce the demand for cancer surveillance and prophylactic surgery.

False negative results occur when someone who carries a known mutation is not eligible for the genetic testing service. As above, "false" refers to the eligibility criteria as an indication of genetic susceptibility. People who are false negative in this sense will not receive any of the benefits of a population-based program. Indeed, they will not be eligible for the program and hence never aware they are false negative. However few people are expected to use a genetic testing service if the false negative rate is high.

The definitions of sensitivity, etc. refer to the carrier status of the patient and not the carrier status of his or her family. Measures that refer to the carrier status of the family are easy to define, but their interpretation can be very different than those of measures that refer to someone's own status. In particular, false positive and false negative results will affect everyone in a family.

SIMULATION MODEL

A simulation model was written in the computer language Java. That model considers two principal objects: *probands* and *pedigrees*. A *proband* is the person who is considering genetic testing and whose family history is being simulated. Input for the simulation model includes the proband's age, gender and genotype, and the model uses this information to determine the same data for the first and second degree relatives in the proband's family. First degree relatives include the proband's parents, siblings, and children; second degree relatives include the proband's grandparents, uncles, aunts, nephews, nieces, grandchildren, and half-siblings. A *pedigree* is the collection of information about a proband and his or her family.

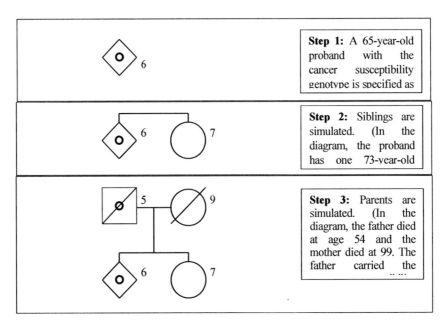

Figure 1. The simulation model

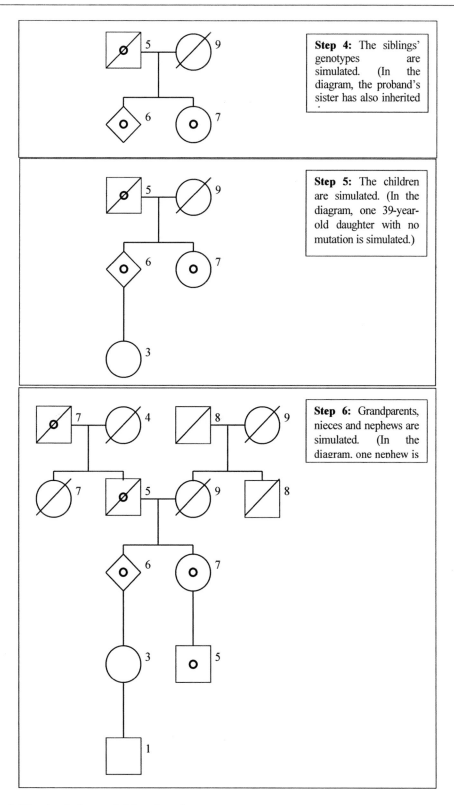

Figure 1. The simulation model (continued)

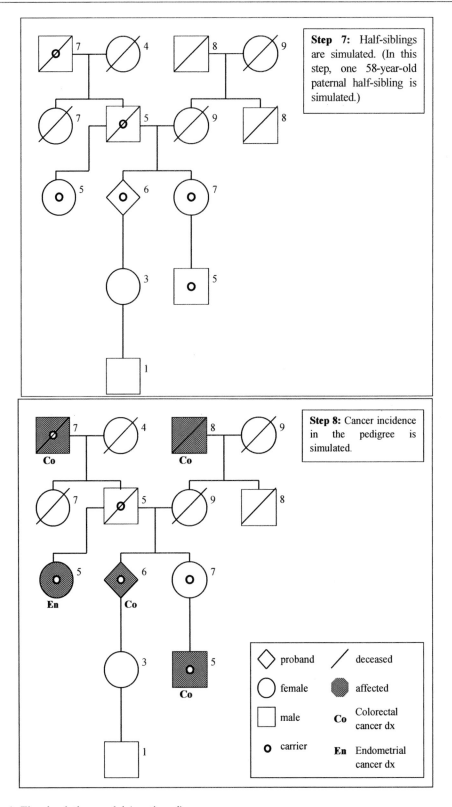

Figure 1. The simulation model (continued)

Figure 1 shows how a proband and his or her family history is simulated. The proband's age and gender, and the number of his or her siblings is determined. Each sibling's age is calculated based on the proband's. (Twins are not allowed, although siblings can have the same age when measured in years.) Figure 2 shows the age distribution of a simulated sibling for 10,000 25-year-old probands. Each sibling's gender is also determined by the model. The proband's parents are considered next, and their ages are calculated based on those of the proband and his or her siblings. Figure 3 shows the parents' age distributions for 10,000 25-year-old probands with an average of two siblings. Each parent's genotype is based on that of the proband according to Mendelian inheritance. The model assumes that cancer susceptibility is a heterozygous condition and, if the proband carries susceptibility, then so does exactly one of the parents. With the parents' genotypes now available, the model simulates each sibling's genotype according to Mendelian inheritance. The proband's number of children is determined by the model based on government statistics, and each child's age is based on the proband's. Figure 4 shows the age distributions of children for 10,000 65-year-old probands assuming each proband has an average of two children. Each child's gender is determined randomly. A child's genotype is based on his or her parents assuming Mendelian inheritance. The simulation model uses similar steps to determine the age and genotype of the parents' parents (i.e., the proband's grandparents), children's children (i.e., the proband's grandchildren), parents' siblings (i.e., the proband's aunts and uncles), and parents' siblings' children (i.e., the proband's nieces and nephews).

Government statistics indicate that about 5.7% of Canadian families include step-children. Accordingly, 5.7% of the simulated probands are assigned maternal and/or paternal half-siblings. The half-siblings are simulated in similar fashion as the siblings, except for their genotypes. Each paternal half-sibling's genotype is inherited from the father and someone with a wild-type genotype. The genotypes of maternal half-siblings are similarly determined.

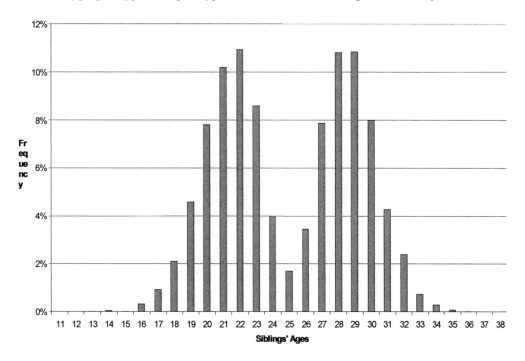

Figure 2. Siblings' age distribution for 10,000 25-year-old probands.

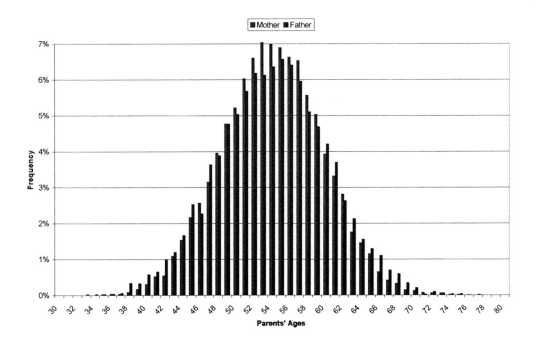

Figure 3. Parents' age distribution for 10,000 25-year-old probands with an average of two siblings.

Finally, according the person's age, gender and genotype, the diagnosis of cancer in a family member is determined according to the corresponding population and carrier rates.

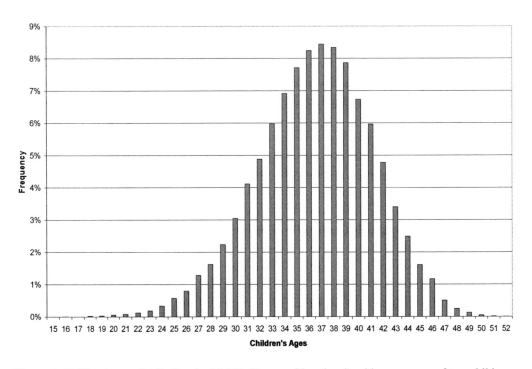

Figure 4. Children's age distribution for 10,000 65-year-old probands with an average of two children.

ESTIMATING THE PERFORMANCE OF A GENETIC TESTING SERVICE

We will consider probands of each gender and various age groups, and a spectrum of eligibility criteria. We will estimate the genetic testing program's sensitivity, specificity and post-test likelihoods. We can restrict the proband's age, gender and family structure so that particular subgroups in a population can be studied separately. We can also specify broad options for these parameters and allow the program to randomly determine them. For example, we might consider probands age 25–50 and allow the simulation model to randomly determine whether the proband is a male or female.

As an example, consider a genetic testing service that identifies BRCA1 mutation carriers based on their family history of breast cancer. People who meet any of the following criteria are eligible:

- a woman with breast cancer diagnosed at age ≤35
- anyone with a family history that includes two or more of the following:

  - breast cancer in two or more closely-related family members (parents, siblings, children, grandparents, aunts, uncles) on the same side of the family
  - multiple primary cancers in one relative
  - male breast cancer

Notice that the eligibility criteria refer to "closely-related family members" and this includes all 1st-degreee and some 2nd-degree relatives.

We simulated the incidence of BRCA1 mutations and cancer family histories for 1,000,000 people. The simulated population was assigned the same age and gender distribution as the BC population, and the same incidence of breast cancer. The model also assumed that 0.112% of probands carry a BRCA1 mutation. The simulated population was classified according to the service's eligibility criteria and whether the probands carried a mutation. (Table 1).

Table 1. Results of simulating 1,000,000 people, classified according to their age, their eligibility for the BRCA1 genetic testing service and whether they carry a BRCA1 mutation

Age	Eligible Carrier	Ineligible Carrier	Eligible Non-Carrier	Ineligible Non-Carrier
< 15	1	203	76	190,240
15-24	10	131	242	133,423
25-34	20	135	663	132,210
35-44	34	175	1,903	167,606
45-54	39	94	2,692	144,668
55-64	37	68	2,414	92,834
65-74	22	48	2,360	68,997
> 74	30	28	2,428	56,088
Total	193	823	12,778	986,146

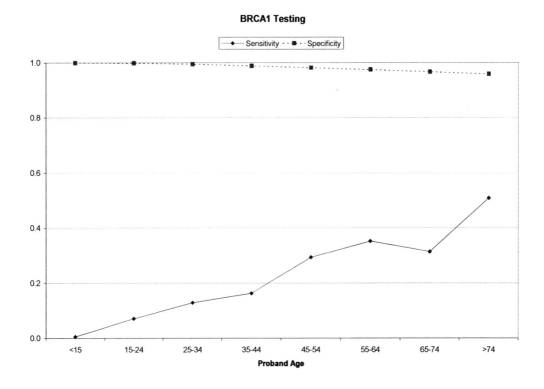

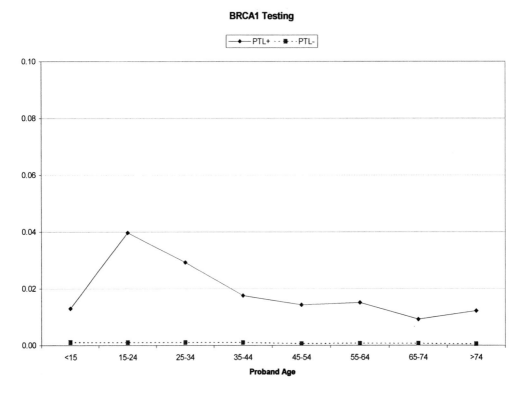

Figure 5. Sensitivity, specificity and post-test likelihoods for the BRCA1 testing example and the original eligibility criteria.

From this table, we calculated the sensitivity, specificity and post-test likelihoods of the eligibility criteria as a predictor of people carrying a BRCA1 mutation. Plots of these parameters for people of different ages are shown in Figure 5.

The sensitivity of the eligibility criteria is greater for older probands. This happens because people are more likely to have breast cancer, and relatives with breast cancer, as they become older. The result is that older probands are more likely to satisfy the eligibility criteria regardless of whether they carry a BRCA1 mutation. For the same reason that sensitivity increases, the specificity of the eligibility criteria decreases for older probands. Ignoring the service's eligibility criteria, the probability that someone in the population has a BRCA1mutation is 0.112%. Someone who satisfies the service's eligibility criteria has a much higher probability of carrying a BRCA1 mutation: 1.49%. Someone who does not meet the criteria has a much lower probability of carrying a mutation: 0.09%. The post-test likelihoods are also affected by the proband's age and both parameters are lower as a proband's age increases. The simulation model assumes that cancer genetic susceptibility does not affect overall mortality in the population. This might be untrue, but there is little evidence of it. However, changes to the sensitivity and specificity will generally affect the post-test likelihoods.

Now consider revised eligibility criteria for the service that considers an extra restriction that if only one affected woman in a family has breast cancer, then the cancer must be pre-menopausal. Formally, people who use the service must now meet one or more of the following eligibility criteria:

- be a woman with breast cancer diagnosed at age≤35
- be anyone with a family history that includes two or more of the following:

  - breast cancer in two or more closely-related family members (parents, siblings, children, grandparents, aunts, uncles) on the same side of the family
  - breast cancer diagnosed before menopause (or age<50 if menopausal status is unknown)
  - multiple primary cancers in one relative
  - male breast cancer

Recall that probands in the simulation have the same age and gender distribution as the BC population, and the same incidence of breast cancer. The added eligibility rule considers cancer family histories in which there are early diagnoses of breast cancer as defined by a woman's menopausal status, but uses an age restrictions if her menopausal status is unknown. The simulated population was classified according to the revised eligibility criteria and the results are shown in Table 2.

From this table, we calculated the sensitivity, specificity and post-test likelihoods of the criteria as predictors of who has a BRCA1 mutation. Plots of these parameters are shown in Figure 6.

As before, the sensitivity of the eligibility criteria increases for older probands, and the specificity decreases, but the sensitivity and specificity in an age group are higher than the corresponding values for the earlier eligibility criteria. As before, the probability that someone in the population has a BRCA1 mutation is 0.112%. However, someone who satisfies the service's revised eligibility criteria has a 1.23% probability of carrying a BRCA1 mutation, and someone who does satisfy the eligibility criteria has a 0.07% probability. For each agegroup, the post-test likelihoods are lower than the corresponding values using the original eligibility criteria. Despite improving the sensitivity of the service, the revised eligibility criteria decreased the service's specificity and post-test likelihoods. This illustrates the sometimes-unintuitive effects of changing the eligibility criteria for a genetic testing service.

Table 2. Results of simulating 1,000,000 people, classified according to their age, the revised eligibility criteria for the BRCA1 genetic testing service and whether they carry a BRCA1 mutation

Age	Eligible Carrier	Ineligible Carrier	Eligible Non-Carrier	Ineligible Non-Carrier
< 15	13	191	639	189,677
15-24	27	114	1,257	132,408
25-34	50	105	2,349	130,624
35-44	76	133	4,840	164,669
45-54	66	67	5,936	141,424
55-64	49	56	4,912	90,336
65-74	42	28	4,472	66,865
> 74	37	22	4,481	54,035
Total	360	716	128,886	970,038

The example considers a genetic testing service for BRCA1-related breast cancer susceptibility, and illustrates some general points. Firstly, the sensitivity and specificity of the service depended on the age of the proband, but the post-test likelihoods did not. Secondly, the choice of eligibility criteria for the service affects all aspect of the service's performance, and the simulation model allows us to predict these effects.

A genetic testing service might consider cancer susceptibility that is determined by one gene. This is the same as a service that offers testing for two or more genes using the same eligibility criteria. (E.g., a service offering genetic testing for both BRCA1 and BRCA2, but using a single set of eligibility criteria.) We can also consider the effect of eligibility criteria if cancer genetic susceptibility encompasses more than one type of cancer. To simulate someone's family history, the model requires the risk of each cancer type associated with a mutation. Another extension occurs if genetic susceptibility is defined by more that one gene (or equivalently, more than one type of mutation in a single gene) and the cancer risks associated with each mutation are different from one another. This is precisely the case for MSH2 and MLH1 genetic susceptibility that affects both the risk of colorectal and endometrial cancers. If more that one gene is being tested by the service, the simulation model requires the cancer risks be specified for each gene. The same situation arises if different mutations confer different levels of cancer susceptibility, in which case different mutations in a gene are equivalent to mutations in separate genes.

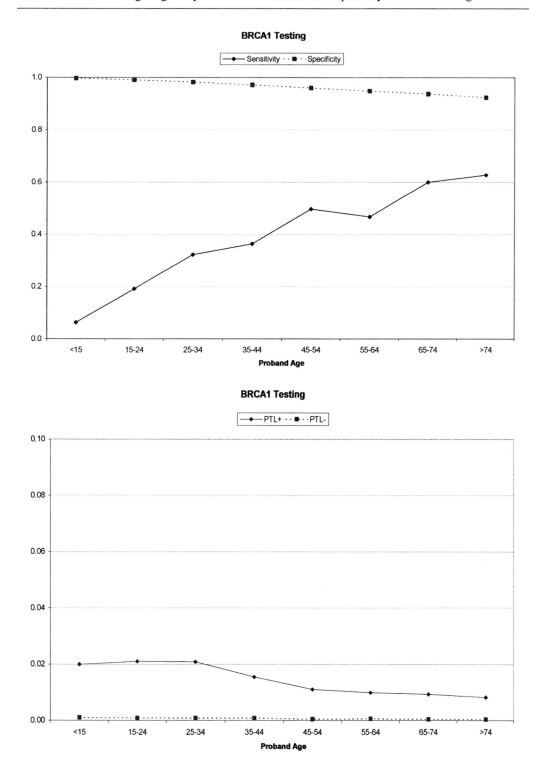

Figure 6. Sensitivity, specificity and post-test likelihoods for the BRCA1 testing example and the revised eligibility criteria.

DISCUSSION

This chapter describes statistical measures for evaluating the performance of a genetic testing service and its eligibility criteria. The sensitivity of a genetic testing service describes how well the service identifies people with genetic susceptibility. The specificity describes how well the service identifies people that do not have genetic susceptibility. Sensitivity is not directly relevant to people without genetic susceptibility and specificity is not directly relevant to people with genetic susceptibility. Of course, before receiving a genetic test, a user of the service doesn't know whether they are genetically susceptible. Unlike sensitivity and specificity, post-test likelihoods may be most interesting to the group that provides a genetic testing service. PTL+ indicates the proportion of service users who will be found to carry genetic susceptibility. PTL- indicates the proportion of people who are ineligible for the service, yet they carry genetic susceptibility. If a service considers everyone to be eligible, then PTL- is 0% and PTL+ is the base population's prevalence of genetic susceptibility. (The base population refers to people for who the service is available. This is the general population if a service is population-based, but might instead be a geographic area or socio-demographic population for a clinic-based service.) A user-pay service is usually of this type, but a service sponsored by an insurer or provided by a government is likely to restrict eligibility.

Some predictions from the simulation model can be compared with observed outcomes if an appropriate genetic testing service exists. However, a simulation model can also estimate the parameters that cannot be observed. For example, it is impossible to calculate the observed sensitivity and specificity at a genetic testing service because ineligible people are never seen. Likewise, it is impossible to observe PTL- because genetic test results for the ineligible people are unknown. The only parameter that can be observed at a genetic testing service is PTL+ because it only considers the "eligible" people. But a simulation model allows us to predict unobservable parameters (i.e., sensitivity, specificity and PTL-). Currently, there are many services that consider cancer susceptibility genetic testing for BRCA1 and BRCA2, some services that offer testing for MSH2 and MLH1, and a few services that offer genetic testing for rarer mutations in genes such as ATM and FAP. However, such services can only measure PTL+. If our model's predictions about PTL+ are very similar to observed data, then predictions about the other parameters are likely to be accurate as well.

It is common for a service to provide genetic testing for the blood relatives of known carriers. This is likely to be more effective for identifying carriers in a family than are the usual eligibility criteria, but only benefits a limited subgroup of the population. If this strategy is adopted, people who receive genetic testing because they are related to carriers cannot be considered in the usual measures of sensitivity, specificity, etc. We could alter the definitions of these parameters so that they measure the same things with respect to families instead of individual people. For example, sensitivity might be redefined as the proportion of families in the population for which the family includes a genetic susceptibility carrier that satisfies the service's eligibility criteria. The denominator of the proportion now refers to a number of families and not a number of people.

The prevalence of carriers at a genetic testing is often greater than the prevalence for the general population. This is most likely to occur because users of a genetic testing service often have reasons beyond those specified in the eligibility criteria. The reverse is also true, as many carriers may not use a genetic testing service because, despite evidence they might carry susceptibility, they do not want genetic testing. Even amongst people who are eligible and are considering genetic testing, pre-test genetic counseling or screening can affect the prevalence of genetic susceptibility carriers.

We are currently generalizing our computer simulation software to simulate a testing service for arbitrary definitions of cancer genetic susceptibility, cancer risk in susceptibility carriers (i.e., penetrance rates) and population cancer risks. The software will be freely-available through the BC Cancer Agency website (www.bccancer.bc.ca).

CONCLUSION

This chapter discussed the effect of eligibility criteria on a cancer susceptibility genetic testing service. We showed that the choice of criteria can affects the performance of a service in unintuitive ways, but the use of a simulation model allows us to predict the likely outcome. The sensitivity, specificity and the post-test likelihoods (PTL+ and PTL-) associated with eligibility criteria all depend on someone's age because cancer incidence risk is a function of age and because older probands usually have older relatives. These parameters will also differ according to the proband's gender because cancer risk also depends on gender. Sensitivity and specificity will not depend on the prevalence of genetic susceptibility in the population, but PTL+ and PTL- will.

Why are changes to eligibility criteria important? If the number of people who are eligible for a genetic testing service is reduced, the financial cost of the service is almost certain to be reduced as well. This is obvious. If the number of eligible people can be reduced without affecting the service's sensitivity and specificity, then a change in eligibility criteria may be justified. (The change might not be justified if it incurs additional non-financial costs.) If changing eligibility criteria increases PTL+, there will likely be an increase in the demand for cancer surveillance and prophylactic measures. This will affect the demand for trained people and specialized facilities to provide these measures.

If there is no effective way of changing a carrier's cancer risk, then the main benefit of testing might to improve human research. The importance of the performance measures associated with eligibility depends on the consequence of making a false-positive or false negative prediction. In particular, determinants of these outcomes' relative importance include the costs associated with treating identified carriers and the cost of testing people who do not carry a mutation.

Simulation studies are a useful method for predicting the performance of a genetic testing service. Foremost, the method allows us to generate very large sample sizes. Despite a large number of simulations overall, the sample size for a particular subset of the population may be substantially smaller. This was illustrated in the example where we simulated one million people in total, but less than 200,000 were under age 15 and only 204 were carriers of a BRCA1 mutation. This can be improved by restricting the simulation so that the entire population is under age 15. These sample sizes might be impossible to achieve in a study that uses observations from a real testing service. There are just over 4 million people in BC, but a simulation study can consider population sizes that are larger than this.

REFERENCES

ASCO (2003). American Society of Clinical Oncology policy statement update: genetic testing for cancer susceptibility. *J Clin Oncology* 21:2397-406.

Begg C.B., Hummer, A., Mujumdar, U., et al. (2004). Familial aggregation of melanoma risks in a large population-based sample of melanoma cases. *Cancer Causes Control* 15: 957-65.

Emery J., Lucassen A., Murphy M. (2001). Common hereditary cancers and implications for primary care. *The Lancet* 358:56-63.

Gallagher, R.P., Huchcroft, S., Phillips, N., et al. (1995). Physical activity, medical history, and risk of testicular cancer (Alberta and British Columbia, Canada). *Cancer Causes Control* 6:398-406.

Ghadirian, P., Howe, G.R., Hislop, T.G., Maisonneuve, P. (1997). Family history of prostate cancer: a multi-center case-control study in Canada. *Int J Cancer* 70:679-81.

Hemminki K., Eng C. (2004). Clinical genetic counselling for familial cancers requires reliable data on familial cancer risks and general action plans. *J Med Genetics* 41:801-7.

The International Collaborative Group on Hereditary Nonpolyposis Colorectal Cancer (ICG-HNPCC) (1991). *Dis Colon Rectum* 34:424-5.

McBride, M.L., Gallagher, R.P., Theriault, G., et al. (1999). Power-frequency magnetic fields and risk of childhood leukemia in Canada. *Am J Epidemiol* 149:831-42.

McDuffie, H.H., Puhwa, P., McLaughlin, J.R., et al. (2001). Non-Hodgkin's lymphoma and specific pesticide exposure in men: cross-country study of pesticides and Health. *Cancer Epi Biom Prev* 10:155-63.

NCIC (2005). *Canadian Cancer Statistics.* Toronto (Canada): National Cancer Institute of Canada .

Yang, C.P., Daling, J.R., Band, P.R., et al. (1992). Noncontraceptive hormone use and breast cancer. *Cancer Causes Control* 3:475-9.

In: Leading Topics in Cancer Research
Editor: Lee P. Jeffries pp. 143-191

ISBN 1-60021-332-4
© 2007 Nova Science Publishers, Inc.

Chapter 6

TUMOR RESISTANCE TO CELL DEATH AND ITS RELATIONSHIP WITH PRION PROTEIN

Maryam Mehrpour[1,2]*, *Franck Meslin*[2] *and Ahmed Hamaï*[2]

[1]Chinese Academy of Sciences, The Laboratory of Apoptosis and Cancer Biology,
The National Key Laboratory of Biomembrane and Membrane Biotechnology,
Institute of Zoology, Beijing, P.R. China
[2]INSERM, U 753, Laboratoire d'Immunologie des Tumeurs Humaines :
Interaction effecteurs cytotoxiques-système tumoral, Institut Gustave Roussy PR1
and IFR 54, Villejuif, France

ABSTRACT

Cancer is an insidious disease, in which virtually every aspect of cellular control can be subverted to allow the uncontrolled, invasive cellular growth that defeats multicellular cooperation and kills an organism. In testimony to the essential role for proper execution of cell death in tumor suppression, apoptosis is widely recognized as an essential tumor-suppressor system. Indeed, defects in apoptosis are considered a hallmark of cancer, and are known to render the tumor resistant to immunosurveillance and therapy. Prion infections represent a fascinating biological phenomenon which has elicited at the interface between neuroscience and immunology. Although Prion protein (PrPc) is well known for its implication in transmissible spongiform encephalopathy, recent data indicated that PrPc may participate in programmed cell death regulation. PrPc would be correlated to the acquisition of a resistance phenotype by tumor cells to cytotoxic effectors or antitumor drugs. This review revisits the molecular mechanisms of tumor resistance to apoptosis and the implication of the PrPc in this phenomenon.

Keywords: Prion protein, tumor resistance to cell death, breast cancer, normal human myoepithelial breast cells.

---

* Correspondence concerning this article should be addressed to Maryam Mehrpour, E-mail: mehrpour@ioz.ac.cn. Tel : (8610) – 62521552.

ABBREVIATIONS

ABC transporter	ATP-Binding Cassette transporter
AIF	Apoptosis-Inducing Factor
AKT	v-akt murine thymoma viral oncogene homolog
ALPS	Autoimmune lymphoproliferative system
ANT	Adenine Nucleotide Translocator
Apaf	Apoptosis protease activation factor
ARF	Alternate Open Reading Frame
A-Smase	acid sphingomyelinase
ASPP	Apoptosis-Stimuling Protein of p53
ATM	Ataxia-Telangiectasia Mutated
ATR	ATM- and Rad3-related
BAD	BCL2-antagonist of cell death
BAK	BCL2-antagonist/killer
BAX	BCL2-associated X protein
BCL2	B-cell leukemia/lymphoma 2
BCL-X_L/BCL2L1	BCL2-like 1
BCL-w/BCL2L2	BCL2-like 2
BFL1/BCL2A1	BCL2-related protein A1
BH	BCL2 Homology
BID	BH3 interacting domain death agonist
BIM/BCL2L11	BCL2-like 11
BIR	Baculoviral IAP repeat
BOK	BCL2-related Ovarian Killer
BOO/DIVA/BCL2L10	BCL2-like 10
CD95L	CD95 Ligand
CDKN2a	Cyclin-Dependent Kinase Inhibitor 2a
CTSD	endolysosomal aspartate protease cathepsin D
DED	Death Effector Domain
DD	Death Domain
DcR	decoy receptor
DISC	Death-inducing signaling complex
DR	Death Receptor
EBV	Epstein-Barr Virus
EGFR	Epidermial Growth Factor
ERK	Extracellular signal-Regulated Kinase
FADD	Fas-associated DD Kinase
FLICE	FADD-like interleukin-1 β-converting enzyme
FLIP	FLICE-like inhibitory Protein
GPI	Glycosyl-phosphatidylinositol
HR	Homologous Recombination
IAP	Inhibitor of Apoptosis protein
c-IAP	Inhibitor of cellular Apoptosis
I-κB	Inhibitor of κB

JMY	Junction-meditaing and regulatory protein
MALT	Mucosa-Associated Lymphoid Tissue
MCL1	Myeloid Cell Leukemia sequence 1
MDM2	Double Minute 2 protein
MOMP	Mitochondrial Outer Membrane Permeabilization
MRP	Multidrug resistance-associated protein
MSH2	MutS homolog 2
NAIP	Neuronal Apoptosis Inhibitory Protein
NHEJ	Non-Homologous End Joining
NF-κB	nuclear factor-κB
NK	Natural Killer Cell
PI-9/SPI-9	Protease Inhibitor 9
PIDD	P53-induced protein with a death domain
PIPLC	phosphoinositol phospholipase C
PrPc	Cellular Prion Protein
PrP^{Sc}	Scrapie Prion Protein
PTP	Permeability Transition Pore
PI3K	Phosphoinositide 3-Kinase
PIP	Phosphoinoisitol Phosphate
PTEN	Phosphatase and Tensin homolog
RAIDD	receptor-interacting protein (RIP)-associated ICH-1/CED-3 homologous protein with a death domain
RIP	Receptor-Interacting Protein
ROS	reactive oxygen species
SAPK	Stress Activated Protein Kinase
Smac/Diablo	Second Mitochondria-derived Activator of Caspase/direct IAP binding protein
STAT3	Signal Transducer and Activator of Transcription 3
TNF	Tumor Necrosis Factor
TNFR	TNF receptor
TRADD	TNFR-associated DD
TRAF	TNFR-associating factor
TRAIL	Tumor Necrosis Factor-Related Apoptosis-Inducing Ligand
TRAIL-R	TRAIL Receptor
TRID	TNF-R1 internalization domain
VDAC	Voltage-dependent anion channel
XAF 1	XIAP-Associated Factor.

INTRODUCTION

New genetic and biochemical approaches have fostered remarkable progress in our understanding of cancer biology during the past decade [1]. One of the most important advances has been the recognition that resistance to cell death, particularly apoptotic cell death, is an important aspect of both tumorigenesis and the development of resistance to anticancer drugs [1-3]. In addition to apoptosis, cells can be effectively eliminated by necrosis, mitototic catastrophe or autophagic cell death. In addition, premature senescence causes reversible arrests of cell division. Some of the characteristics of these different modes of cell death are summarized in Table 1. Much recent research on new cancer therapies has therefore focused on devising ways to overcome this resistance and to trigger the cell death of tumor cells. Although the detailed mechanisms underlying tumor cell's resistance to apoptosis remain to be characterized, some important components and steps in this process have already been elucidated. A simple look at the wide range of antineoplastic treatments that are ineffective at killing cancer cells (Table 2) implies that the tumor resistance mechanisms are complex. For decades, clinicians and basic scientists have been puzzled by the fact that tumor cells simultaneously acquire the capability to escape immune surveillance mechanisms and evade the cytotoxic action of diverse cytotoxic insults, for example, DNA damage (e.g. by irradiation, alkylation, methylation or crosslinking), microtubule destabilization or topoisomerase inhibition. Complete treatment responses after chemotherapeutic regimens rarely benefit more than 20% of the melanoma patients, and the term 'remission' is rarely used with the melanoma. Moreover, new genetic and biochemical approaches in breast cancer indicate also that drug resistance is likely not a primary consequence of acquired genetic alterations selected *during* or *after* therapy, but rather inherent to the malignant behavior of cancer cells at diagnosis. Various mechanisms including genetic instability, oncogene overexpression, tumor suppressor downregulation, epigenetic modifications, loss of cell cycle control and impact of tumor microenvironnement result in development of tumor resistance to cell death. Understanding these mechanisms at the molecular level provides deeper insight into carcinogenesis, influences therapeutic strategy and might, ultimately, lead to new therapeutic approaches based on modulation of apoptosis sensitivity.

Prion diseases are a group of transmissible neurodegenerative disorders, including Creutzfeldt-Jakob disease, Gerstmann-Sträussler syndrome, kuru, and fatal familial insomnia in humans as well as scrapie and bovine spongiform encephalopathy in animals [4]. These diseases are caused by the conversion of PrPc (cellular Prion protein), a normal cell surface glycoprotein, into PrP^{Sc}, a β-sheet-rich conformer that is infectious in the absence of nucleic acid [5-6]. Although a great deal is known about the role of PrP^{Sc} in the disease process, the normal function of PrPc has remained elusive. A variety of functions have been proposed for PrPc, including roles in metal ion trafficking [7], cell adhesion [8], and transmembrane signaling. Identifying the function of PrPc may provide important clues to the pathogenesis of prion diseases, since there is evidence that PrPc plays an essential role in mediating the neurotoxic effects of PrP^{Sc} [9]. Several intriguing lines of evidence have emerged recently indicating that PrPc may function to protect cells from various kinds of internal or environmental stress. PrPc overexpression rescues not only cultured neurons but also tumor cell lines from pro-apoptotic stimuli, including BAX expression, serum withdrawal, DNA damage, cytokine and anti-cancer drug treatments [10-17]. This review revisits the molecular mechanisms of tumor resistance to apoptosis in cancer and the implication of the cellular prion protein PrPc in this phenomena.

Apoptosis can be initiated by two alternative pathways: either through death receptors on the cell surface (extrinsic pathway) or through mitochondria (intrinsic pathway). In both pathways (Figure 1), cysteine aspartyl-specific proteases (caspases) are activated that cleave cellular substrates, and this leads to the biochemical and morphological changes that are characteristic of apoptosis (Table 1). Finally, the contents of dead cells are packaged into apoptotic bodies, which are recognized by neighboring cells or macrophages and cleared by phagocytosis.

Table 1. Characteristics of different types of cell death

| Type of cell death | General characteristics of death | | | | Detection methods |
| | Morphological changes | | | Cellular and Biochemical features | |
	Nucleus	Cell membrane	Cytoplasm		
Apoptosis	Chromatin condensation, nuclear margination, DNA laddering	Blebbing is often seen	Formation of apoptotic bodies	Caspase dependent	Annexin-V staining; TUNEL staining; DNA laddering; caspase activation; flow cytommetry to detect cells in sub G1 content; detection of change in mitochondrial membrane potential, detection of ROS levels electron microscopy.
Autophagy	Partial chromatin condensation, No DNA laddering	Blebbing	Formation of double membrane vacuoles which sequester mitochondria and ribosomes	Caspase and p53 independent. The cell digest itself	Lack of marginated condensed nuclear chromatin by electron microscopy; protein degradation assays; exclusion of vital dyes until late stages. Prominent cytoplasmic vacuoles detected with monodansylcadavenine.
Mitotic catastrophe	Multiple micronuclei, nuclear fragmentation	-	-	Occurs after or during mitosis and is probably caused by mis-segregation of chromosomes and /or cell fusion. Giant cell formation. Caspase independent (at early stage). Abnormal CDK1/cyclin B activation. Can lead to apoptosis and is p53-independent	Multinucleated cells detected by light or electron microscopy.
Necrosis	Clumping and random degradation of nuclear DNA	Swelling, rupture	Increased vacuolation; organelle degeneration, mitochondrial swelling	Typically not genetically determined	Early permeability to vital dyes such as trypan blue, flow cytommetry for vital dye staining.
Senescence	Distinct heterochromatic structure	-	Flattening and increased granularity	Cells are metabolically active but non-dividing and show an increase in cell size; Cells express senescence-associated b-galactosidase and this process is p53-dependent.	Electron microscopy, Staining for senescence-associated b-galactosidase

**Table 2. Wide spectrum of chemotherapeutic drugs cancer cells
show resistance against *in vivo***

Alkylating agents		

Cyclophosphamide
Triazenes
   Dacarbazine
   Temozolomide
	Alkylation and methylation of nucleic acids	Inhibition of nucleic acid and protein synthesis

Nitosoureas
   Carmustine
   Lomustine
   Semustine
	Alkylation of nucleic acids and protein	ssDNA Breaks
		DNA crosslinking
		Carbamoylation of proteins

Nitrogen mustard	Alkylation of nucleic acids	DNA crosslinking
Antibiotics		

Anthracyclines
   Adriamycin
   Doxorubicin
   Epirubicin
	DNA intercalating agent
	Free radicals
		ssDNA Breaks
		DNA crosslinking
		Inhibition of DNA and RNA synthesis

Plant-dervived products		
Epipodophyllotoxins *Etoposide*	Inhibition of topoisomerase II	DNA breaks

Taxanes
   Taxol
   Paclitaxel
   Docetaxel
	Microtubule disruption (prevent depolymerisation)	Altered cell division, motility
		Intracellular transport

Vinca alkaloids
   Vincristine
   Vinblastine
	Microtubule disruption (prevent assembly)	Altered cell division, motility
		Intracellular transport

Hormonal analogs Antiestrogen *Tamoxifen*	Competitive inhibitor of endogenous estrogens	Altered estrogen signaling
Platinum Drugs Cisplatin Carboplatin	DNA and protein crosslink	ssDNA and dsDNA breaks Changes in DNA structure Inhibition of DNA and RNA synthesis

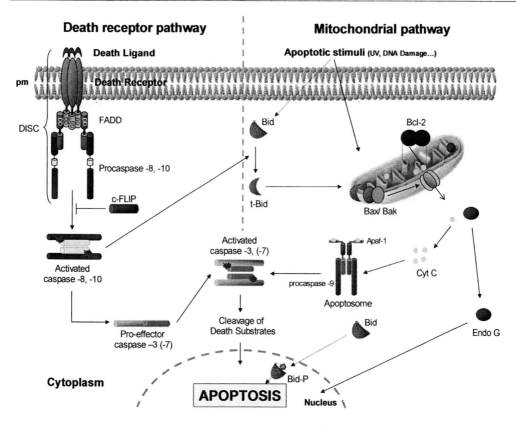

Figure 1. The two main apoptotic signalling pathways. Death receptors are members of the tumor-necrosis factor (TNF) receptor superfamily and comprise a subfamily that is characterized by an intracellular domain — the death domain (DD). Death receptors are activated by their natural ligands. When ligands bind to their respective death receptors the death domains attract the intracellular adaptor protein FADD (Fas-associated death domain protein, also known as MORT1), which, in turn, recruits the inactive proforms of certain members of the caspase protease family. The caspases that are recruited to this death-inducing signalling complex (DISC) — caspase-8 and caspase-10 — function as 'initiator' caspases. At the DISC, procaspase-8 and procaspase-10 are cleaved and yield active initiator caspases. In some cells — known as type I cells — the amount of active caspase-8 formed at the DISC is sufficient to initiate apoptosis directly, but in type II cells, the amount is too small and mitochondria are used as 'amplifiers' of the apoptotic signal. Activation of mitochondria is mediated by the BCL2 family member BID. BID is cleaved by active caspase-8 and translocates to the mitochondria. Then cytochrome *c* is released from mitochondria and interacts with Apaf-1, procaspase- 9 and dATP to form the apoptosome. This causes the caspase- 9 activation, which then activates effector caspase- 3. Active executioner caspases (caspase- 3, -7) cleave the death substrates, which eventually results in apoptosis and causes morphological changes. There is crosstalk between these two pathways.

I. APOPTOSIS PATHWAYS

The main effector cells against tumors are cytotoxic T cells and Natural killer (NK) cells. These immune cells use two mains mechanisms to kill tumor cells: the granule exocytosis (perforin/granzymes) pathway and the death receptors pathways.

1. The Death Receptor Family: Extrinsic Pathway

Death receptors are members of the Tumor Necrosis Factor receptor (TNFR) superfamily, which consists of 32 members and 19 ligands (a downloadable table can be accessed at http://www.niams.nih.gov/rtbc/ImageStore/Test/WORD/AB/IRG/tnfchart.doc.) with a broad range of biological functions including the regulation of cell death, survival, differentiation or immune regulation [18-22]. Members of the TNF receptor family share similar cysteine-rich extracellular domains. In addition, death receptors are defined by a cytoplasmic domain of about 80 amino acids called 'death domain', which plays a crucial role in transmitting the death signal from the cell's surface to intracellular signaling pathways. The best-characterized death receptors comprise CD95 (APO-1Fas), TNF receptor 1 (TNFRI), the two agonistic-receptors TRAIL-R1 (DR4) and TRAIL-R2 (DR5), while the role of three antagonistic decoy receptors TRAIL-R3 (DcR1), TRAIL-4 (DcR2), and osteoprotegrin has not exactly been defined.

The corresponding ligands comprise death receptor ligands such as CD95 ligand, TNF, lymphotoxin (the latter two bind to TNFRI), and Tumor Necrosis Factor-Related Apoptosis-Inducing Ligand (TRAIL). With the exception of lymphotoxin, all ligands are type II transmembrane proteins, which also exist as soluble molecules after cleavage by metalloproteases present in the microenvironment. Death receptors are activated upon oligomerization in response to ligand binding.

1.1. CD95 Receptor-CD95 Ligand System

The CD95 receptor-CD95 ligand system is a key signal pathway involved in the regulation of apoptosis in different cell types [21-23]. CD95, a 48 kDa type I transmembrane receptor, is expressed in activated lymphocytes, in a variety of tissues of lymphoid or nonlymphoid origin, as well as in tumor cells. CD95L, a 40 kDa type II transmembrane molecule, occurs in a membrane-bound and in a soluble form, generated through cleavage by metalloproteases. CD95L is produced by activated T cells and plays a crucial role in the regulation of the immune system by triggering autocrine suicide or paracrine death in neighboring lymphocytes or other target cells. Also, CD95L is constitutively expressed in several tissues and has been implied in immune privilege of certain organs such as the testis or the eye [25]. Moreover, CD95L expression on cancer cells has been implicated in immune escape of tumors [26]. By constitutive expression of death receptor ligands such as CD95L, tumors may adopt a killing mechanism from cytotoxic lymphocytes to delete the attacking antitumor T cells through the induction of apoptosis via CD95/CD95L interaction [26]. However, this model of tumor counterattack has also been challenged, since no study has so far conclusively demonstrated that tumor counterattack is a relevant immune escape mechanism *in vivo*.

Links between the receptor and the mitochondrial pathway exist at different levels [27]. Upon death receptor triggering, activation of caspase-8 may result in cleavage of BID, which in turn translocates to mitochondria to release cytochrome *c*, thereby initiating a mitochondrial amplification loop [27]. The activated death receptors recruit and activate an adaptor protein called Fas-associated death domain (FADD) through interactions between the death domain (DD) on the death receptors and FADD. The death effector domain (DED) of FADD recruits and activates caspase-8, leading to the formation of the death-inducing signaling complex (DISC). In type I cells, the presence of activated caspase-8, a so-called initiator caspase, is sufficient to induce activation of one or more effector caspases (e.g., caspase-3 or -7), which then act on final death substrates in apoptosis [28-29]. However, in type II cells, even a small amount of activated caspase-8, although not enough to activate the effector caspases, is sufficient to trigger a mitochondria-dependent apoptotic amplification loop by activating BID, which induces the accumulation of BAX in mitochondria, the release of cytochrome c from mitochondria, the activation of caspase-9, caspase-3, and caspase-7, and finally, programmed cell death. In addition, cleavage of caspase-6 downstream of mitochondria may positively feed-back to amplify the receptor pathway by cleaving caspase-8 [30].

Recently, an unexpected role for BID was found in the ATM pathway that responds to DNA damage [31-32] and BID can be a target for ATM/ATR. Although BID clearly induces apoptosis following activation of death receptors, its role in controlling apoptosis following DNA damage need to be clarified.

1.2. TRAIL Receptor and TRAIL/Apo-2 Ligand System

TRAIL/Apo-2L was identified based on its sequence homology to other members of the TNF superfamily [18, 33]. Similar to CD95L, TRAIL is a type II transmembrane protein, but can be proteolytically cleaved from the cell surface. TRAIL is constitutively expressed in a wide range of tissues. Interestingly, the TRAIL receptor system is rather complex [34-35]. TRAIL-R1 (DR4) and TRAIL-R2 (DR5), the two agonistic TRAIL receptors, contain a conserved cytoplasmic death domain motif, which engages the apoptosis machinery upon ligand binding [23, 36-42] (reviewed in Refs [43 ,36]). TRAIL-R3 (DcR1), and TRAIL-R4 (DcR2) are antagonistic decoy receptors that bind TRAIL but do not transmit a death signal [35, 39, 44-45]. DcR1 is a glycosyl-phosphatidylinositol GPI-anchored cell surface protein, which lacks a cytoplasmic tail, while DcR2 harbors a substantially truncated cytoplasmic death domain. In addition to these four membrane-associated receptors, osteoprotegerin is a soluble decoy receptor, which is involved in the regulation of osteoclastogenesis [46]. Similar to CD95L, TRAIL rapidly triggers apoptosis in many tumor cells [18,35]. Ligation of the agonistic TRAIL receptors DR4 and DR5 by TRAIL or agonistic antibodies results in receptor trimerization and clustering of the receptors' death domains [47].

In addition to inducing apoptosis by DISC formation (Figure 2), TRAIL binding to its receptors also leads to activation of the transcription factor nuclear factor-kappa B (NF-κB) (Figure 2). TRAIL death receptors, like the TNF receptor 1 (TNFR1) [48], activate NF-κB through the TNFR1-associated death domain protein (TRADD) [37]. Activated TRADD recruits the DD-containing protein RIP and TNF receptor-associated factor-2 (TRAF2), leading to activation of the NF-κB pathway; in contrast, dominant-negative TRADD can block the NF-κB activation induced by TRAIL receptors [37, 49]. In TNFR1 signaling, TRADD is believed to be upstream of FADD. However, in TRAIL signaling, TRADD may be mediated by FADD, because TRADD recruitment to the DISC is observed only in the presence of FADD [49].

The death-inducing signaling complexes of both TRAIL and Fas receptors contain FADD and caspase-8. In addition to caspase-8, also caspase-10 is recruited to the TRAIL DISC. However, the importance of caspase-10 in the TRAIL DISC for apoptosis induction has been controversially discussed [18]. The TRAIL system has attracted considerable attention for cancer therapy since TRAIL has been shown to kill cancer cells predominantly, while sparing normal cells (see below). The underlying mechanisms for the differential sensitivity of malignant *vs* nonmalignant cells is not well understood. Screening of various different tumor cell types in normal cells did not reveal a consistent association between TRAIL sensitivity and expression of agonistic or antagonistic TRAIL receptors as suggested [50]. Instead, susceptibility for TRAIL-induced cytotoxicity has been suggested to be regulated intracellularly.

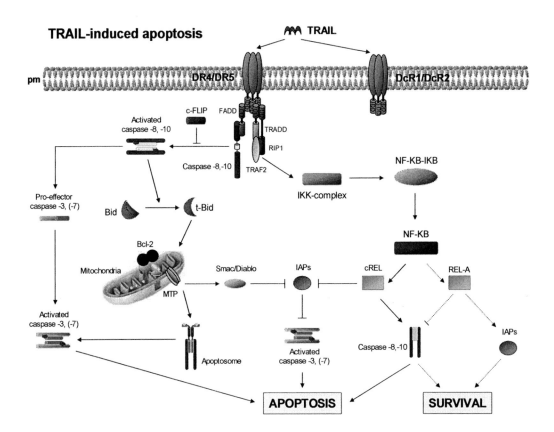

Figure 2. Apoptosis signalling through TRAIL receptors. Binding of TRAIL to their receptor (TRAIL-R1/DR4 and TRAIL-R2/DR5) may transduce via activated caspase-8 directly by activating effector caspase-3 or indirectly by activating BID, which in turn translocated into mitochondria and cause cytochrome *c* and Smac release to cytosol. The released cytochrome *c* interacts with Apaf-1 and cause caspase-9 activation, which then activates effector caspase-3. The released Smac inhibits IAPs by preventing their binding to caspase-9 and caspase-3. Flip bind to the DISC and prevent the activation of caspase-8. Apoptosis pathways induced by TRAIL can also activate NF-κB. Different subunit activation of NF-κB determines whether NF-κB favors apoptosis or survival.

1.3. TNF Receptor and TNF Ligand System

Tumor necrosis factor alpha (TNF) is a highly pleiotropic cytokine that elicits diverse cellular responses ranging from proliferation and differentiation to activation of apoptosis [19, 51]. The different biological activities are mediated by two distinct cell surface receptors: TNF receptor 1 (TNF-R1) and TNF-R2. TNF-R1 appears to be the key mediator of TNF signaling. Recent reports indicated that one possible clue to the basic mechanisms of

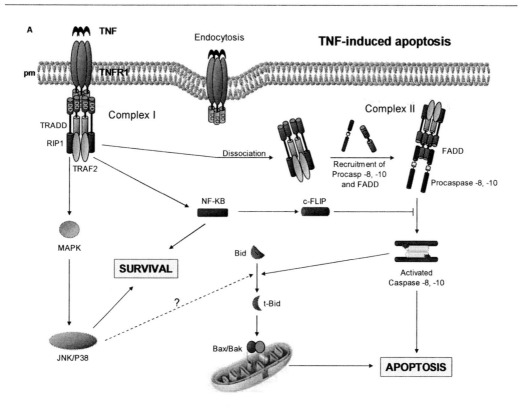

Figure 3A. Signalling through TNF receptor. First model of TNFR1-Mediated Apoptosis. After binding of TNF to TNFR1, rapid recruitment of TRADD, RIP1, and TRAF2 occurs (complex I). Subsequently TNFR1, TRADD, and RIP1 become modified and dissociate from TNFR1. The liberated death domain (DD) of TRADD (and/or RIP1) now binds to FADD, resulting in caspase-8/10 recruitment (forming complex II) and resulting in apoptosis. If NF-κB activation triggered by complex I is successful, cellular FLIP$_L$ levels are sufficiently elevated to block apoptosis and cells survive.

TNF-R1 signal diversification may lie in a compartmentalization of TNF signaling (see comment in [52]). Based on pharmacological inhibitor studies, authors proposed that induction of apoptosis requires internalization of TNF-R1 [53]. In addition, TNF-mediated NF-κB activation was recently linked to the recruitment of TNF-R1 to lipid rafts on the cell surface [54]. Along this line, Micheau and Tschopp [48] have proposed a model describing induction of TNF-R1-mediated apoptosis via two sequential signaling complexes: a plasma membrane-located NF-κB signaling complex I consisting of TNF-R1, TRADD, RIP-1, and TRAF-2 and a cytosolic apoptosis signaling complex II, which is composed of TRADD, FADD, and caspase-8 but is not associated with TNF-R1 (Figure 3A). Since the first complex can activate survival signals and influence the activity of the second complex, this mechanism provides a checkpoint to control the execution of apoptosis. In contrast to this model, recent report from Schütze's group [55] shows existence of a ligand-induced establishment of a TNF-R1-associated DISC within the first minutes after receptor internalization on endocytic vesicles (Figure 3B). In this model, within minutes internalized TNF-R1 (TNF receptosomes) recruits TRADD, FADD, and caspase-8 to establish the DISC. In addition, the authors identified the TNF-R1 internalization domain (TRID) required for receptor endocytosis and showed that TNF-R1 internalization, DISC formation, and apoptosis are inseparable events. Furthermore, fusion of TNF receptosomes with trans-Golgi vesicles results in activation of acid sphinomylinase and cathepsin D (Figure 3B). In addition to inducing apoptosis by receptosome trafficking TNF-receptor binding also leads to NF-κB activation. This is initiated by TRADD-dependent recruitment of RIP-1 and TRAF-2. This conclusion is based on the fact that when the authors used the TNF-R1 deleted TRID cells, they obtained the complex containing of RIP1 and TRAF2. If NF-κB activation is successful cellular factors are sufficiently elevated to block apoptosis and cells survive.

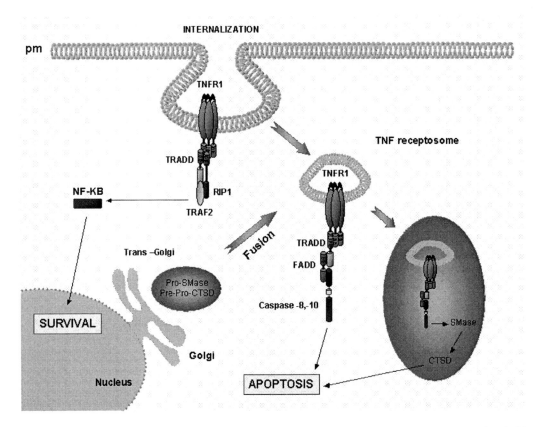

Figure 3B. Signalling through TNF receptor. Second model of TNFR1-Mediated signaling: After TNF binding internalization of TNF-R1 (TNF receptosome) precedes formation of TNF-R1-associated DISC containing TRADD, FADD, and caspase-8. Caspase-8 is autocatalytically cleaved during receptosome trafficking. TNF receptosomes fuse with trans-Golgi vesicles containing pro-A-SMase and pre-pro-CTSD to form multivesicular endosomes in which A-SMase and CTSD (Cathepsin D) activation is induced trigger apoptosis. This differs from the situation with FAS, where the DISC assembles rapidly and receptor internalization can be prevented by caspase inhibitors. In addition to inducing apoptosis by receptosome trafficking TNF receptor binding also leads to NF-κB activation. This is initiated by TRADD-dependent recruitment of RIP-1 and TRAF-2. If NF-κB activation is successful and cellular factors are sufficiently elevated to block apoptosis cells survive.

2. Mitochondria Intrinsic Pathway

Chemotherapy, irradiation and other stimuli can initiate apoptosis through the mitochondrial intrinsic pathway. The regulation of this pathway is complex. The inducers include oncogene, low oxygen (hypoxia), growth factor deprivation, cell-cell detachment (anoïkis) and other stress signals. Pro-apoptotic BCL2 family proteins (reviewed in Refs [56-57]) — for example, BAX, BID, BAD and BIM — are important mediators of these signals. The pro-apoptotic members can be subdivided into the BAX subfamily (BAX, BAK, BOK) and the BH3-only proteins (for example, BID, BAD and BIM) [58]. Activation of mitochondria leads to release of apoptogenic factors such as cytochrome c, Smac/Diablo (second mitochondria-derived activator of caspase/direct IAP binding protein), Omi/HtrA2, endonuclease G and AIF (Apoptosis-inducing factor) from the mitochondrial intermembrane space [59-64]. The release of cytochrome c into the cytosol triggers caspase-3 activation through the formation of the cytochrome c/Apaf-1/caspase-9-containing apoptosome complex, while Smac/Diablo and Omi/HtrA2 promote caspase activation through neutralizing the inhibitory effects to inhibitor of apoptosis proteins (IAPs). The concomitant events are the mitochondrial outer membrane permeabilization (MOMP), disruption of electron transport, loss of mitochondrial transmembrane potential ($\Delta\psi$m, DeltaPsim), decline in ATP levels, production of reactive oxygen species (ROS), and loss of mitochondrial structural integrity. In addition, some of the mitochondrial proteins (AIF, HtrA2/Omi, endonuclease G) released as a result of MOMP can promote caspase-independent cell death through mechanisms that are relatively poorly defined. Caspase-independent cell death can also result from stimuli that cause lysosomal membrane permeabilization with the consequent release of cathepsin proteases [64-66]. Although the impact of BCL2 family members on apoptosis is well known, the biochemical mechanism of their function is not entirely clear. Currently, there are different nonexclusive models that have been proposed to explain how cytohrome c release is regulated. One potential mechanism involved mitochondrial swelling, either due to the opening of mitochondrial permeability transition pore (mPTP), or to mitochondrial hyperpolarization, both of which result in the rupture of the outer mitochondrial membrane, thereby the release of cytochrome c and the loss of mitochondrial membrane potential. This is questionable since there are evidence showing that cytochrome c release and apoptosis occur in the absence of mitochondrial swelling. Recent report from Tsujimoto's group suggests that mPTP is more related to necrosis than to apoptosis [67]. According to one model, mitochondrial membrane permeabilization involves the permeability transition pore complex (PTPC), a multiprotein complex that consists of the adenine nucleotide translocator (ANT) of the inner membrane, the voltage-dependent anion channel (VDAC) of the outer membrane and various other proteins [56]. BCL2 proteins might interact with the PTPC and regulate its permeability. Accoding to the another model the pro-apoptotic molecules in BCL2 family proteins are activated to create discontinuity or pore at the outer membrane of mitochondria to mediate cytochrome c release [68-70]. In this model, BH3-only proapoptotic proteins (such as BID, Bim, Noxa etc.) induce mitochondrial membrane permeabilization either through activation of BAX/BAK or directly neutralize anti-apoptotic molecules such as BCl2/BCL-X_L, two structurally and functionally identical molecules [71-73].

II. TUMOR RESISTANCE MECHANISMS

Tumor cells can acquire resistance to apoptosis by various mechanisms that interfere at different levels of apoptosis signaling (summarized in Table 3).

Table 3. Mechanisms of tumor resistance to apoptosis

Molecules		References
Death receptors		
Expression of soluble receptors for death ligands	Soluble CD95 DcR3	[85-88] [89-91]
TRAIL-R1/ TRAIL-R2 ratio		[107]
Deficient receptor redistribution		[19]
Downregulation and mutation of Death receptors	CD95 TNF TRAIL-R1 TRAIL-2	[92-95] [96] [97-100] [74-77] [78]
Expression of anti-apoptotic molecules		
BCL2 family members	BCL2/ BCL-Xl MCL1	[138-140,142-146,259] [140,147-150] [151,260]
Flip		[112,114,116-119,261-267]
IAPs	Survivin CIAP2 ML-IAP	[133,134,268,269] [135, 136]
PI-9/SPI-6		[137,270,271]
Prion protein		[15,16,272]
Downregulation and mutation of pro-apoptotic		
Bax		[153-156,273-275]
APAF1		[214]
Caspase 8		[152]
XAF1		[130]
Alterations of p53 pathway		
P53		[164-166,168,169,276-280]
INK4A/ARF		[172]
ASPP		[173, 281]
Further mechanisms		
Alterations of the survival pathways		
PI3K		[177]
PTEN		[179-187]
AKT		[178]
NF-kB activity		[188-190] [191, 192]-[194]
MAP kinases		[146], [11]
Chemoresistance mechanisms		
Expression of transporters	MDR1/PglycoproteinMRP	[200]; [196]
Expression of nuclear enzyme	topoisomerase II	[205, 206]
DNA repair mechanisms	MSH2	[210]- [211]
Extracellular matrix		[215]

1. Defective Death Receptor Signaling

1.1. Loss of Function of Receptor Genes by Mutations or Methylation

Death receptors expression may vary between different cell types and can be downregulated or absent in resistant tumor cells. Their inactivation by, e.g. mutations or gene methylation, will probably result in less immune surveillance-induced apoptosis and, consequently, contribute to a malignant phenotype. Deletions and mutations of the death receptors TNF receptors, Fas and TRAIL-R1 and TRAIL-R2 have also been observed in tumors [74-78]. The fact that loss of chromosome 8p21–22, where the TRAIL-receptor genes are mapped [44, 79-82] is a frequent event in various cancers.

Methylation of the Fas promotor and enhancer region was found in colon cancer cell lines and in colon carcinomas. It contributed to the down-regulation of Fas expression and subsequent loss of sensitivity to Fas-induced apoptosis in colon carcinoma cells [83-84].

1.2. Expression of Soluble Receptors

One mechanism by which tumors interfere with death-receptor-mediated apoptosis might be the expression of soluble receptors that act as decoys for death ligands. Two distinct soluble receptors soluble CD95 (sCD95) and decoy receptor 3 (DcR3) have been shown to competitively inhibit CD95 signaling. sCD95 is expressed in various malignancies, and elevated levels can be found in the sera of cancer patients. High sCD95 serum levels were associated with poor prognosis in melanoma patients [85-88]. DcR3 binds to CD95L and the TNF family member LIGHT and inhibits CD95L-induced apoptosis. It is genetically amplified in several lung and colon carcinomas and is overexpressed in several adenocarcinomas, glioma cell lines and glioblastomas [89-91]. Ectopic expression of DcR3 in a rat glioma model resulted in decreased immune-cell infiltration, which indicates that DcR3 is involved in immune evasion of malignant glioma [91]. Moreover, death receptors are downregulated or inactivated in many tumors. The expression of the death receptor CD95 is reduced in some tumor cells for example, in hepatocellular carcinomas, neoplastic colon epithelium, melanomas and other tumors [92-95] compared with their normal counterparts. Loss of CD95, probably by downregulation of transcription, might contribute to chemoresistance and immune evasion. Oncogenic RAS seems to downregulate CD95 [96], and in hepatocellular carcinomas loss of CD95 expression is accompanied by p53 aberrations [95].

Several CD95 gene mutations have been reported in primary samples of myeloma and T-cell leukaemia [97-99]. The mutations include point mutations in the cytoplasmic death domain of CD95 and a deletion that leads to a truncated form of the death receptor. These mutated forms of CD95 might interfere in a dominant-negative way with apoptosis induction by CD95. In families with germ-line CD95 mutations, which usually result in autoimmune lymphoproliferative syndrome (ALPS), the risk of developing lymphomas is increased [100].

1.3. The Importance of TRAIL-R1/ TRAIL-R2 Ratio

Originally, the regulation of TRAIL induced apoptosis was suggested to be especially controlled by the membrane expression of TRAIL-receptors. Although membrane expression of TRAIL-R1 and TRAIL-R2 is clearly necessary to induce the death signal of TRAIL, membrane expression of DcR1 or DcR2, however, does not necessarily correlate with cell sensitivity to TRAIL [101-102].

Besides the importance of the balance of death receptors and decoy receptor membrane expression, the ratio between may play a role in determining TRAIL-sensitivity. Although this has not been studied very well, there are some indications that in some situations or cell lines, one of the two death receptors is more efficient in death signaling than the other. TRAIL can induce apoptosis through TRAIL-R1 and TRAIL-R2 independently [103-104], but at physiological conditions (37 °C) it binds with a higher affinity to TRAIL-R2 than to TRAIL-R1 [105]. Additionally, in order to induce apoptosis, TRAIL-R1 and TRAIL-R2 have distinct cross-linking requirements. TRAIL-R1 equally responds to cross-linked (e.g. membrane bound) TRAIL and non-cross-linked (soluble) rhTRAIL, whereas TRAIL-R2 signals only in response to cross-linked soluble rhTRAIL [106]. Thus, depending on the type of TRAIL used for apoptosis induction, TRAIL-R1/TRAIL-R2 ratio can determine TRAIL-sensitivity [107].

1.4. Deficient Receptor Redistribution

Studies in melanoma cells have demonstrated that binding of TRAIL to the TRAIL-receptors on the membrane causes a redistribution of the TRAIL-receptors within the cell [108]. The movement of decoy-receptors was dependent on signals from TRAIL-R1 and TRAIL-R2. Reduced decoy receptor relocalization may, therefore, contribute to sensitivity of melanoma cells (and possibly other cancer cells) to TRAIL-induced apoptosis [109].

In colon cancer cells, it was found that a deficient TRAIL death receptor transport to the cell surface resulted in TRAIL-resistant cells. TRAIL-resistant clones were isolated after exposure of a TRAIL-sensitive cell line to TRAIL. Although total cellular mRNA and protein levels were similar in TRAIL-sensitive parental and TRAIL-resistant clones, TRAIL-R1 surface expression and TRAIL-R1 recruitment to the DISC were not detected in the TRAIL-resistant clones. Glycosylation inhibitor tunicamycin increased TRAIL-R1 (and TRAIL-R2) expression and resensitized the resistant clones to TRAIL [110].

Redistribution of death receptors in lipid rafts, which are plasma membrane microdomains enriched in cholesterol and glycosphingolipids, can regulate the efficacy of signaling by death receptors [19]. In colon cancer cells, resveratrol induced TRAIL-R1 and TRAIL-R2 (and FAS) redistribution in lipid rafts and this sensitized the cells to TRAIL-induced apoptosis [111]. This indicates that not only the basic expression levels on the cell surface, but also redistribution/relocalization of TRAIL-receptors to the cell membrane and formation of lipid rafts determine TRAIL-sensitivity.

2. Expression of Anti-Apoptotic Proteins

Various proteins inhibit the apoptotic process at different levels (see Figure 1 and 2)

FLIPs (FADD-like interleukin-1 β-converting enzyme-like protease (FLICE/ caspase-8)-inhibitory proteins) interfere with the initiation of apoptosis directly at the level of death receptors [112]. Two splice variants a long form (cFLIP$_L$) and a short form (cFLIP$_S$) have been identified in human cells. Although the role of c-FLIP$_S$ as an inhibitor of death receptor-mediated apoptosis is well understood and resembles the activity of viral analogues of FLIP, called viral FLIPs proteins (v-FLIPs) [112, 116], the specific role of cFLIP$_L$ in death receptor-mediated apoptosis remains unclear. The overexpression of cFLIP$_L$ may either induce or inhibit apoptosis, depending on protein levels and cell type. Both forms share structural homology with procaspase-8, but lack its catalytic site. This structure allows them to bind to the DISC, thereby inhibiting the processing and activation of the initiator caspase-8. High FLIP expression that has been found in many tumor cells has been correlated with resistance to CD95- and TRAIL-induced apoptosis [113]. In addition, FLIP expression was associated with tumor escape from T-cell immunity and enhanced tumor progression in experimental studies *in vivo* pointing to a role of FLIP as a tumor progression factor [113]. However, the impact of FLIP on apoptosis sensitivity towards cytotoxic drugs may vary between cell types. Thus, overexpression of FLIP did not confer protection against cytotoxic drugs in T-cell leukemia cells, while it inhibits chemotherapy-induced cell death in colorectal cancer [114]. FLIP antisense oligonucleotides or downregulation of FLIP expression by metabolic inhibitors sensitized various tumor cells for death receptor-induced apoptosis [104, 114-115]. v-FLIPs are encoded by some tumorigenic viruses, including HHV8 [116-118]. In cells that are latently infected with HHV8, v-FLIP is expressed at low levels, but its expression is increased in advanced Kaposi's sarcomas or on serum withdrawal from lymphoma cells in culture [119]. Therefore, v-FLIPs might contribute to the persistence and oncogenicity of v-FLIP-encoding viruses.

The IAPs (inhibitor of apoptosis proteins) are cellular caspase inhibitors, which are characterized by the presence of one to three baculoviral IAP repeats (BIRs). Through these BIR domains the IAP proteins bind to and inhibit caspases. IAPs inhibit directly active caspase-3 and -7 and to block caspase-9 activation. Members of the IAP-family include XIAP, cIAP1, cIAP2, NAIP, livin, BRUCE and survivin [120]. Increasing evidence demonstrates that IAPs, especially survivin and XIAP, are upregulated in several tumor types. Recently, it is demonstrated that survivin binds to Smac/Diablo, which is released from the mitochondria. By binding to Smac/Diablo, survivin prevents binding of Smac/Diablo to IAPs. Free IAPs, such as XIAP may then directly bind to caspases to prevent apoptosis. In addition to the regulation of apoptosis, IAP members such as survivin have been found to be involved in the regulation of mitosis [121-122]. Inhibition of apoptosis by IAPs in response to cytotoxic therapy has been suggested by several experimental studies to be an important mechanism of resistance [64, 123-125]. A mutation in the promotor region of survivin was detected in several cancer cell lines and causes (at least in part) overexpression of survivin [126]. Although it is clear from studies in several cancer cell lines that down-regulation of survivin enhances TRAIL-induced apoptosis [127-128]. Since caspase 3 is regulated by XIAP, upregulation of XIAP is a likely mechanism of TRAIL-resistance. Recently, it was shown that disruption of the gene encoding XIAP in human colon cancer cells did not interfere with basal proliferation, but indeed caused a remarkable sensitivity to TRAIL [129]. This suggests that XIAP (and other IAPs) may be important for the modulation of TRAIL-sensitivity in many tumor types. Recently, a XIAP-interacting protein named XIAP-associated factor 1 (XAF1) has been identified [130]. XAF1 antagonizes the ability of XIAP to suppress caspase activity and cell death *in vitro*. It is not known how XAF1 interacts with XIAP to inhibit its activity. In contrast to Smac/Diablo, XAF1 does not need to be processed and seems to be constitutively able to interact with and inhibit XIAP. However, unlike XIAP which is found primarily in the cytoplasm, endogenous XAF1 is localized in the nucleus. The different compartmentalization between XIAP and XAF1 raises the question of how these two proteins can interact: does XAF1 translocate into the cytoplasm where it inhibits XIAP, or does XIAP enter the nucleus where it is sequestered by XAF1? It is conceivable that XIAP could be transported into the nucleus within the caspase-3 protein complex, where it would continue to inhibit caspase-3 activity. This caspase-inhibiting activity could then be relieved by nuclear XAF1, in a fashion similar to the cytoplasmic inhibition of XIAP by Smac/Diablo.

Expression of survivin is highly tumor specific [131,132]. It is found in most human tumors but not in normal adult tissues [131-132]. In neuroblastoma, expression correlates with a more aggressive and unfavorable disease [123]. Survivin inhibited UVB-induced apoptosis *in vitro* and *in vivo*, whereas it did not affect CD95-induced cell death [123]. Expression of a non-phosphorylatable mutant of survivin induces cytochrome *c* release and cell death. In xenograft tumor models, this mutant suppressed tumor growth and reduced intra-peritoneal tumor dissemination [133-134]. The frequent translocation t(11;18)(q21;q21) that is found in about 50% of marginal cell lymphomas of the mucosa-associated lymphoid tissue (MALT) affects cIAP2 gene [135]. This indicates a role for cIAP2 in the development of MALT lymphoma. ML-IAP is expressed at high levels in melanoma cell lines but not in primary melanocytes. Melanoma cell lines that express ML-IAP are significantly more resistant to drug-induced apoptosis than those that do not express ML-IAP [136].

PI-9/SPI-6 expression of this serine protease inhibitor, which inhibits granzyme B, results in the resistance of tumor cells to cytotoxic lymphocytes, leading to immune escape [137].

Anti-apoptotic BCL2 family members (BCL2, BCL-X$_L$, BCL-w, MCL1, A1/BFL1, BOO/DIVA, NRH) can inhibit apoptosis through mitochondria on different levels. Most anti-apoptotic members contain the BCL2 homology (BH) domains 1, 2 and 4, whereas the BH3 domain seems to be crucial for apoptosis induction. Moreover, it has been shown *in vitro* and *in vivo* models that BCL2 expression confers resistance to many kinds of chemotherapeutic drugs and irradiation [138-140]. A characteristic feature of BCL2 proteins is the formation of homodimers and heterodimers with other members of the family. For example, BCL2 can form heterodimers with BAX, BAD or other proapoptotic molecules, and may thus block their proapoptotic activity. In some types of tumors, a high level of BCL2 expression is associated with a poor response to chemotherapy and seems to be predictive of shorter, disease-free survival [140-143]. The tumor-associated viruses Epstein–Barr virus (EBV) and human herpesvirus 8 (HHV8 or Kaposi's sarcoma-associated herpesvirus) encode proteins that are homologues of BCL2. Both proteins BHRF1 from EBV and KSBCL2(vBCL2) from HHV8 have an anti-apoptotic function and enhance survival of the infected cells [144-146]. In this way, they might contribute to tumor formation after virus infection, and to resistance of these tumors to therapy. In addition, other anti-apoptotic BCL2 family members also seem to be involved in resistance of tumors to apoptosis. For example, BCL-X$_L$ can confer resistance to multiple apoptosis-inducing pathways in cell lines and seems to be upregulated by a constitutively active mutant epidermal growth factor receptor (EGFR) *in vitro* [147-150]. MCL1 (myeloid cell leukaemia sequence 1) can also render cell lines resistant to chemotherapy [151]. In some leukaemia patients, MCL1 expression was increased at the time of relapse, which indicates that some anticancer drugs might select for leukaemia cells that have elevated MCL1 levels.

3. Inactivation of Pro-Apoptotic Genes

Caspase-8

Convincing evidence is accumulating which shows caspase-8 to be a key and irreplaceable molecule in TRAIL-induced as well as Fas-L and TNF alpha-induced apoptosis. Caspase-8 is deleted or silenced preferentially in childhood neuroblastomas with amplification of MYCN [152]. In these tumors, the gene for the initiator caspase-8 is frequently inactivated by gene deletion or methylation. Caspase-8-deficient neuroblastoma cells are resistant to death receptor- and doxorubicin -mediated apoptosis.

BAX and BAK

Besides overexpression of anti-apoptotic genes, tumors can acquire apoptosis resistance by down-regulating or mutating pro-apoptotic molecules. In certain types of cancer, the pro-apoptotic BCL2 family member BAX or BAK are mutated [153-155]. Reduced *BAX* expression is associated with a poor response rate to chemotherapy and shorter survival in some situations [156]. Several studies in mice have confirmed the function of BAX as a tumor suppressor. The importance of BAX, BAK or both in death receptor signaling or chemotherapy drug-induced apoptosis seems to depend on the cell type. However this is the ratio between BAX or BAK/BCL2 or BC-X_L may play a role in determining cell death sensitivity.

APAF-1

Metastatic melanomas have found another way to escape mitochondria-dependent apoptosis. These tumors often do not express APAF-1, which forms an integral part of the apoptosome [157], and the *APAF-1* locus shows a high rate of allelic loss. The remaining allele is transcriptionally inactivated by gene methylation. *APAF1*-negative melanomas fail to respond to chemotherapy a situation that is commonly found in this type of tumor.

4. p53-Dependent Pathways

Defects in DNA repair including defects in non-homologous end joining (NHEJ) and homologous recombination (HR), in DNA-damage checkpoints or in telomere maintenance lead to genomic instability and a predisposition to cancer (Figure 4) [1]. This genetic instability provides a way in which a normal cell can accumulate sufficient mutations to become malignant, and is the basis for the so-called 'mutator hypothesis' of cancer [158]. However, the cell has important mechanisms to protect against genomic instability driven by the loss of cell-cycle checkpoints, persistent DNA damage or telomere dysfunction. Central to this mechanism is the tumor-suppressor protein p53, which acts as a 'guardian of the genome' in protecting cells against cancer. *TP53* is the most commonly mutated gene in human cancer, a finding that reflects its crucial anticancer activity [159]. p53 acts to obstruct tumorigenesis by serving as a cellular-stress and DNA-damage sentinel.

In response to a variety of stress signals such as DNA damage, oncogene activation, hypoxia or nucleotide depletion, p53 undergoes post translational modification (phosphorylation, acetylation and sumoylation) that allows its stabilization and accumulation in the nucleus. Then, p53 activates the transcription of genes involved in cell cycle arrest, apoptosis, and DNA repair [160]. p53 is inhibited by MDM2, a ubiquitin ligase that targets p53 for its destruction by the proteasome. MDM2 is inactivated by binding to ARF (alternate open reading frame). Cellular stress, including that induced by chemotherapy or γ-irradiation, activates p53 either directly, by inhibition of MDM2, or indirectly by activation of ARF. ARF can also be induced by proliferative oncogenes such as RAS. p53 can induce the expression of numerous apoptotic genes such as CD95, TRAIL-R2, BAX, Bam, Puma and Noxa that can contribute to the activation of both death-receptor and mitochondrial apoptotic pathways. The choice of response to p53 activation is determined, in part, by differential regulation of p53 activity in normal and tumor cells. In this model, activation of p53 in normal cells leads to the selective expression of cell-cycle-arrest target genes (such as *CDKN1A*, which encodes WAF1), resulting in a reversible or permanent inhibition of cell proliferation. In tumor cells, phosphorylation of p53 at Ser46 (through activation of kinases, expression of co-activators such as p53DINP1 or repression of phosphatases such as WIP1) and/or functional interaction with apoptotic cofactors, such as ASPP (apoptosis-stimulating protein of p53), JMY (Junction-mediating and regulatory protein) and the other p53-family members p63 and p73 allows for the activation of apoptotic target genes. These cofactors can bind p53 (directly or indirectly) as shown for ASPP and JMY or as shown for p63 and p73 assist p53 DNA binding by directly interacting with p53-responsive promoters.

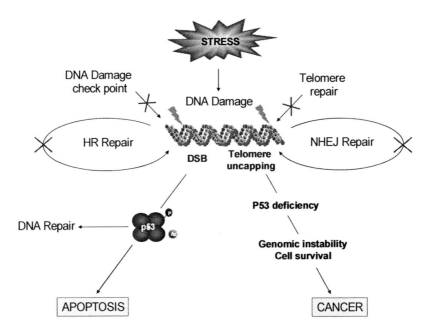

Figure 4. p53-dependent apoptosis, malignancy and resistance to cancer treatments. Defects in several processes, including DNA-damage checkpoint function, telomere maintenance, and DNA double-strand break (DSB) repair including non-homologous end joining (NHEJ) and homologous recombination (HR), result in DSBs or exposed chromosomal ends. In the presence of p53, cells with DSBs or uncapped telomeres are predisposed to apoptosis, which limits tumorigenesis. If, however, p53 is absent, cells with DSBs or eroded telomeres can survive inappropriately, creating a permissive environment for the generation of genomic instability that can drive carcinogenesis. Defects in apoptosis underlie not only tumorigenesis, but also resistance to cancer treatments.

In parallel, p53 can possess a non nuclear proapoptotic function that is independent of its transcriptional activity. This pathway occur through transcriptional upregulation of PIDD protein (P53-induced protein with a death domain) [161]. PIDD can promote assembly of a complex between itself, RAIDD (receptor-interacting protein (RIP)-associated ICH-1/CED-3 homologous protein with a death domain) and caspase- 2 ('the piddosome'). It remains unclear how assembly of the piddosome can promote cell death, but this may involve caspase 2−dependent MOMP [66]. More recent evidence has also revealed a function for p53 as a binding partner of antiapoptotic members of the BCL2 family in the outer membrane such as BCL2 and Bcl-XL [162-163].

As in tumor cells p53 is a key element in stress-induced apoptosis, alterations of the p53 pathway influence the sensitivity of tumors to apoptosis. Tumors that are deficient in Trp53 (the gene that encodes p53 in mice) in immunocompromised mice and cell lineages from transgenic mice that express mutant *Trp53* showed a poor response to γ-irradiation or chemotherapy [164]. Specific mutations in *TP53* (the gene that encodes p53 in humans) have been linked to primary resistance to doxorubicin treatment and early relapse in patients with breast cancer [165]. In cancer cell lines, the specific disruption of the *TP53* gene conferred resistance to 5-FU, but greater sensitivity to adriamycin or radiation *in vitro* [166]. Adenoviral transfer of the wild-type *Trp53* gene into tumor cells with mutated p53 induced apoptosis and suppressed tumor growth in nude mice [167-171]. Mutations of *CDKN2A* (also named Ink4a/Arf locus encodes two tumor suppressor genes, p16^{Ink4a} and p19^{Arf}) are almost as widespread in tumors as are *TP53* mutations [172]. Lymphomas from *Trp53*-knockout mice and from *Cdkn2a*-knockout mice are highly invasive, display apoptotic defects and are markedly resistant to chemotherapy *in vitro* and *in vivo* [173].

In addition to the fact that most human cancers have either mutations in p53 or defects in the pathway, p53-null mice are highly prone to developing cancers. Moreover, crosses of most tumor-prone strains to p53-null mice result in increased tumorigenesis that is clearly correlated with, at least in some cases, loss of the apoptotic function of p53 [174]. Therefore, inactivation of the apoptosis pathway allows cancer cells to develop (Figure 4). So important is this inactivation of apoptosis to cancer development that evasion of apoptosis is considered to be one of the six fundamental hallmarks of cancer. A corollary of this is that if the apoptotic pathway inactivated in tumor development is the same as, or overlaps, that leading to cell death by DNA damage, most cancers would be expected to be resistance to apoptosis in response to DNA damage [175] ; most tumors lose the ability to die by apoptosis. For example, apoptosis has a relatively modest role in the tumor response to radiation. The anti-tumor effect of radiation is realized through mitotic catastrophe or in senescence-like irreversible growth arrest [176].

5. Further Mechanisms

Among the main forces limiting cell death to its appropriate and physiological level are survival signals derived from the activation of the PI3K/AKT/PTEN, the NF-κB and MAPK pathways. These signaling cascades are organized in intricate networks, and a detailed description of their regulation and outcome is outside the scope of this review. Below is a summary of how these pathways may contribute to tumor resistance.

5.1. Altered Several Signaling Pathways

PI3K/AKT/PTEN

This pathway is typically engaged in response to multiple mitogens (including oncogenes such as Ras) that bind to receptor kinases at the plasma membrane and lead to the activation of the phosphoinositide 3-kinase (PI3K) [177]. Once activated, PI3K converts the lipid PIP$_2$ into PIP$_3$. PIP$_3$ activates the protein kinase B/AKT which, in turn, targets multiple factors involved in cell proliferation, migration and survival. Regarding survival functions, AKT promotes the transcription of Bcl-X_L, and the inactivation of the proapoptotic protein BAD, caspase- 9, and the transcription factor FKHRL1 (an inducer of a number of proapoptotic factors). In addition, AKT can activate NF-κB and potentiate its survival functions, illustrating the intricate crosstalk between both pathways [177].

Such a prosurvival force is too dangerous to be unchecked [178], and thus mammalian cells have developed intrinsic mechanisms to regulate AKT activity. At the center of these protective mechanisms is the tumor suppressor PTEN, a phosphatase that targets PIP_3 and prevents the activation of AKT [179]. Therefore, PTEN counteracts survival signals and promotes apoptosis. Moreover, feedback loops have been recently found between PTEN and the p53 tumor suppressor pathway [180-181]. One-third of primary melanomas and about 50% of metastatic melanoma cell lines showed reduced expression of PTEN as a result of allelic deletion, mutation or transcriptional silencing [182-183], suggesting that inactivation of PTEN is a late, but frequent, event on melanomagenesis [184-187].

The NF-κB Pathway

NF-κB is a transcription factor considered 'at the crossroads of life and death' by its function as a modulator of inflammation, angiogenesis, cell cycle, differentiation, adhesion, migration and survival [188]. In the context of cell death control, NF-kB modulates the expression of a plethora of survival factors that interfere with mitochondrial and death receptor-mediated apoptosis [188] (Figure 2). In melanoma cells, the NF-kB pathway can be altered by upregulation of the NF-κB subunits p50 and Rel A [189- 190] and downregulation of the NF-κB inhibitor IκB [191-192]. Consequently, downstream NF-κB targets like c-*myc*, cyclin D1, the antiapoptotic factor TRAF2, the invasion-associated proteins Mel-CAM or the proangiogenic chemokine GRO are also frequently upregulated in melanoma [178]. Depending on the stimulus and the cellular context, NF-κB can activate pro-apoptotic genes, such as those encoding CD95, CD95L, and TRAIL receptors, and anti-apoptotic genes, such as those encoding IAPs and BCL-X_L. Genes encoding NF-κB or IκB proteins are amplified or translocated in human cancer [193]. In Hodgkin's disease cells, constitutive activity of NF-κB has been observed [194].

The MAP Kinases Pathways

The MAP kinases are a superfamily of proteins that transmit signaling cascades from extracellular stimuli into cells ; examples of MAP kinases include extracellular signal-regulated kinases (ERKs), SAPK, stress-activated protein kinase (also known c-jun N-terminal protein kinases, JNKs), and p38 MAP kinases. Like NF-κB, MAP kinases participate in a wide variety of cellular processes, including immunoregulation, inflammation, cell growth, cell differentiation, and cell death. SAPK can regulate the activity of AP-1 transcription factors. Usually, activation of ERKs in response to death stimuli is believed to have an antiapoptotic effect. In support of this conclusion were findings that TRAIL induced rapid ERK1/2 activation in a group of melanoma cell lines, and the inhibition of that activation sensitized TRAIL-resistant melanoma cells to TRAIL-induced apoptosis, suggesting that ERK1/2 activation can itself protect against TRAIL-induced cell death in these TRAIL-resistant cell lines. However, TRAIL also induced rapid ERK1/2 activation in TRAIL-sensitive melanoma cell lines, indicating that ERK1/2 activation by itself is not sufficient to protect against TRAIL-induced cell death in these TRAIL-sensitive cell lines. Zhang et al. hypothesize that TRAIL treatment involves different MAP kinases, different cell environments, and different cytokines, all of which interact to tip the balance in favor of cell survival or cell death [79]. In TNF-resistant human breast carcinoma cells several mechanisms contribute to protect cells to TNF-α-induced cell death including abnormal cleavage of cytosolic phospholipase A2, alteration the cellular redox state and the loss of p53 wild-type function. However, the effect elicited by TNF-α on cell death was NF-kappaB- and SAPK/JNK-independent [195]. Probably, the implication of MAP Kinase pathway engaged in tumor resistance depends on the stress stimulus, the cell type, the tumor environment and many other factors.

5.2. Chemoresistance Mechanisms

Cancer treatment by chemotherapy and γ-irradiation kills target cells primarily by inducing apoptosis. Therefore, key elements of resistance to apoptosis influences resistance to chemotherapy and γ-irradiation. Traditionally, chemoresistance was attributed to a failure of drug-target interactions either due to a reduction of the effective concentration of the drug, via enhanced drug efflux pumps [196], or to detoxification enzymes or the drug's target(s) itself(s) [197-199]. Classical multidrug resistance is attributed to the elevated expression of ATP-dependent drug-efflux pumps ABCB1 [also known as P-glycoprotein (Pgp)], ABCC1 [also known as multidrug resistance-associated protein (MRP1)] and ABCG2 [also known as breast cancer-resistance protein (BCRP) and mitoxantrone-resistance protein (MXR)], all of which belong to the superfamily of ATP-binding cassette (ABC) transporters [for review see 200]. P-glycoprotein protects cells not only from chemotherapy-induced apoptosis, but also from other caspase-dependent death stimuli such as CD95L, TNF and UV-radiation. However, it does not confer resistance to the perforin/granzymes pathway [196, 201-202]. In addition to their role in drug resistance, there is substantial evidence that these efflux pumps have overlapping functions in tissue defense. Collectively, these proteins are capable of transporting a vast and chemically diverse array of toxicants including bulky lipophilic cationic, anionic, and neutrally charged drugs and toxins as well as conjugated organic anions that encompass dietary and environmental carcinogens, pesticides, metals, metalloids, and lipid peroxidation products. ABC transporters are expressed in tissues important for absorption (e.g., lung and gut) and metabolism and elimination (liver and kidney). In addition, these transporters have an important role in maintaining the barrier function of sanctuary site tissues (e.g., blood–brain barrier, blood–cerebral spinal fluid barrier, blood–testis barrier and the maternal–fetal barrier or placenta). Thus, these ABC transporters are increasingly recognized for their ability to modulate the absorption, distribution, metabolism, excretion, and toxicity of xenobiotics [203].

How these mechanisms contribute to drug resistance in melanoma is a matter of controversy [204]. For example, although some reports indicate an upregulation of drug pumps such as P-glycoprotein and the multidrug resistance-associated protein MPR-1 upon treatment, others fail to do so [204]. Similar contradictory results have been reported detoxification factors such as the glutathione/glutathione S transferase, associated with the inactivation of alkylating drugs. For drugs like etoposide, it has been argued that tumor cells may avoid DNA damage by actually downregulating its target, topoisomerase II [205-206]. Specifically, topoisomerase II has been found to be downregulated or mutated in melanoma cells [207-208], although its levels may not necessarily correlate with drug sensitivity [209]. Another possible mechanism to counteract the deleterious effects of DNA-damaging drugs could be a hyperactivation of DNA repair mechanisms, either by upregulating mismatch repair genes or by potentiating enzymes that remove DNA-alkylation damage. Again, reports in the melanoma literature come in different flavors. MSH2 and other mismatch repair genes can be found upregulated [210] or downregulated [211]. Therefore, the melanoma field is in great need of standardized pharmacological studies that unequivocally determine how chemotherapeutic cells are incorporated into tumor and normal melanocytes. However, the fact that chemotherapeutic drugs do activate classical DNA damage sensors in melanoma, for example, related to the p53 pathway [21, 212-214] and that restoring apoptotic defects increases drug sensitivity, indicates that melanoma cells actually *sense* the drugs but have developed clever escape alternatives to prevent or compensate for their action.

The extracellular matrix might also contribute to drug resistance *in vivo* [215]. Small-cell lung cancer is surrounded by an extensive stroma of extracellular matrix, and adhesion of the cancer cells to the extracellular matrix suppresses chemotherapy-induced apoptosis through integrin signalling. Furthermore, in myeloma, constitutive activation of STAT3 signalling upregulates BCL-X_L and so confers resistance to apoptosis [216].

III. PRION PROTEIN

The prion hypothesis (proteinaceous infectious particles) that spongiform encephalopathies are caused and transmitted by a misfolded prion protein, a protease-resistant protein referred to as PrP^{Sc}, has been accepted for some time, but has not yet been proved. Recent data lead us a step closer to proving the infectivity of prion protein [217-220]. These authors report for the first time that synthetic mammalian prions cause disease when they are transferred to transgenic mice [217]. Two recent papers using yeast system provide also the strongest evidence yet to support the protein-only hypothesis for the transmission of prion diseases. Similar to the events that occur in prion diseases, Sup35 can be converted into an 'infectious' form that can propagate itself and form aggregates — known as amyloids. Cells in which this has occurred are known as [*PSI*$^+$] cells, and can be distinguished from their normal counterparts, [*psi*] cells, by alterations in their colour under certain conditions. The authors used *Escherichia coli* to overexpress a region of Sup35 that is sufficient to stimulate amyloid formation and purified aggregates of this protein. Expression in a bacterial system ensured the absence of any virus from the yeast cells that might be responsible for infectivity. They then used novel methods to deliver the aggregates into [*psi*] cells and showed that this resulted in conversion to the [*PSI*$^+$] state. Protease treatment greatly decreased the infectivity of the aggregates, whereas nuclease treatment had no effect, providing the strongest evidence so far that prion proteins, in the absence of genetic material, are sufficient for infectivity. In addition, it confirms that distinct 'strains' of prion arise in the absence of genetic alterations owing to differences in protein conformation [218-219]. This conformational conversion and subsequent pathologies absolutely require the presence of PrPc since the absence of endogenous PrPc totally precludes the PrP^{Sc}-mediated infectivity and neurotoxicity [220]. We believe that the issue of identifying PrPc function is important because understanding these functions have an impact on the pathophysiological manifestation of prion disease and cancer.

Structure and Location of PrPc

The gene *PRNP* that encodes prion protein is located on human chromosome 20pter-p12, approximately 20 kbp upstream of *PRND* gene which encodes a biochemically and structurally similar protein (Doppel) to the prion protein. *PRNP* gene spans 20 kbp and composed of 2 exons. Mutations in the repeat region as well as elsewhere in *PRNP* gene have been associated with Creutzfeldt-Jakob disease, fatal familial insomnia, Gerstmann-Straussler disease, Huntington disease-like 1, and kuru. Two transcript variants (2479 nucleotides) encoding the same protein have been found for this gene (Sanger Institute- Ensembl Protein Report, 2005). This gene code for the cellular prion protein (PrPc) consists of 253 amino acids (Figure 5), an ubiquitous protein of 32-35 kDa expressed by all known mammals predominantly in the brain, lymphocytes and stroma cells of lymphoid organs [6].

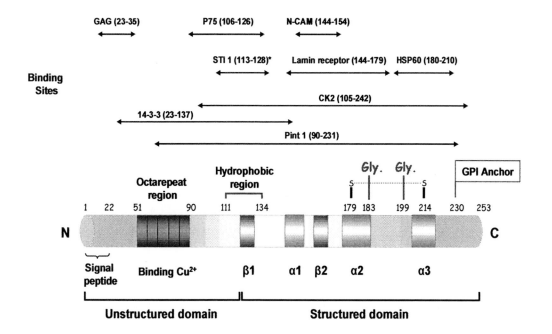

PrPc

Figure 5. Representation of the binding domains of PrPc ligands on the human PrPc molecule. The human PrPc molecule contains a signal peptide (1-22), five octapeptide repeats (51-91), highly conserved hydrophobic domain (106-126), three peptide sequences responsable for α-helix structure (α1-α2-α3), two peptide sequences responsable for β-helix structure, and a signal sequence for GPI anchor (231-254). Double arrows indicated the binding site for each PrPc-binding molecule, which is also represented by amino acid numbers in parentheses and correspond to the mouse PrPc amino acid sequence and to the bovine sequence [242]. Highly conserved octapeptide repeats of PrPc are similar to the BCL2 homology domain 2 (BH2) of BCL2 family proteins. Recently, the 14-3-3-binding domain was located in the N-terminal half of PrPc spanning amino acid residues 23-137[258].

Trafficking of Cellular Prion Proteins

In cells, PrPc is post-translationally processed (posttranslational GPI anchoring, disulfide bonding, glycosylation) and transported along the secretory pathway to the plasma membrane, where it is attached to the cell surface by a glycosylphosphatidylinositol anchor. The PrPc can adopt multiple membrane topologies, including a fully translocated form two transmembrane forms (^{Ntm}PrP and ^{Ctm}PrP), and a cytosolic form [221]. At the plasma membrane PrPc can be constitutively internalised. The route and mechanism of internalization of PrPc are controversial [222]. Seminal studies by Harris and colleagues showed that ectopic expression of chicken PrPc into mouse N2a neuroblastoma cells was internalized via coated pits in a process dependent upon its N-terminal domain [223]. However, the concept that the GPI-anchor determines PrPc trafficking has been challenged. Indeed, Nunziante et al.[224] have shown that mouse PrP in which the N-terminal domain has been substituted by the non-Cu^{2+}-binding *Xenopus* homologue is endocytosed on N2a cells. PrPc endocytosis can also be increased by intercellular Cu^{2+} [223]. In neuronal cells, a major pathway for internalization of PrPc appears to use clathrin-mediated endocytosis. PrPc seems to coexist in the cell surface in raft and non raft components of the membrane (lipid rafts are defined as region of membranes resistant to cold detergent extraction), and it has been suggested that PrPc may leave rafts to be internalizes by coated-pits [225]. In contrast, subsequent studies [226-227], also using N2a cells, have argued that mammalian PrPc is internalized by one of the non-coated pit mechanisms characterized for raft-associated proteins [228-229]. Peters *et al.* using immunoelectron microscopy analysis in CHO cells have shown that PrPc uses an atypical endocytic pathway to reach the lysosomes. This pathway does not involve clathrin-coated vesicles, but contains caveolin-1, a protein that is characteristic of caveolae [230]. Particularly interesting was the demonstration that PrPc interacts functionally with Fyn, in a caveolin-1 manner in 1C11 cells, leading to activation of this tyrosine kinase activity [231]. More recently, Sunyach and collaborators have shown that experimental conditions aimed at blocking endocytosis prevent PrPc internalization and concomitantly abolish PrPc-mediated p53-dependent caspase-3 activation in human cells. Thus, it can be concluded that p53-dependent caspase-3 activation triggered by PrPc is directly dependent upon its endocytosis in human cells lines [232].

It is still unclear whether caveolae-mediated endocytosis is involved in PrPc trafficking in epithelial or/and tumor cells. However, the data raise the possibility that transit through this unusual pathway might be involved in the implication of PrPc in tumor resistance to cell death induced by death receptor ligand.

Signal Transduction of Cellular Prion Proteins

Recent studies have advanced the hypothesis that PrPc may a role in signal transduction (Figure 6). Antibody-mediated PrP dimerization elicits rapid phosphorylation of extracellular regulated kinases 1 and 2 (ERK1/2) in neuron-like cell line and BW5147 lymphoid cells [231]. Particularly interesting was the demonstration that PrPc interacts functionally with Fyn, in a caveolin-1 manner in 1C11 differentiated neuronal cells leading to activation of this tyrosine kinase activity [231-233]. Here it is argued that since ERK1/2 are fully controlled through NADPH oxidase-dependent reactive oxygen species production, PrPc basically functions in maintaining the cellular redox homeostasis [231-233]. In another study, a PrPc binding peptide activated both the ERK- and cAMP-dependent protein kinase A pathway in retinal explants from neonatal mice [9]. Finally, mouse primary cerebellar granule neurons seeded either onto PrPc-coated dishes or onto Chinese hamster ovary cells overexpressing PrPc at their cell surface have increased neurite outgrowth and neuronal survival [234]. Neuronal survival involves the activation of the phosphatidyl-inositol-3-kinase/Akt and the mitogen-activated protein kinase/ERK kinases pathways. PrPc also binds to laminin and this interaction promotes neuritogenesis by a mechanism that could involve the mitogen-activated protein kinase/ERK pathway [234-,35]. Laminin is a major adhesive molecule, and the interaction with PrPc may promote neuronal adhesion. Intracellular endocytosed PrPc may interact with proteins involved in signaling pathways including Grb2, an adaptor protein involved in neuronal survival [236]. As with other GPI-anchor proteins, PrPc can transfer from cell to cell and may transduce signals to a large number of cells [237]. Furthermore, recent findings in neuronal and non-neuronal cell models indicate prion protein association with secreted exosomes. Exosomes are membrane vesicles released into the extracellular environment upon exocytic fusion of multivesicular endosomes with the cell surface. Exosome secretion can be used by cells to eject molecules targeted to intraluminal vesicles of multivesicular bodies, but particular cell types may exploit exosomes as intercellular communication devices for transfer of proteins and lipids among cells [238].

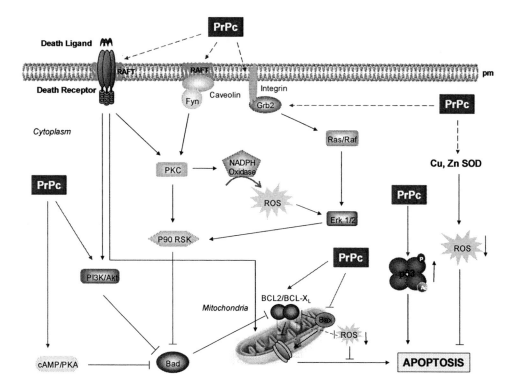

Figure 6. Signaling through PrPc. PrPc by interaction with various partners is involved in apoptosis. PrPc would inhibit the apoptotic process through multiple mechanisms, such as death receptor ligand pathway through interaction with lipid rafts and the endocytosis event, mitochondria pathway through its anti-BAX function and cellular redox homeostasis through decrease of ROS production. Dotted lines indicate the hypothetic involvement of PrPc.

Taken together, these studies indicate that endogenously expressed PrPc can change several intracellular signaling pathways specially involving in cell adhesion, cell trafficking, and transmembrane signaling those to determine cellular survival.

PrPc Protects Human Neurons against Cell Death

Several intriguing lines of evidence have emerged recently indicating that PrPc may function to protect human neurons from various kinds of internal or environmental stress (for review see [12]). The original of a possible PrPc participation in programmed cell death came from the identification of a significant similarity with the BCL2 homology domain 2 (BH2) and its ability to bind to BCL2 in yeast double hybrid approach [239-240]. Particularly, interesting studies from Kuwahara laboratory indicated that PrPc could protect human neurons from serum withdrawal [241] and BAX-induced apoptosis [10]. The octapeptide repeat domain that displays some similarity with the BH2 domain of BCL2 is essential for PrP's neuroprotective function against BAX. Furthermore, familial PrPc mutations D178N and T183A associated with the human prion diseases fatal familial insomnia and familial atypical spongiform encephalopathy partially or completely abolish PrPc anti-BAX function [12]. Therefore, the authors propose that the normal structure of the PrPc is likely important for the anti-BAX function. While PrPc needs to achieve some form of maturity (glycosylation and transport) in for its anti-BAX function, the GPI anchor of PrPc is not required for this function [10]. Furthermore, PrPc expressed uniquely in the cytosol is also able to inhibit BAX [12]. Recently the same laboratory show that PrPc is very specific for BAX and cannot prevent BAK -, tBID-, staurosporine- caspase- or thapsigargin-mediated cell death. PrPc does not colocalize with BAX in normal or apoptotic primary neurons and cannot prevent BAX-mediated cytochrome c release in a mitochondrial cell-free system. PrPc could protects against BAX-mediated cell death by preventing the BAX proapoptotic conformational change that occurs initially in BAX activation [11]. The authors propose that both BCL2 and PrPc maintain BAX in an inactive state and confer neuroprotection. The conversion of PrP into PrP^{Sc} would inactivate antiapoptotic PrP, leaving BCL2 as the only major BAX inhibitor. At this stage the balance between BAX and BCL2 is equilibrated, but neurons would be more sensitive to apoptotic insults . Any further event leading to decreased expression of BCL2 as observed in the aging CNS and loss of PrPc neuroprotective function would increase neurotoxicity [12]. However, expression of PrPc can prevents the release of cytochrome c induced by serum deprivation in hippocampal cell lines HW8-2 and HpL3-4 [242]. Li and collaborators used mouse PrPc containing a modified signal peptide and yeast system to analyse the implication of PrPc in BAX-induced cell death in yeast [243]. The authors found that this PrPc potently suppressed the death of yeast cells expressing mammalian BAX. In contrast, cytosolic PrP-(23–231) failed to rescue growth of BAX-expressing yeast, indicating that protective activity requires targeting of PrPc to the secretory pathway. In opposite to the data of Leblanc's group in neuron cells; the octapeptide repeat domain is not essential for PrPc's neuroprotective function against BAX in yeast system, while a charged region encompassing residues 23–31 is essential for this function. Although *S. cerevisiae* does not contain endogenous *BCL2* family members or caspases, the initial events underlying BAX activity in yeast and mammalian cells are similar, including translocation of the protein to mitochondria, release of cytochrome c, and alterations in mitochondrial function [244]. How does PrPc protect yeast from BAX-induced cell death? In contrast of PrPc's neuroprotective function against BAX which it become from conformational change of Bax directly and its inactivation, in yeast the protective effect of PrPc seems to be related to its interacts with endogenous yeast proteins that lie downstream of BAX in a cellular stress or toxicity pathway.

Another studies show that the PrPc binds to a heat-shock-related protein, stress-inducible protein 1 (STI1) (Figure 5), and that the interaction between these two proteins at the cell surface can rescue cultured retinal cells from apoptosis induced by treatment with anisomycin. A functional role for this interaction is supported by the finding of both proteins on neuronal cell surfaces in the central nervous system. The same research group shows that binding of PrPc by a peptide that recognizes the STI1-binding site (known as PrR) also protects neurons against apoptosis *in vitro*. It goes further to demonstrate that this protection depends on an increase in the levels of cyclic AMP that activates protein kinase A. the first question is how the binding of PrPc at the outer membrane activates adenylyl cyclase, which is normally regulated by G proteins on the inner membrane. We can find a beginning of explanation in the data of Mouillet-Richard *et al* [245]. The authors propose recently that the antibody-mediated ligation of PrPc affects the potency or dynamics of G-protein activation by agonist-bound serotonergic receptors. The PrPc-dependent modulation of 5-HT receptor couplings is restricted to 1C115-HT cells expressing a complete serotonergic phenotype. It critically involves a PrPc-caveolin platform implemented on the neurites of 1C115-HT cells during differentiation. In addition, PrPc-null mice are more susceptible to neuronal loss after experimental brain injury [246]. Examination the phenotype of PrPc-null mice show increased levels of nuclear factor NF-κB and Mn superoxide dismutase, COX-IV, decreased levels of Cu/Zn superoxide dismutase activity, decreased p53, and altered melatonin levels. Additionally, neurons cultured from these animals display abnormalities related to increased susceptibility to oxidative stress [247]. Finally, expression of wild-type PrPc completely abrogates the neurodegenerative phenotype of mice expressing the PrP paralogue, Doppel, or N-terminally truncated forms of PrP (Δ32–121 and Δ32–134) [12, 248-249]. Contradictory results have been reported on phenotype of PrP-null mice. Some studies found no significant abnormalities whereas others reported impairments in neuronal functioning, loss of cerebellar Purkinje cells and defects in sleep patterns and circadian activity. The divergences among PrP-null mice arise from differences in the methods used to suppress protein expression, and more specifically whether the expression of an adjacent PrP homologue protein, Doppel, has been artificially induced in the brain [250]; for more detail see [12].

PrPc and Tumor Resistance

In order to define genetic determinants of tumor cell resistance to the cytotoxic action of TNF, we have applied cDNA microarrays to a human breast carcinoma TNF-sensitive MCF7 cell line and its established TNF-resistant clone. A great number of genes involved in the PI3K/Akt signalling pathway were differentially expressed. Unexpected, endogenous PrPc was found overexpressed at both mRNA (17 fold) and protein levels (10 fold) in TNF-resistant derivative cells as compared to TNF-sensitive MCF7 cell line. The confocal scanning fluorescence analysis showed that PrPc was highly expressed in the Golgi apparatus of TNF-resistant MCF7 cell line (Figure 7A, left). In addition, TNF-resistant MCF7 cells is sensitive to phosphoinositol phospholipase C (PIPLC) treatment confirming that PrPc form is overexpressed at the surface of this tumor cells (Figure 7A, right).

A

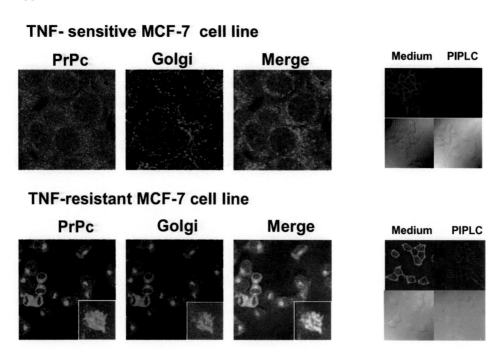

Figure 7A. PrPc protein expression in breast carcinoma cell lines. Confocal microscopy analysis for PrPc localization in breast carcinoma cell line. Left, TNF-sensitive MCF7 and TNF-resistant cell lines were immunostained with either with mouse Pri 308 anti-human PrPc monoclonal antibody (gift from Dr Grassi, CEA, France) or the rabbit RM130 Golgi-specific antibody (gift from Dr Bornons, Institut curie, France). Right: Cells were treated (PIPLC) or not (Medium) with 1 unit/ml PIPLC for 1 h at 37°C, followed by immunofluorescence staining with Pri 308 antibody. Nuclei were counterstained with Topro-3. The confocal scanning fluorescence micrographs are representative for the vast majority of the cells analyzed.

Immunohistochemical staining for PrPc in human breast carcinoma (one hundred patients) showed that PrPc was highly expressed in the tumor cells of 30 % of breast carcinoma and in the myoepithelial cells of all of normal tissue while it was absent in normal luminal cells (Figure 7B).

Examine of a panel of human breast carcinoma cell lines for their sensitivity to TNF and their PrPc expression show a good correlation between susceptibility to the cytotoxic action of TNF and expression for PrPc (Figure 7 C). Furthermore, ectopic expression of human PrPc converted TNF sensitive MCF7 cells into TNF resistant, by a mechanism involving alteration of cytochrome c release from mitochondria and nuclear condensation. These data show for the first time that ectopic expression of PrPc protects breast cancer cell line from TNF mediated cell death, by interfering with mitochondrial pathway and also its involvement in tumor resistance. More recently, Du *et al.* using the adriamycin-senstivie gastric carcinoma cell line SGC7901/ADR and its derivative resistance clone reported that PrPc is also involved in multidrug resistance. Overexpression of PrPc conferred resistance of both P-glycoprotein

(P-gp)-related and P-gp-nonrelated drugs on SGC7901. PrPc knock down expression partially reverse multidrug-resistant phenotype of SGC7901/ADR. PrPc significantly upregulated the expression of the classical MDR-related molecule P-gp but not multidrug resistance associated protein and glutathione S-transferase pi. PrPc could also suppress adriamycin-induced apoptosis and alter the expression of BCL2 and BAX [15].

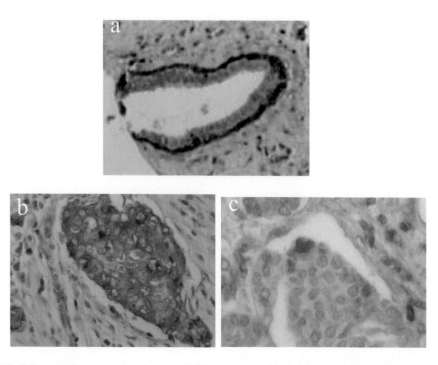

Figure 7B. PrPc protein expression in normal human myoepithelial breast cells and breast carcinoma. Immunohistochemistry analysis for PrPc. Tumor samples were obtained from 100 patients at Institue Gustave Roussy and were immunostained with SAF 69 anti-human PrPc antibody (gift from Dr Grassi, CEA, France). a, normal human breast tissue showing myoepithelial cells positive and luminal negative cells for PrPc. b, tumor tissue showing cancer cells and stromal cells positive for PrPc. c, tumor tissue showing cancer cells negative and stromal cells positive for PrPc. Photomicrographs are representative for the vast majority of the samples analyzed.

On the other hand, we did not observed that PrPc could also suppress adriamycin-induced apoptosis in breast human breast carcinoma cell line (manuscript in preparation). The molecular target of PrPc is unknown. It is quite possible that the antiapoptotic function of PrPc observed in breast adenocarcinoma cells after TNF treatment occurs through its anti-BAX function through BCL2 interaction and BAX conformation change. We can also imagine their involvement in early events in TNFR family signalling, particularly in lipid rafts. More recently, Sunyach and collaborators show that experimental conditions aimed at blocking endocytosis prevent PrPc internalization and concomitantly abolish PrPc-mediated p53-dependent caspase- 3 activation in human cells. Thus, they propose that p53-dependent caspase- 3 activation triggered by PrPc is directly dependent upon its endocytosis in human cells lines [232]. PrPc like 14-3-3 chapron protein and p53 seems to be involved in multiple cellular processes.

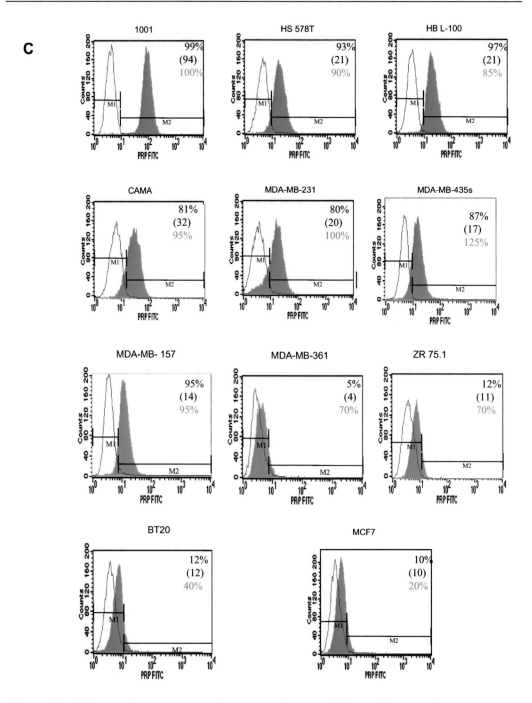

Figure 7C. PrPc protein expression in breast carcinoma cell lines. PrPc protein expression as determined by indirect immunofluorescence analysis using Pri 308 anti-human PrPc monoclonal antibody (green curve). Isotypic IgG1 control was included (open curve). The level of cell surface expression is indicated by the shift of the green curve to the right from the open control curve. Black numbers indicate percentages of positive cells. Numbers in parentheses correspond to mean fluorescence intensity. Cells were also treated or not with TNF (100 ng/ml) for 72 hours and the MTT assays were performed in replicate of three samples. Red numbers indicate percentages of MTT activity.

Nucleus	PrPc	Merge

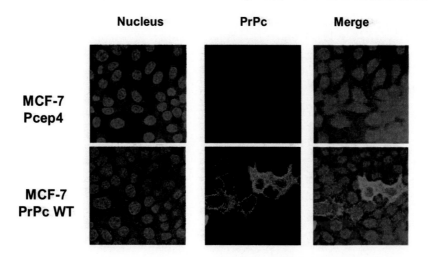

Figure 8. Overexpression of PrPc is not toxic for human breast carcinoma cell-line. The PrPc was expressed by the PrPc Wild type (WT) Pcep4 recombinant vector which encodes the human *PRNP* gene. MCF7 cell line was transfected for 24 hours, followed by immunofluorescence staining using Pri308 monoclonal antibody. Nuclei were counterstained with Topro-3. The confocal scanning fluorescence micrographs are representative for the vast majority of the cells analyzed.

The Protective Function of PrPc: Controversy Story

To our knowledge, normal PrPc has never been shown to be toxic upon overexpression in tumor sample or transfected cells. Therefore, PrPc is not toxic by itself and tumor cell endogenously, transiently or stably overexpressing PrPc can be routinely obtained in laboratories (Figure 8). However, in human embryonic kidney 293 cell line, rabbit epithelial Rov9 cell line, and murine cortical TSM1 cell line, PrPc overexpression increases the susceptibility of these cells to the apoptotic inducer, staurosporine. The authors showed that this cellular response was due to activation of caspase- 3 via transcriptional and post-transcriptional control of the proapoptotic oncogene *p53* [251-252]. These results are in contradiction with reports indicating that the absence of PrPc sensitizes cells to apoptotic stimuli, and also with the fact that activation of ERKs in response to death stimuli is believed to have an antiapoptotic effect. The major cause to explain this discrepancy is that the effect of PrPc may depend on cell type and death stimuli. Recent reports show that BCL2 conformational change occurs during the onset of apoptosis, although it is suggested that this conformational change may be integral property for its antiapoptotic function [253]. Interaction of BCL2 with nuclear orphan receptor may convert the BCL2 from a protector to a killer molecule via conformational change [254]. We propose (Figure 9) that in the cell with BCL2 and PrPc protector both PrPc and BCL2 maintain BAX in an inactive state and confer cell protection. Interaction of BCL2 with PrPc or other factor convert BCL2 from a protector to a killer molecule via conformational change. Among others, BCL2 and BCL-X_L can be cleaved by endogenous caspases to give a potent proapoptotic carboxy-terminal fragment. As a consequence, overexpression of these proteins would accelerate cell death after caspase activation [255]. This hypothesis is in agreement with other reports indicating that the transfection of the BCL2 gene in MCF-7 did not reduce TNF sensitivity [256]. While BCL2 was overexpressed in TNF-sensitive MCF7 cell line, it is downregulated in TNF-resistant MCF7 cell lin [167]. Adenovirus-mediated transfer of wild type p53 gene sensitizes TNF-resistant MCF7 cell line to the cytotoxic action of TNF without affecting the expression of BCL2 level [167]. PrPc like BCL2 may be converted into a lethal protein. PrPc has a caspase-like site at amino acid 145, and it may generate a potent proapoptotic PrPc fragment as seen with the 145 STOP codon mutation that is associated with a vascular form of prion disease [257]. Lastly, it is possible that unknown factors convert PrPc from a protector to a killer molecule via conformational change that induces cell death.

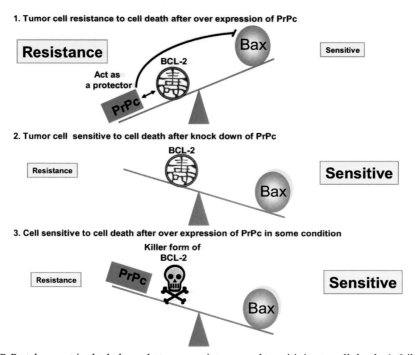

Figure 9. PrPc takes part in the balance between resistance and sensitivity to cell death. 1. Like Roucou et al.[13] we propose that both Bcl-2 and overexpression of PrPc maintain Bax in an inactive form and protect cancer cell from cell death. In some conditions, including Bax expression, serum withdrawal, TNF and anti-cancer drug PrPc overexpression confers resistance to cell death. 2. Cells deficient of PrPc are sensitive to cell death because BCL2 alone can not maintain Bax in an inactive form and protect cancer cell from cell death. 3. In some cells and/or under some death stimuli (for example staursporine), in the presence of PrPc and interaction with some partenaires (for example nuclear orphan recptor), Bcl-2 conformational change, convert the BCL2 protector form to killer form. Cells become sensitives to cell death. In the cell's deficience for PrPc, Bcl-2 conformational change does not happen and cells continue to resist to apoptosis.

CONCLUSION

PrPc, originally considered only involved in prions diseases, now emerges as an important actor that participating in cell death of human normal epithelial and cancer cells. PrPc would regulate the tumor resistance to cell death process through multiple mechanisms, such as death receptor ligand pathway through interaction with lipid rafts and the endocytosis event, mitochondria pathway through its anti-BAX function and cellular redox homeostasis through decrease of ROS production. The challenge is to disentangle this complexity.

ACKNOWLEDGMENTS

We apologize to those investigators whose work was not cited or discussed because of space limitations. We thank the members of our laboratories, past and present, for their support and advice. This work was supported by grants from INSERM, Association pour la Recherche sur le Cancer (grant 3520 to MD). Franck Melin and Ahmed Hamaï are recipients of fellowship from Ligue Nationale Contre le Cancer and canceropole Ile de France, respectively.

REFERENCES

[1]   Hanahan, D. and R.A. Weinberg, The hallmarks of cancer. *Cell,* 2000. 100: p. 57-70.

[2]   Green, D.R. and G.I. Evan, A matter of life and death. *Cancer Cell,* 2002. 1: p. 19-30.

[3]   Johnstone, R.W., A.A. Ruefli, and S.W. Lowe, Apoptosis: a link between cancer genetics and chemotherapy. *Cell,* 2002. 108: p. 153-164.

[4]   Prusiner, S.B., Early evidence that a protease-resistant protein is an active component of the infectious prion. *Cell,* 2004. 116(2 Suppl): p. S109, 1 p following S113.

[5]   Prusiner, S.B., Prions. *Proc Natl Acad Sci U S A,* 1998. 95(23): p. 13363-83.

[6]   Aguzzi, A. and M. Polymenidou, Mammalian prion biology: one century of evolving concepts. *Cell,* 2004. 116(2): p. 313-27.

[7]   Pauly, P.C. and D.A. Harris, Copper stimulates endocytosis of the prion protein. *J Biol Chem,* 1998. 273(50): p. 33107-10.

[8]   Mange, A., et al., PrP-dependent cell adhesion in N2a neuroblastoma cells. *FEBS Lett,* 2002. 514(2-3): p. 159-62.

[9]   Chiarini, L.B., et al., Cellular prion protein transduces neuroprotective signals. *Embo J,* 2002. 21(13): p. 3317-26.

[10]   Bounhar, Y., et al., Prion protein protects human neurons against Bax-mediated apoptosis. *J Biol Chem,* 2001. 276(42): p. 39145-9.

[11]   Roucou, X., et al., Cellular prion protein inhibits proapoptotic Bax conformational change in human neurons and in breast carcinoma MCF-7 cells. *Cell Death Differ,* 2005. 12(7): p. 783-95.

[12]   Roucou, X. and A.C. LeBlanc, Cellular prion protein neuroprotective function: implications in prion diseases. *J Mol Med,* 2005. 83(1): p. 3-11.

[13]   Roucou, X., M. Gains, and A.C. LeBlanc, Neuroprotective functions of prion protein. *J Neurosci Res,* 2004. 75(2): p. 153-61.

[14]   Roucou, X., et al., Cytosolic prion protein is not toxic and protects against Bax-mediated cell death in human primary neurons. *J Biol Chem,* 2003. 278(42): p. 40877-81.

[15] Du, J., et al., Overexpression and significance of prion protein in gastric cancer and multidrug-resistant gastric carcinoma cell line SGC7901/ADR. *Int J Cancer*, 2005. 113(2): p. 213-20.

[16] Diarra-Mehrpour, M., et al., Prion protein prevents human breast carcinoma cell line from tumor necrosis factor alpha-induced cell death. *Cancer Res*, 2004. 64(2): p. 719-27.

[17] Senator, A., et al., Prion protein protects against DNA damage induced by paraquat in cultured cells. *Free Radic Biol Med*, 2004. 37(8): p. 1224-30.

[18] Walczak, H. and P.H. Krammer, The CD95 (APO-1/Fas) and the TRAIL (APO-2L) Apoptosis Systems. *Exp. Cell Res.*, 2000. 256(1): p. 58-66.

[19] Muppidi, J.R., J. Tschopp, and R.M. Siegel, Secondary Complexes and Lipid Rafts in TNF Receptor Family Signal Transduction. *Immunity*, 2004. 21(4): p. 461-465.

[20] Walczak, H., Tumoricidal activity of tumor necrosis factor-related apoptosis- inducing ligand in vivo. *Nature Med.*, 1999. 5: p. 157-163.

[21] Krammer, P.H., CD95(APO-1/Fas)-mediated apoptosis: live and let die. *Adv. Immunol.*, 1999. 71: p. 163-210.

[22] Ashkenazi, A. and V.M. Dixit, Apoptosis control by death and decoy receptors. *Curr Opin Cell Biol*, 1999. 11(2): p. 255-60.

[23] Debatin, K., and and P. Krammer, Death receptors in chemotherapy and cancer. *Oncogene*, 2004. 23(16): p. 2950-66.

[24] Kischkel, F.C., Cytotoxicity-dependent APO-1 (Fas/CD95)-associated proteins form a death-inducing signaling complex (DISC) with the receptor. 1995. 14: p. 5579-5588.

[25] Green, D.R. and T.A. Ferguson, The role of Fas ligand in immune privilege. *Nat Rev Mol Cell Biol*, 2001. 2(12): p. 917-24.

[26] Igney, F.H.a. and P.H. Krammer, Death and anti-death: tumor resistance to apoptosis. *Nature Reviews Cancer Nat Rev Cancer*, 2002. 2(4): p. 277-288.

[27] Roy, S. and D.W. Nicholson, Programmed cell-death regulation: basic mechanisms and therapeutic opportunities. American Association for Cancer Research Special Conference: Lake Tahoe, CA, USA, 27 February-2 March 2000. *Mol Med Today*, 2000. 6(7): p. 264-6.

[28] Eggert A, Grotzer MA , and Z. TJ, Resistance to tumor necrosis factor-related apoptosis-inducing ligand (TRAIL)-induced apoptosis in neuroblastoma cells correlates with a loss of caspase-8 expression. *Cancer Res*, 2001. 61: p. 1314-1319.

[29] Daniel, P.T., et al., The kiss of death: promises and failures of death receptors and ligands in cancer therapy. *Leukemia*, 2001. 15(7): p. 1022-32.

[30] Cowling, V. and J. Downward, Caspase-6 is the direct activator of caspase-8 in the cytochrome *c*-induced apoptosis pathway: absolute requirement for removal of caspase-6 prodomain. *Cell Death Differ*, 2002. 9(10): p. 1046-56.

[31] Zinkel, S.S., A role for proapoptotic BID in the DNA-damage response. *Cell*, 2005. 122: p. 579-591.

[32] Kamer, I., Proapoptotic BID is an ATM effector in the DNA-damage response. *Cell*, 2005. 122: p. 593-603.

[33] Wiley, S.R., et al., Identification and characterization of a new member of the TNF family that induces apoptosis. *Immunity*, 1995. 3(6): p. 673-82.

[34] Danial, N.N. and S.J. Korsmeyer, *Cell*, 2004. 116: p. 205-219.

[35] LeBlanc, H.N. and A. Ashkenazi, Apo2L/TRAIL and its death and decoy receptors. *Cell Death Differ*, 2003. 10(1): p. 66-75.

[36] Van Geelen, C.M.M., E.G.E. de Vries, and S. de Jong, Lessons from TRAIL-resistance mechanisms in colorectal cancer cells: paving the road to patient-tailored therapy. *Drug Resistance Updates*, 2004. 7(6): p. 345-358.

[37] Chaudhary, P.M., et al., Death receptor 5, a new member of the TNFR family, and DR4 induce FADD-dependent apoptosis and activate the NF-kappaB pathway. *Immunity*, 1997. 7(6): p. 821-30.

[38] McDonnell, T.J., BCL-2-immunoglobulin transgenic mice demonstrate extended B cell survival and follicular lymphoproliferation. *Cell*, 1989. 57: p. 79-88.

[39] Pan, G., et al., An antagonist decoy receptor and a death domain-containing receptor for TRAIL. *Science*, 1997. 277(5327): p. 815-8.

[40] MacFarlane, M., et al., Identification and molecular cloning of two novel receptors for the cytotoxic ligand TRAIL. *J Biol Chem*, 1997. 272(41): p. 25417-20.

[41] Walczak, H., et al., TRAIL-R2: a novel apoptosis-mediating receptor for TRAIL. *Embo J*, 1997. 16(17): p. 5386-97.

[42] Wu, G.S., KILLER/DR5 is a DNA damage-inducible p53-regulated death receptor gene. *Nature Genet.*, 1997. 17: p. 141-143.

[43] Debatin, K.M. and P.H. Krammer, Death receptors in chemotherapy and cancer. *Oncogene*, 2004. 23(16): p. 2950-66.

[44] Degli-Esposti, M.A., et al., The novel receptor TRAIL-R4 induces NF-kappaB and protects against TRAIL-mediated apoptosis, yet retains an incomplete death domain. *Immunity*, 1997. 7(6): p. 813-20.

[45] Degli-Esposti, M.A., et al., Cloning and characterization of TRAIL-R3, a novel member of the emerging TRAIL receptor family. *J Exp Med*, 1997. 186(7): p. 1165-70.

[46] Emery, J.G., et al., Osteoprotegerin is a receptor for the cytotoxic ligand TRAIL. *J Biol Chem*, 1998. 273(23): p. 14363-7.

[47] Kischkel FC, et al., Apo2L/TRAIL-dependent recruitment of endogenous FADD and caspase-8 to death receptors 4 and 5. *Immunity*, 2000. 12: p. 611-20.

[48] Micheau, O. and J. Tschopp, Induction of TNF receptor I-mediated apoptosis via two sequential signaling complexes. *Cell*, 2003. 114(2): p. 181-90.

[49] Schneider, P., et al., TRAIL receptors 1 (DR4) and 2 (DR5) signal FADD-dependent apoptosis and activate NF-kappaB. *Immunity*, 1997. 7(6): p. 831-6.

[50] Ozoren, N. and W.S. El-Deiry, Cell surface Death Receptor signaling in normal and cancer cells. *Semin Cancer Biol*, 2003. 13(2): p. 135-47.

[51] Wajant, H., Death receptors. *Essays Biochem*, 2003. 39: p. 53-71.

[52] Barnhart, B.C. and M.E. Peter, The TNF receptor 1: a split personality complex. *Cell*, 2003. 114(2): p. 148-50.

[53] Schutze, S., et al., Inhibition of receptor internalization by monodansylcadaverine selectively blocks p55 tumor necrosis factor receptor death domain signaling. *J Biol Chem*, 1999. 274(15): p. 10203-12.

[54] Legler, D.F., et al., Recruitment of TNF receptor 1 to lipid rafts is essential for TNFalpha-mediated NF-kappaB activation. *Immunity*, 2003. 18(5): p. 655-64.

[55] Schneider-Brachert, W., et al., Compartmentalization of TNF receptor 1 signaling: internalized TNF receptosomes as death signaling vesicles. *Immunity*, 2004. 21(3): p. 415-28.

[56]   Zamzami, N. and G. Kroemer, The mitochondrion in apoptosis: how Pandora's box opens. *Nature Rev. Mol. Cell Biol.*, 2001. 2: p. 67-71.

[57]   Martinou, J.C. and D.R. Green, Breaking the mitochondrial barrier. *Nature Rev. Mol. Cell Biol.*, 2001. 2: p. 63-67.

[58]   Huang, D.C. and A. Strasser, BH3-only proteins-essential initiators of apoptotic cell death. *Cell*, 2000. 103: p. 839-842.

[59]   Du, C., et al., Smac, a mitochondrial protein that promotes cytochrome *c*-dependent caspase activation by eliminating IAP inhibition. *Cell,* 2000. 102(1): p. 33-42.

[60]   Kroemer, G. and J.C. Reed, Mitochondrial control of cell death. *Nat Med*, 2000. 6(5): p. 513-9.

[61]   Li, L.Y., X. Luo, and X. Wang, Endonuclease G is an apoptotic DNase when released from mitochondria. *Nature*, 2001. 412(6842): p. 95-9.

[62]   van Loo, G., et al., The role of mitochondrial factors in apoptosis: a Russian roulette with more than one bullet. *Cell Death Differ*, 2002. 9(10): p. 1031-42.

[63]   Fulda, S., et al., Smac agonists sensitize for Apo2L/TRAIL- or anticancer drug-induced apoptosis and induce regression of malignant glioma in vivo. *Nat Med*, 2002. 8(8): p. 808-15.

[64]   Li, J., et al., Human ovarian cancer and cisplatin resistance: possible role of inhibitor of apoptosis proteins. *Endocrinology*, 2001. 142(1): p. 370-80.

[65]   Ferri, K.F. and G. Kroemer, Control of apoptotic DNA degradation. *Nat Cell Biol*, 2000. 2(4): p. E63-4.

[66]   Kroemer, G. and S.J. Martin, Caspase-independent cell death. 2005. 11(7): p. 725-730.

[67]   Nakagawa, T., et al., Cyclophilin D-dependent mitochondrial permeability transition regulates some necrotic but not apoptotic cell death. *Nature*, 2005. 434(7033): p. 652-8.

[68]   Annis, M.G., et al., Bax forms multispanning monomers that oligomerize to permeabilize membranes during apoptosis. *Embo J*, 2005. 24(12): p. 2096-103.

[69]   Kandasamy, K., et al., Involvement of proapoptotic molecules Bax and Bak in tumor necrosis factor-related apoptosis-inducing ligand (TRAIL)-induced mitochondrial disruption and apoptosis: differential regulation of cytochrome *c* and Smac/DIABLO release. *Cancer Res*, 2003. 63(7): p. 1712-21.

[70]   De Giorgi, F., et al., The permeability transition pore signals apoptosis by directing Bax translocation and multimerization. *Faseb J,* 2002. 16(6): p. 607-9.

[71]   Desagher, S., et al., Bid-induced conformational change of Bax is responsible for mitochondrial cytochrome *c* release during apoptosis. *J Cell Biol*, 1999. 144(5): p. 891-901.

[72]   Kuwana, T., et al., BH3 domains of BH3-only proteins differentially regulate Bax-mediated mitochondrial membrane permeabilization both directly and indirectly. *Mol Cell*, 2005. 17(4): p. 525-35.

[73]   Korsmeyer, S.J., et al., Pro-apoptotic cascade activates BID, which oligomerizes BAK or BAX into pores that result in the release of cytochrome *c*. *Cell Death Differ*, 2000. 7(12): p. 1166-73.

[74]   Shin, M.S., Mutations of tumor necrosis factor-related apoptosis-inducing ligand receptor 1 (TRAIL-R1) and receptor 2 (TRAIL-R2) genes in metastatic breast cancers. *Cancer Res.*, 2001. 61: p. 4942-4946.

[75]   Pai, S.I., Rare loss-of-function mutation of a death receptor gene in head and neck cancer. *Cancer Res*, 1998. 58: p. 3513-3518.

[76] Fisher, M.J., Nucleotide substitution in the ectodomain of trail receptor DR4 is associated with lung cancer and head and neck cancer. *Clin. Cancer Res.*, 2001. 7: p. 1688-1697.

[77] Lee, S.H., Alterations of the DR5/TRAIL receptor 2 gene in non-small cell lung cancers. *Cancer Res.*, 1999. 59: p. 5683-5686.

[78] Mullauer, L., et al., Mutations in apoptosis genes: a pathogenetic factor for human disease. *Mutat Res*, 2001. 488(3): p. 211-31.

[79] Zhang, L. and B. Fang, Mechanisms of resistance to TRAIL-induced apoptosis in cancer. *Cancer Gene Ther*, 2005. 12(3): p. 228-37.

[80] Held, J. and K. Schulze-Osthoff, Potential and caveats of TRAIL in cancer therapy. *Drug Resist Updat*, 2001. 4(4): p. 243-52.

[81] Marsters, S.A., et al., Activation of apoptosis by Apo-2 ligand is independent of FADD but blocked by CrmA. *Curr Biol*, 1996. 6(6): p. 750-2.

[82] Wu, D., H.D. Wallen, and G. Nunez, Interaction and regulation of subcellular localization of CED-4 by CED-9. *Science*, 1997. 275(5303): p. 1126-9.

[83] Petak, I., et al., Hypermethylation of the gene promoter and enhancer region can regulate Fas expression and sensitivity in colon carcinoma. *Cell Death Differ*, 2003. 10(2): p. 211-7.

[84] Hopkins-Donaldson, S., et al., Silencing of death receptor and caspase-8 expression in small cell lung carcinoma cell lines and tumors by DNA methylation. *Cell Death Differ*, 2003. 10(3): p. 356-64.

[85] Cheng, J., Protection from Fas-mediated apoptosis by a soluble form of the Fas molecule. *Science*, 1994. 263: p. 1759-1762.

[86] Midis, G.P., Y. Shen, and L.B. Owen-Schaub, Elevated soluble Fas (sFas) levels in nonhematopoietic human malignancy. *Cancer Res.*, 1996. 56: p. 3870-3874.

[87] Ugurel, S., et al., Increased soluble CD95 (sFas/CD95) serum level correlates with poor prognosis in melanoma patients. *Clin. Cancer Res.*, 2001. 7: p. 1282-1286.

[88] Gerharz, C.D., Resistance to CD95 (APO-1/Fas)-mediated apoptosis in human renal cell carcinomas: an important factor for evasion from negative growth control. *Lab. Invest.*, 1999. 79: p. 1521-1534.

[89] Pitti, R.M., Genomic amplification of a decoy receptor for Fas ligand in lung and colon cancer. *Nature*, 1998. 396: p. 699-703.

[90] Yu, K.Y., A newly identified member of tumor necrosis factor receptor superfamily (TR6) suppresses LIGHT-mediated apoptosis. *J. Biol. Chem.*, 1999. 274: p. 13733-13736.

[91] Roth, W., Soluble decoy receptor 3 is expressed by malignant gliomas and suppresses CD95 ligand-induced apoptosis and chemotaxis. *Cancer Res.*, 2001. 61: p. 2759-2765.

[92] Strand, S., Lymphocyte apoptosis induced by CD95 (APO-1/Fas) ligand-expressing tumor cells - a mechanism of immune evasion? *Nature Med.*, 1996. 2: p. 1361-1366.

[93] Moller, P., Expression of APO-1 (CD95), a member of the NGF/TNF receptor superfamily, in normal and neoplastic colon epithelium. *Int. J. Cancer*, 1994. 57: p. 371-377.

[94] Leithauser, F., Constitutive and induced expression of APO-1, a new member of the nerve growth factor/tumor necrosis factor receptor superfamily, in normal and neoplastic *cells. Lab. Invest.*, 1993. 69: p. 415-429.

[95] Volkmann, M., Loss of CD95 expression is linked to most but not all p53 mutants in European hepatocellular carcinoma. *J. Mol. Med.*, 2001. 79: p. 594-600.

[96] Peli, J., Oncogenic Ras inhibits Fas ligand-mediated apoptosis by downregulating the expression of Fas. *EMBO J.*, 1999. 18: p. 1824-1831.

[97] Maeda, T., Fas gene mutation in the progression of adult T cell leukemia. *J. Exp. Med.*, 1999. 189: p. 1063-1071.

[98] Landowski, T.H., et al., Mutations in the Fas antigen in patients with multiple myeloma. *Blood*, 1997. 90: p. 4266-4270.

[99] Cascino, I., et al., Fas/Apo-1 (CD95) receptor lacking the intracytoplasmic signaling domain protects tumor cells from Fas-mediated apoptosis. *J. Immunol.*, 1996. 156: p. 13-17.

[100] Straus, S.E., The development of lymphomas in families with autoimmune lymphoproliferative syndrome with germline Fas mutations and defective lymphocyte apoptosis. *Blood*, 2001. 98: p. 194-200.

[101] Griffith, T.S., et al., Intracellular regulation of TRAIL-induced apoptosis in human melanoma cells. *J Immunol*, 1998. 161(6): p. 2833-40.

[102] Hao, C., et al., Induction and intracellular regulation of tumor necrosis factor-related apoptosis-inducing ligand (TRAIL) mediated apotosis in human malignant glioma cells. *Cancer Res*, 2001. 61(3): p. 1162-70.

[103] Sprick, M.R., FADD/MORT1 and caspase-8 are recruited to TRAIL receptors 1 and 2 and are essential for apoptosis mediated by TRAIL receptor 2. *Immunity*, 2000. 12: p. 599-609.

[104] Kischkel, F.C., et al., Apo2L/TRAIL-dependent recruitment of endogenous FADD and caspase-8 to death receptors 4 and 5. *Immunity,* 2000. 12(6): p. 611-20.

[105] Truneh, A., et al., Temperature-sensitive differential affinity of TRAIL for its receptors. DR5 is the highest affinity receptor. *J Biol Chem*, 2000. 275(30): p. 23319-25.

[106] Wajant, H., et al., Differential activation of TRAIL-R1 and -2 by soluble and membrane TRAIL allows selective surface antigen-directed activation of TRAIL-R2 by a soluble TRAIL derivative. *Oncogene,* 2001. 20(30): p. 4101-6.

[107] Muhlenbeck, F., et al., The tumor necrosis factor-related apoptosis-inducing ligand receptors TRAIL-R1 and TRAIL-R2 have distinct cross-linking requirements for initiation of apoptosis and are non-redundant in JNK activation. *J Biol Chem*, 2000. 275(41): p. 32208-13.

[108] Zhang, X.D., et al., Differential localization and regulation of death and decoy receptors for TNF-related apoptosis-inducing ligand (TRAIL) in human melanoma cells. *J Immunol,* 2000. 164(8): p. 3961-70.

[109] Zhang, X.D., et al., Mechanisms of resistance of normal cells to TRAIL induced apoptosis vary between different cell types. *FEBS Lett*, 2000. 482(3): p. 193-9.

[110] Jin, Z., et al., Deficient tumor necrosis factor-related apoptosis-inducing ligand (TRAIL) death receptor transport to the cell surface in human colon cancer cells selected for resistance to TRAIL-induced apoptosis. *J Biol Chem*, 2004. 279(34): p. 35829-39.

[111] Delmas, D., et al., Redistribution of CD95, DR4 and DR5 in rafts accounts for the synergistic toxicity of resveratrol and death receptor ligands in colon carcinoma cells. *Oncogene*, 2004. 23(55): p. 8979-86.

[112] Krueger, A., et al., FLICE-inhibitory proteins: regulators of death receptor-mediated apoptosis. *Mol. Cell. Biol.*, 2001. 21: p. 8247-8254.

[113] French, L.E. and J. Tschopp, Defective death receptor signaling as a cause of tumor immune escape. *Semin Cancer Biol*, 2002. 12(1): p. 51-5.

[114] Longley, D.B., et al., c-FLIP inhibits chemotherapy-induced colorectal cancer cell death. *Oncogene*, 2005.

[115] Fulda, S., E. Meyer, and K.M. Debatin, Metabolic inhibitors sensitize for CD95 (APO-1/Fas)-induced apoptosis by down-regulating Fas-associated death domain-like interleukin 1-converting enzyme inhibitory protein expression. *Cancer Res*, 2000. 60(14): p. 3947-56.

[116] Thome, M., Viral FLICE-inhibitory proteins (FLIPs) prevent apoptosis induced by death receptors. *Nature*, 1997. 386: p. 517-521.

[117] Hu, S., et al., I-FLICE, a novel inhibitor of tumor necrosis factor receptor-1- and CD-95-induced apoptosis. *J. Biol. Chem.*, 1997. 272: p. 17255-17257.

[118] Bertin, J., Death effector domain-containing herpesvirus and poxvirus proteins inhibit both Fas- and TNFR1-induced apoptosis. *Proc. Natl Acad. Sci. USA*, 1997. 94: p. 1172-1176.

[119] Sturzl, M., Expression of K13/v-FLIP gene of human herpesvirus 8 and apoptosis in Kaposi's sarcoma spindle cells. J. Natl Cancer Inst., 1999. 91: p. 1725-1733.

[120] Vaux, D.L. and J. Silke, Iaps, Rings and ubiquitylation. Nature Reviews Molecular Cell Biology *Nat Rev Mol Cell Biol, 2005.* 6(4): p. 287-297.

[121] Altieri, D.C., The molecular basis and potential role of survivin in cancer diagnosis and therapy. *Trends Mol. Med.*, 2001. 7: p. 542-547.

[122] Altieri, D.C., Survivin, versatile modulation of cell division and apoptosis in cancer. *Oncogene*, 2003. 22: p. 8581-8589.

[123] Adida, C., et al., Anti-apoptosis gene, survivin, and prognosis of neuroblastoma. *Lancet*, 1998. 351: p. 882-883.

[124] Datta, R., et al., XIAP regulates DNA damage-induced apoptosis downstream of caspase-9 cleavage. *J Biol Chem*, 2000. 275(41): p. 31733-8.

[125] Tamm, I., et al., Peptides targeting caspase inhibitors. *J Biol Chem*, 2003. 278(16): p. 14401-5.

[126] Xu, Y., et al., A mutation found in the promoter region of the human survivin gene is correlated to overexpression of survivin in cancer cells. DNA Cell Biol, 2004. 23(7): p. 419-29.

[127] Chawla-Sarkar, M., et al., Downregulation of Bcl-2, FLIP or IAPs (XIAP and survivin) by siRNAs sensitizes resistant melanoma cells to Apo2L/TRAIL-induced apoptosis. *Cell Death Differ*, 2004. 11(8): p. 915-23.

[128] Griffith, T.S., et al., Induction and regulation of tumor necrosis factor-related apoptosis-inducing ligand/Apo-2 ligand-mediated apoptosis in renal cell carcinoma. *Cancer Res*, 2002. 62(11): p. 3093-9.

[129] Cummins, J.M., et al., X-linked inhibitor of apoptosis protein (XIAP) is a nonredundant modulator of tumor necrosis factor-related apoptosis-inducing ligand (TRAIL)-mediated apoptosis in human cancer cells. *Cancer Res*, 2004. 64(9): p. 3006-8.

[130] Liston, P., Identification of XAF1 as an antagonist of XIAP anti-caspase activity. *Nature Cell Biol.*, 2001. 3: p. 128-133.

[131] Reed, J.C., The Survivin saga goes in vivo. *J. Clin. Invest.*, 2001. 108: p. 965-969.

[132] Ambrosini, G., C. Adida, and D.C. Altieri, A novel anti-apoptosis gene, survivin, expressed in cancer and lymphoma. *Nature Med.*, 1997. 3: p. 917-921.

[133] Grossman, D., Transgenic expression of survivin in keratinocytes counteracts UVB-induced apoptosis and cooperates with loss of p53. *J. Clin. Invest.*, 2001. 108: p. 991-999.

[134] Mesri, M., et al., Cancer gene therapy using a survivin mutant adenovirus. *J. Clin. Invest*, 2001. 108: p. 981-990.

[135] Dierlamm, J., The apoptosis inhibitor gene API2 and a novel 18q gene, MLT, are recurrently rearranged in the t(11;18)(q21;q21) associated with mucosa-associated lymphoid tissue lymphomas. *Blood*, 1999. 93: p. 3601-3609.

[136] Vucic, D., et al., ML-IAP, a novel inhibitor of apoptosis that is preferentially expressed in human melanomas. *Curr. Biol.*, 2000. 10: p. 1359-1366.

[137] Medema, J.P., Blockade of the granzyme B/perforin pathway through overexpression of the serine protease inhibitor PI-9/SPI-6 constitutes a mechanism for immune escape by tumors. *Proc. Natl Acad. Sci. USA*, 2001. 98: p. 11515-11520.

[138] Miyashita, T. and J.C. Reed, BCL-2 gene transfer increases relative resistance of S49.1 and WEHI7.2 lymphoid cells to cell death and DNA fragmentation induced by glucocorticoids and multiple chemotherapeutic drugs. *Cancer Res.*, 1992. 52: p. 5407-5411.

[139] Schmitt, C.A., C.T. Rosenthal, and S.W. Lowe, Genetic analysis of chemoresistance in primary murine lymphomas. *Nature Med.*, 2000. 6: p. 1029-1035.

[140] Findley, H.W., et al., Expression and regulation of BCL-2, BCL-XL, and BAX correlate with p53 status and sensitivity to apoptosis in childhood acute lymphoblastic leukemia. *Blood*, 1997. 89: p. 2986-2993.

[141] Coustan-Smith, E., Clinical relevance of BCL-2 overexpression in childhood acute lymphoblastic leukemia. *Blood*, 1996. 87: p. 1140-1146.

[142] Campos, L., High expression of BCL-2 protein in acute myeloid leukemia cells is associated with poor response to chemotherapy. *Blood*, 1993. 81: p. 3091-3096.

[143] Hermine, O., Prognostic significance of BCL-2 protein expression in aggressive non-Hodgkin's lymphoma. Groupe d'Etude des Lymphomes de l'Adulte (GELA). *Blood*, 1996. 87: p. 265-272.

[144] Tarodi, B., T. Subramanian, and G. Chinnadurai, Epstein-Barr virus BHRF1 protein protects against cell death induced by DNA-damaging agents and heterologous viral infection. *Virology*, 1994. 201: p. 404-40.

[145] Henderson, S., Epstein-Barr virus-coded BHRF1 protein, a viral homologue of Bcl-2, protects human B cells from programmed cell death. *Proc. Natl Acad. Sci. USA*, 1993. 90: p. 8479-8483.

[146] Sarid, R., et al., Kaposi's sarcoma-associated herpesvirus encodes a functional bcl-2 homologue. *Nature Med.*, 1997. 3: p. 293-298.

[147] Boise, L.H., BCL-X, a BCL-2-related gene that functions as a dominant regulator of apoptotic cell death. *Cell*, 1993. 74: p. 597-608.

[148] Dole, M.G., BCL-XL is expressed in neuroblastoma cells and modulates chemotherapy-induced apoptosis. *Cancer Res.*, 1995. 55: p. 2576-2582.

[149] Nagane, M., et al., Drug resistance of human glioblastoma cells conferred by a tumor-specific mutant epidermal growth factor receptor through modulation of BCL-XL and caspase-3-like proteases. *Proc. Natl Acad. Sci. USA*, 1998. 95: p. 5724-5729.

[150] Minn, A.J., et al., Expression of BCL-XL can confer a multidrug resistance phenotype. *Blood*, 1995. 86: p. 1903-1910.

[151] Zhou, P., et al., MCL-1, a BCL-2 family member, delays the death of hematopoietic cells under a variety of apoptosis-inducing conditions. *Blood*, 1997. 89: p. 630-643.

[152] Teitz, T., Caspase-8 is deleted or silenced preferentially in childhood neuroblastomas with amplification of MYCN. *Nature Med.*, 2000. 6: p. 529-535.

[153] Rampino, N., Somatic frameshift mutations in the BAX gene in colon cancers of the microsatellite mutator phenotype. *Science*, 1997. 275: p. 967-969.

[154] Meijerink, J.P., Hematopoietic malignancies demonstrate loss-of-function mutations of BAX. *Blood*, 1998. 91: p. 2991-2997.

[155] Molenaar, J.J., Microsatellite instability and frameshift mutations in BAX and transforming growth factor-[beta] RII genes are very uncommon in acute lymphoblastic leukemia in vivo but not in cell lines. *Blood*, 1998. 92: p. 230-233.

[156] Krajewski, S., Reduced expression of proapoptotic gene BAX is associated with poor response rates to combination chemotherapy and shorter survival in women with metastatic breast adenocarcinoma. *Cancer Res.*, 1995. 55: p. 4471-4478.

[157] Soengas, M.S., Apaf-1 and caspase-9 in p53-dependent apoptosis and tumor inhibition. *Science*, 1999. 284: p. 156-159.

[158] Sarasin, A., An overview of the mechanisms of mutagenesis and carcinogenesis. *Mutat. Res.*, 2003. 544: p. 99-106.

[159] Levine, A.J., p53, the cellular gatekeeper for growth and division. *Cell*, 1997. 88: p. 323-331.

[160] Vousden, K.H. and X. Lu, Live or let die: the cell's response to p53. *Nature Rev. Cancer*, 2002. 2: p. 594-604.

[161] Berube, C., et al., Apoptosis caused by p53-induced protein with death domain (PIDD) depends on the death adapter protein RAIDD. *Proc Natl Acad Sci U S A*, 2005. 102(40): p. 14314-20.

[162] Erster, S. and U.M. Moll, Stress-induced p53 runs a transcription-independent death program. *Biochem Biophys Res Commun*, 2005. 331(3): p. 843-50.

[163] Chipuk, J.E., et al., PUMA couples the nuclear and cytoplasmic proapoptotic function of p53. *Science*, 2005. 309(5741): p. 1732-5.

[164] Lee, J.M. and A. Bernstein, p53 mutations increase resistance to ionizing radiation. *Proc. Natl Acad. Sci. USA*, 1993. 90: p. 5742-5746.

[165] Aas, T., Specific P53 mutations are associated with de novo resistance to doxorubicin in breast cancer patients. *Nature Med.*, 1996. 2: p. 811-814.

[166] Bunz, F., Disruption of p53 in human cancer cells alters the responses to therapeutic agents. *J. Clin. Invest.*, 1999. 104: p. 263-269.

[167] Ameyar, M., et al., Adenovirus-mediated transfer of wild-type p53 gene sensitizes TNF resistant MCF7 derivatives to the cytotoxic effect of this cytokine: relationship with c-myc and Rb. *Oncogene*, 1999. 18(39): p. 5464-72.

[168] Ameyar-Zazoua, M., et al., Wild-type p53 induced sensitization of mutant p53 TNF-resistant cells: role of caspase-8 and mitochondria. *Cancer Gene Ther*, 2002. 9(3): p. 219-27.

[169] Thiery, J., et al., Role of p53 in the sensitization of tumor cells to apoptotic cell death. *Mol Immunol*, 2002. 38(12-13): p. 977-80.

[170] Asgari, K., Inhibition of the growth of pre-established subcutaneous tumor nodules of human prostate cancer cells by single injection of the recombinant adenovirus p53 expression vector. *Int. J. Cancer*, 1997. 71: p. 377-382.

[171] Wang, C.Y., et al., Control of inducible chemoresistance: enhanced anti-tumor therapy through increased apoptosis by inhibition of NF-[kappa]B, *Nature Med.*, 1999. 5: p. 412-417.

[172] Sherr, C.J., The INK4A/ARF network in tumor suppression. *Nature Rev. Mol. Cell Biol.*, 2001. 2: p. 731-737.

[173] Schmitt, C.A., et al., INK4A/ARF mutations accelerate lymphomagenesis and promote chemoresistance by disabling p53. *Genes Dev.*, 1999. 13: p. 2670-2677.

[174] Attardi, L.D., The role of p53-mediated apoptosis as a crucial anti-tumor response to genomic instability: lessons from mouse models. *Mutat. Res.*, 2005. 569: p. 145-157.

[175] Brown, J.M. and L.D. Attardi, The role of apoptosis in cancer development and treatment response. *Nature Reviews Cancer Nat Rev Cancer*, 2005. 5(3): p. 231-237.

[176] Gudkov, A.V. and E.A. Komarova, The role of p53 in determining sensitivity to radiotherapy. *Nature Rev. Cancer*, 2003. 3: p. 117-129.

[177] Cantley, L.C., The phosphoinositide 3-kinase pathway. *Science*, 2002. 296(5573): p. 1655-7.

[178] Baldwin, A.S., Control of oncogenesis and cancer therapy resistance by the transcription factor NF-kappaB. *J Clin Invest*, 2001. 107(3): p. 241-6.

[179] Maehama, T., G.S. Taylor, and J.E. Dixon, PTEN and myotubularin: novel phosphoinositide phosphatases. *Annu Rev Biochem*, 2001. 70: p. 247-79.

[180] Mayo, L.D., et al., PTEN protects p53 from Mdm2 and sensitizes cancer cells to chemotherapy. *J Biol Chem*, 2002. 277(7): p. 5484-9.

[181] Stambolic, V., et al., Regulation of PTEN transcription by p53. *Mol Cell*, 2001. 8(2): p. 317-25.

[182] Birck, A., et al., Mutation and allelic loss of the PTEN/MMAC1 gene in primary and metastatic melanoma biopsies. *J Invest Dermatol*, 2000. 114(2): p. 277-80.

[183] Zhou, X.P., et al., Epigenetic PTEN silencing in malignant melanomas without PTEN mutation. *Am J Pathol*, 2000. 157(4): p. 1123-8.

[184] Whiteman, D.C., et al., Nuclear PTEN expression and clinicopathologic features in a population-based series of primary cutaneous melanoma. *Int J Cancer*, 2002. 99(1): p. 63-7.

[185] Poetsch, M., T. Dittberner, and C. Woenckhaus, PTEN/MMAC1 in malignant melanoma and its importance for tumor progression. *Cancer Genet Cytogenet*, 2001. 125(1): p. 21-6.

[186] Celebi, J.T., et al., Identification of PTEN mutations in metastatic melanoma specimens. *J Med Genet*, 2000. 37(9): p. 653-7.

[187] Guldberg, P., et al., Disruption of the MMAC1/PTEN gene by deletion or mutation is a frequent event in malignant melanoma. *Cancer Res*, 1997. 57(17): p. 3660-3.

[188] Karin, M. and A. Lin, NF-kappaB at the crossroads of life and death. *Nat Immunol*, 2002. 3(3): p. 221-7.

[189] Meyskens, F.L., Jr., et al., Activation of nuclear factor-kappa B in human metastatic melanomacells and the effect of oxidative stress. *Clin Cancer Res*, 1999. 5(5): p. 1197-202.

[190] McNulty, S.E., N.B. Tohidian, and F.L. Meyskens, Jr., RelA, p50 and inhibitor of kappa B alpha are elevated in human metastatic melanoma cells and respond aberrantly to ultraviolet light B. *Pigment Cell Res*, 2001. 14(6): p. 456-65.

[191] Yang, J. and A. Richmond, Constitutive IkappaB kinase activity correlates with nuclear factor-kappaB activation in human melanoma cells. *Cancer Res*, 2001. 61(12): p. 4901-9.

[192] Dhawan, P. and A. Richmond, A novel NF-kappa B-inducing kinase-MAPK signaling pathway upregulates NF-kappa B activity in melanoma cells. *J Biol Chem*, 2002. 277(10): p. 7920-8.

[193] Rayet, B. and C. Gelinas, Aberrant REL/NF-[kappa]B genes and activity in human cancer. *Oncogene*, 1999. 18: p. 6938-6947.

[194] Wood, K.M., M. Roff, and R.T. Hay, Defective I[kappa]B[alpha] in Hodgkin cell lines with constitutively active NF-[kappa]B. *Oncogene*, 1998. 16: p. 2131-2139.

[195] Bentires-Alj, M., et al., Stable inhibition of nuclear factor kappaB in cancer cells does not increase sensitivity to cytotoxic drugs. *Cancer Res*, 1999. 59(4): p. 811-5.

[196] Smyth, M.J., et al., The drug efflux protein, P-glycoprotein, additionally protects drug-resistant tumor cells from multiple forms of caspase-dependent apoptosis. *Proc. Natl Acad. Sci. USA*, 1998. 95: p. 7024-7029.

[197] Gottesman, M.M. and I. Pastan, Biochemistry of multidrug resistance mediated by the multidrug transporter. *Annu Rev Biochem*, 1993. 62: p. 385-427.

[198] Soengas, M. and S. Lowe, Apoptosis and melanoma chemoresistance. *Oncogene*, 2003. 22: p. 3138-3151.

[199] Zhang, K., P. Mack, and K.P. Wong, Glutathione-related mechanisms in cellular resistance to anticancer drugs. *Int J Oncol*, 1998. 12(4): p. 871-82.

[200] Cole, S.P., Overexpression of a transporter gene in a multidrug-resistant human lung cancer cell line. *Science*, 1992. 258: p. 1650-1654.

[201] Ambudkar, S. V., Kimchi-Sarfaty, C., Sauna, Z. E., and Gottesman, M. M. P-glycoprotein: from genomics to mechanism. Oncogene, *22:* 7468-7485, 2003.

[202] Johnstone, R.W., E. Cretney, and M.J. Smyth, P-glycoprotein protects leukemia cells against caspase-dependent, but not caspase-independent, cell death. *Blood*, 1999. 93: p. 1075-1085.

[203] Leslie, E.M., R.G. Deeley, and S.P.C. Cole, Multidrug resistance proteins: role of P-glycoprotein, MRP1, MRP2, and BCRP (ABCG2) in tissue defense. *Toxicology and Applied Pharmacology*, 2005. 204(3): p. 216-237.

[204] Helmbach, H., et al., Drug-resistance in human melanoma. *Int J Cancer*, 2001. 93(5): p. 617-22.

[205] Withoff, S., et al., Human DNA topoisomerase II: biochemistry and role in chemotherapy resistance (review). *Anticancer Res*, 1996. 16(4A): p. 1867-80.

[206] Larsen, A.K. and A. Skladanowski, Cellular resistance to topoisomerase-targeted drugs: from drug uptake to cell death. *Biochim Biophys Acta*, 1998. 1400(1-3): p. 257-74.

[207] Campain, J.A., et al., Acquisition of multiple copies of a mutant topoisomerase IIalpha allele by chromosome 17 aneuploidy is associated with etoposide resistance in human melanoma cell lines. *Somat Cell Mol Genet*, 1995. 21(6): p. 451-71.

[208] Lage, H., et al., Modulation of DNA topoisomerase II activity and expression in melanoma cells with acquired drug resistance. *Br J Cancer*, 2000. 82(2): p. 488-91.

[209] Satherley, K., et al., Relationship between expression of topoisomerase II isoforms and chemosensitivity in choroidal melanoma. *J Pathol*, 2000. 192(2): p. 174-81.

[210] Rass, K., et al., DNA mismatch repair enzyme hMSH2 in malignant melanoma: increased immunoreactivity as compared to acquired melanocytic nevi and strong mRNA expression in melanoma cell lines. *Histochem J*, 2001. 33(8): p. 459-67.

[211] Korabiowska, M., et al., Comparative study of the expression of DNA mismatch repair genes, the adenomatous polyposis coli gene and growth arrest DNA damage genes in melanoma recurrences and metastases. *Melanoma Res*, 2000. 10(6): p. 537-44.

[212] Rieber, M. and M. Strasberg Rieber, Induction of p53 without increase in p21WAF1 in betulinic acid-mediated cell death is preferential for human metastatic melanoma. *DNA Cell Biol*, 1998. 17(5): p. 399-406.

[213] Rieber, M. and M. Strasberg-Rieber, Induction of p53 and melanoma cell death is reciprocal with down-regulation of E2F, cyclin D1 and pRB. *Int J Cancer*, 1998. 76(5): p. 757-60.

[214] Soengas, M.S., Inactivation of the apoptosis effector Apaf-1 in malignant melanoma. *Nature*, 2001. 409: p. 207-211.

[215] Sethi, T., Extracellular matrix proteins protect small cell lung cancer cells against apoptosis: a mechanism for small cell lung cancer growth and drug resistance in vivo. *Nature Med.*, 1999. 5: p. 662-668.

[216] Catlett-Falcone, R., Constitutive activation of STAT3 signaling confers resistance to apoptosis in human U266 myeloma cells. *Immunity*, 1999. 10: p. 105-115.

[217] Legname, G., Synthetic mammalian prions. *Science*, 2004. 305: p. 673-676.

[218] King, C.-Y. and R. Diaz-Avalos, Protein-only transmission of three yeast prion strains. *Nature*, 2004. 428: p. 319-323.

[219] Tanaka, M., et al., Conformational variations in an infectious protein determine prion strain differences. *Nature*, 2004. 428: p. 323-327.

[220] Bueler, H., Mice devoid of PrP are resistant to scrapie. Cell, 1993. 73: p. 1339-1347.

[221] Stewart, G.S., et al., MDC1 is a mediator of the mammalian DNA damage checkpoint. *Nature*, 2003. 421: p. 961-966.

[222] Prado, M.A., et al., PrPc on the road: trafficking of the cellular prion protein. *J Neurochem*, 2004. 88(4): p. 769-81.

[223] Harris, D.A., Trafficking, turnover and membrane topology of PrP. *Br Med Bull*, 2003. 66: p. 71-85.

[224] Nunziante, M., S. Gilch, and H.M. Schatzl, Essential role of the prion protein N terminus in subcellular trafficking and half-life of cellular prion protein. *J Biol Chem*, 2003. 278(6): p. 3726-34.

[225] Sunyach, C., et al., The mechanism of internalization of glycosylphosphatidylinositol-anchored prion protein. *Embo J*, 2003. 22(14): p. 3591-601.

[226] Marella, M., et al., Filipin prevents pathological prion protein accumulation by reducing endocytosis and inducing cellular PrP release. *J Biol Chem*, 2002. 277(28): p. 25457-64.

[227] Kaneko, K., et al., COOH-terminal sequence of the cellular prion protein directs subcellular trafficking and controls conversion into the scrapie isoform. *Proc Natl Acad Sci U S A*, 1997. 94(6): p. 2333-8.

[228] Sabharanjak, S., et al., GPI-anchored proteins are delivered to recycling endosomes via a distinct cdc42-regulated, clathrin-independent pinocytic pathway. *Dev Cell*, 2002. 2(4): p. 411-23.

[229] Johannes, L. and C. Lamaze, Clathrin-dependent or not: is it still the question? *Traffic*, 2002. 3(7): p. 443-51.

[230] Peters, P.J., et al., Trafficking of prion proteins through a caveolae-mediated endosomal pathway. J. Cell Biol., 2003. 162(4): p. 703-717.

[231] Mouillet-Richard, S., Signal transduction through prion protein. *Science,* 2000. 289: p. 1925-1928.

[232] Sunyach, C. and F. Checler, Combined pharmacological, mutational and cell biology approaches indicate that p53-dependent caspase3 activation triggered by cellular prion is dependent on its endocytosis. *Journal of Neurochemistry*, 2005. 92(6): p. 1399-1407.

[233] Schneider, B., et al., NADPH oxidase and extracellular regulated kinases 1/2 are targets of prion protein signaling in neuronal and nonneuronal cells. *Proc Natl Acad Sci U S A*, 2003. 100(23): p. 13326-31.

[234] Chen, S., et al., Prion protein as trans-interacting partner for neurons is involved in neurite outgrowth and neuronal survival. *Mol. Cell. Neurosci.*, 2003. 22: p. 227-233.

[235] Graner, E., Cellular prion protein binds laminin and mediates neuritogenesis. *Mol. Brain Res.*, 2000. 76: p. 85-92.

[236] Spielhaupter, C. and H.M. Schatzl, PrPC directly interacts with proteins involved in signaling pathways. *J Biol Chem*, 2001. 276(48): p. 44604-12.

[237] Liu, T., et al., Intercellular transfer of the cellular prion protein. *J Biol Chem*, 2002. 277(49): p. 47671-8.

[238] Porto-Carreiro, I., et al., Prions and exosomes: from PrPc trafficking to PrPsc propagation. *Blood Cells Mol Dis*, 2005. 35(2): p. 143-8.

[239] Kurschner, C. and J.I. Morgan, Analysis of interaction sites in homo- and heteromeric complexes containing Bcl-2 family members and the cellular prion protein. *Brain Res Mol Brain Res*, 1996. 37(1-2): p. 249-58.

[240] Kurschner, C. and J.I. Morgan, The cellular prion protein (PrP) selectively binds to Bcl-2 in the yeast two-hybrid system. *Brain Res Mol Brain Res*, 1995. 30(1): p. 165-8.

[241] Kuwahara, C., Prions prevent neuronal cell-line death. *Nature*, 1999. 400: p. 225-226.

[242] Kim, B., et al., The cellular prion protein (PrP (C)) prevents apoptotic neuronal cell death and mitochondrial dysfunction induced by serum deprivation. *Brain Res Mol Brain Res*, 2004. 124: p. 40-50.

[243] Li, A. and D.A. Harris, Mammalian prion protein suppresses Bax-induced cell death in yeast. *J Biol Chem*, 2005. 280(17): p. 17430-4.

[244] Zha, H., et al., Structure-function comparisons of the proapoptotic protein Bax in yeast and mammalian cells. *Mol Cell Biol*, 1996. 16(11): p. 6494-508.

[245] Mouillet-Richard, S., et al., Modulation of serotonergic receptor signaling and cross-talk by prion protein. *J Biol Chem*, 2005. 280(6): p. 4592-601.

[246] Hoshino, S., et al., Prions prevent brain damage after experimental brain injury: a preliminary report. *Acta Neurochir Suppl*, 2003. 86: p. 297-9.

[247] Brown, D.R., R.S. Nicholas, and L. Canevari, Lack of prion protein expression results in a neuronal phenotype sensitive to stress. *J Neurosci Res*, 2002. 67(2): p. 211-24.

[248] Shmerling, D., et al., Expression of amino-terminally truncated PrP in the mouse leading to ataxia and specific cerebellar lesions. *Cell,* 1998. 93(2): p. 203-14.

[249] Rossi, D., Onset of ataxia and Purkinje cell loss in PrP null mice inversely correlated with Dpl level in brain. *EMBO J.*, 2001. 20: p. 694-702.

[250] Behrens, A. and A. Aguzzi, Small is not beautiful: antagonizing functions for the prion protein PrP(C) and its homologue Dpl. *Trends Neurosci*, 2002. 25(3): p. 150-4.

[251] Paitel, E., et al., Primary cultured neurons devoid of cellular prion display lower responsiveness to staurosporine through the control of p53 at both transcriptional and post-transcriptional levels. *J Biol Chem*, 2004. 279(1): p. 612-8.

[252] Paitel E, Fahraeus R, and Checler F, Cellular prion protein sensitizes neurons to apoptotic stimuli through Mdm2-regulated and p53-dependent caspase 3-like activation. *J Biol Chem*, 2003. 278: p. 10061-10066.

[253] Kim, P.K., et al., During apoptosis bcl-2 changes membrane topology at both the endoplasmic reticulum and mitochondria. *Mol. Cell*, 2004. 14: p. 523-529.

[254] Lin, B. and e. al., Conversion of Bcl-2 from protector to killer by interaction with nuclear orphan receptor Nur77/TR3. . *Cell* 2004. 116: p. 527-540.

[255] Clem, R., et al., Modulation of cell death by Bcl-XL through caspase interaction. *Proc Natl Acad Sci USA* 1998. 95: p. 554-559.

[256] Vanhaesebroeck, B., et al., Effect of bcl-2 proto-oncogene expression on cellular sensitivity to tumor necrosis factor-mediated cytotoxicity. *Oncogene,* 1993. 8(4): p. 1075-81.

[257] Ghetti B, et al., Vascular variant of prion protein cerebral amyloidosis with tau-positive neurofibrillary tangles: the phenotype of the stop codon 145 mutation in PRNP. *Proc Natl Acad Sci USA* 1996. 93: p. 744-748.

[258] Satoh, J., et al., The 14-3-3 protein detectable in the cerebrospinal fluid of patients with prion-unrelated neurological diseases is expressed constitutively in neurons and glial cells in culture. *Eur. Neurol.*, 1999. 41: p. 216-225.

[259] Weller, M., et al., Protooncogene bcl-2 gene transfer abrogates Fas/APO-1 antibody-mediated apoptosis of human malignant glioma cells and confers resistance to chemotherapeutic drugs and therapeutic irradiation. *J. Clin. Invest.*, 1995. 95: p. 2633-2643.

[260] Kaufmann, S.H., Elevated expression of the apoptotic regulator MCL-1 at the time of leukemic relapse. *Blood,* 1998. 91: p. 991-1000.

[261] Irmler, M., Inhibition of death receptor signals by cellular FLIP. *Nature*, 1997. 388: p. 190-195.

[262] Medema, J.P., Cleavage of FLICE (caspase-8) by granzyme B during cytotoxic T lymphocyte-induced apoptosis. 1997. 27: p. 3492-3498.

[263] Mueller, C.M. and D.W. Scott, Distinct molecular mechanisms of Fas resistance in murine B lymphoma cells. *J. Immunol.*, 2000. 165: p. 1854-1862.

[264] Tepper, C.G. and M.F. Seldin, Modulation of caspase-8 and FLICE-inhibitory protein expression as a potential mechanism of Epstein-Barr virus tumorigenesis in Burkitt's lymphoma. *Blood,* 1999. 94: p. 1727-1737.

[265] Kataoka, T., FLIP prevents apoptosis induced by death receptors but not by perforin/granzyme B, chemotherapeutic drugs, and [gamma] irradiation. J. *Immunol.*, 1998. 161: p. 3936-3942.

[266] Medema, J.P., et al., Immune escape of tumors in vivo by expression of cellular FLICE-inhibitory protein. *J. Exp. Med.*, 1999. 190: p. 1033-1038.

[267] Djerbi, M., The inhibitor of death receptor signaling, FLICE-inhibitory protein defines a new class of tumor progression factors. *J. Exp. Med.*, 1999. 190: p. 1025-1032.

[268] Okada, H. and T.W. Mak, Pathways of apoptotic and non- apoptotic death in tumor cells. *Nature Reviews Cancer Nat Rev Cancer*, 2004. 4(8): p. 592-603.

[269] Amundson, S.A., An informatics approach identifying markers of chemosensitivity in human cancer cell lines. *Cancer Res.*, 2000. 60: p. 6101-6110.

[270] Barrie, M.B., et al., Antiviral cytokines induce hepatic expression of the granzyme B inhibitors, proteinase inhibitor 9 and serine proteinase inhibitor 6. *J Immunol*, 2004. 172(10): p. 6453-9.

[271] Bird, C.H., et al., Selective regulation of apoptosis: the cytotoxic lymphocyte serpin proteinase inhibitor 9 protects against granzyme B-mediated apoptosis without perturbing the Fas cell death pathway. *Mol Cell Biol*, 1998. 18(11): p. 6387-98.

[272] Du, J.P., et al., [The overexpression of prion protein in drug resistant gastric cancer cell line SGC7901/ADR and its significance]. *Zhonghua Yi Xue Za Zhi*, 2003. 83(4): p. 328-32.

[273] Yin, C., et al., Bax suppresses tumorigenesis and stimulates apoptosis in vivo. *Nature,* 1997. 385: p. 637-640.

[274] Bargou, R.C., Overexpression of the death-promoting gene Bax-[alpha] which is downregulated in breast cancer restores sensitivity to different apoptotic stimuli and reduces tumor growth in SCID mice. *J. Clin. Invest.*, 1996. 97: p. 2651-2659.

[275] Ionov, Y., et al., Mutational inactivation of the proapoptotic gene BAX confers selective advantage during tumor clonal evolution. *Proc. Natl Acad. Sci. USA*, 2000. 97: p. 10872-10877.

[276] Ryan, K.M., A.C. Phillips, and K.H. Vousden, Regulation and function of the p53 tumor suppressor protein. *Curr. Opin. Cell Biol.*, 2001. 13: p. 332-337.

[277] Okada, H., Survivin loss in thymocytes triggers p53-mediated growth arrest and p53-independent cell death. *J. Exp. Med.*, 2004. 199: p. 399-410.

[278] Okada, H. and T.W. Mak, Pathways of apoptotic and non-apoptotic death in tumor cells. Nature Rev. *Cancer*, 2004. 4: p. 592-603.

[279] Shatrov, V.A., et al., Adenovirus-mediated wild-type-p53-gene expression sensitizes TNF-resistant tumor cells to TNF-induced cytotoxicity by altering the cellular redox state. *Int J Cancer*, 2000. 85(1): p. 93-7.

[280] Lowe, S.W., p53 status and the efficacy of cancer therapy in vivo. *Science*, 1994. 266: p. 807-810.

[281] Liu, Z.-J., X. Lu, and S. Zhong, ASPP--Apoptotic specific regulator of p53. *Biochimica et Biophysica Acta (BBA) - Reviews on Cancer*, 2005. 1756(1): p. 77-80.

In: Leading Topics in Cancer Research
Editor: Lee P. Jeffries, pp. 193-217

ISBN 1-60021-332-4
© 2007 Nova Science Publishers, Inc.

Chapter 7

POLYUNSATURATED FATTY ACIDS, PEROXIDATION AND CELL DEATH: RELEVANCE TO ATHEROSCLEROSIS AND CANCER

Keri L. H. Carpenter [a], Karin Müller [a], Balaji Muralidhar [a], Iain R. Challis [a], Jeremy N. Skepper [b] and Mark J. Arends [a]*

[a]University of Cambridge, Department of Pathology, Cambridge UK
[b]University of Cambridge, Multi-Imaging Centre, Cambridge, UK

ABSTRACT

Polyunsaturated fatty acids (PUFAs) are necessary for normal cellular function. However PUFAs are prone to peroxidation, which can cause cell death including apoptosis. Susceptibility to peroxidation increases with the degree of unsaturation, i.e. with greater numbers of carbon-carbon double bonds per fatty acid molecule.

Studies of human cancer cell lines treated with PUFAs in vitro demonstrated that apoptosis increased with degree of fatty acid unsaturation. This suggests that the induction of apoptosis is by a peroxidative mechanism. This might translate into an anti-cancer effect in vivo, consistent with epidemiological evidence that diets rich in the highly unsaturated fatty acids, eicosapentaenoic acid (EPA; 20:5, n-3) and docosahexaenoic acid (DHA; 22:6, n-3) correlate with reduced risk of colorectal cancer.

Atherosclerosis is a chronic inflammatory disease. The lipid-rich foam cells of human atherosclerotic lesions are predominantly monocyte-derived macrophages (HMM), and their death contributes to the lipid cores of plaques (advanced lesions). HMM death is implicated in destabilisation of advanced atherosclerotic lesions, leading to plaque rupture with thrombogenic consequences, including cardiovascular events and strokes. In vitro, HMM treated with PUFAs showed a general trend for increasing

---

* Corresponding author. Address for correspondence: University of Cambridge, Department of Neurosurgery, Box 167, Addenbrooke's Hospital, Hills Road, Cambridge CB2 2QQ, UK. Tel: +44 1223 336933; Fax: +44 1223 216926; Email: klc1000@wbic.cam.ac.uk

apoptosis with increasing degree of fatty acid unsaturation, although arachidonic acid (AA; 20:4, n-6) stood out above the trend (in contrast to its behaviour in cancer cell lines) as it induced apoptosis more strongly than both the more highly unsaturated (and more peroxidisable) EPA and DHA. In HMM in vitro, AA-induced apoptosis was diminished by the cyclo-oxygenase inhibitor indomethacin and by the lipoxygenase inhibitor nordihydroguaiaretic acid, suggesting roles for these enzymes in the induction of apoptosis by AA. Moreover 15(S)-hydroperoxy-5,8,11,13-eicosatetraenoic acid was a very strong inducer of apoptosis in HMM, whereas 15(S)-hydroxy-5,8,11,13-eicosatetraenoic acid was innocuous.

A major source of PUFAs in atherosclerosis is plasma low-density lipoprotein (LDL). Much evidence implicates oxidation of LDL in atherogenesis, including the apoptosis-inducing effect of oxidised LDL (oxLDL) on HMM in vitro. LDL oxidation involves peroxidation of the PUFA chains of LDL lipids, which are predominantly esters. Various LDL oxidation products can induce death in HMM in vitro, and radical scavengers such as alpha-tocopherol and BO-653 can prevent both LDL oxidation and the ensuing HMM death. Lipoprotein-associated phospholipase A_2 (Lp-PLA$_2$) is a naturally present LDL-borne enzyme that hydrolyses oxidised phospholipids (but not non-oxidised phospholipids) forming lysophosphatidylcholine and oxidised, non-esterified fatty acids. Treatment of LDL with inhibitors of Lp-PLA$_2$, especially the highly specific inhibitor SB222657, diminished the ensuing HMM death including apoptosis, when the LDL was oxidised and added to HMM in vitro, even though the Lp-PLA$_2$ inhibitors did not diminish LDL oxidation.

These findings may be relevant to potential mechanisms of fatty acid influences on atherosclerosis and cancer and may suggest strategies for combating these diseases.

INTRODUCTION

Cell death, including apoptosis, is an important process in atherosclerosis and cancer, and it also plays an important role in diabetes and a number of obesity-related health problems leading to cardiovascular complications. Whether apoptosis is beneficial or detrimental in atherosclerosis is still debated, whereas in cancer it is the failure of malignant cells to undergo apoptosis that is crucial. In diabetes, the death of pancreatic β-cells is thought to lie at the centre of organ failure. Epidemiological evidence shows that diets rich in polyunsaturated fatty acids (PUFAs), especially eicosapentaenoic acid (EPA) and docosahexaenoic acid (DHA) can protect against cardiovascular risk and cancer, although the mechanisms are often unclear. In contrast, high plasma levels of saturated fatty acids can be toxic, leading to the phenomenon of lipoapoptosis in diabetes and some obesity-related illnesses, which have high risk of cardiovascular complications. Monounsaturated fatty acids (e.g. oleic acid) can in some cases modulate the pro-apoptotic effect of other fatty acids. This article will highlight some of the mechanisms by which PUFAs and saturated fatty acids can induce cell death, including apoptosis, and how this could translate into effects on the above-mentioned diseases, discussing some of the authors' own work as well as that of other researchers.

DIETARY PUFAS: EPIDEMIOLOGICAL EVIDENCE

Polyunsaturated fatty acids (PUFAs) are necessary for normal cellular functions, such as maintaining correct membrane fluidity, cell signalling, and energy storage. However PUFAs are prone to peroxidation, which can cause cell death including apoptosis. Susceptibility to peroxidation increases with the degree of unsaturation, i.e. with greater numbers of carbon-carbon double bonds per fatty acid molecule. Monounsaturates are relatively resistant to peroxidation. PUFAs therefore possess the potential to do harm as well as good in biological systems.

Dietary eicosapentaenoic (EPA; 20:5, n-3) and docosahexaenoic (DHA; 22:6, n-3) have long been considered protective against cardiovascular disease, supported recently by evidence from a patient supplementation study [GISSI-Prevenzione Investigators, 1999], though the mechanisms are not fully understood. Fish oil is a rich source of EPA and DHA. "Mediterranean diets" are also considered to protect against cardiovascular disease. This cuisine traditionally contains olive oil, rich in the monounsaturate oleic acid (OA; 18:1, n-9). Such diets are also rich in natural antioxidants, including vitamin E. Another PUFA component of at least some Mediterranean diets is α-linolenic acid (18:3, n-3), which has been reported to confer protection against cardiovascular disease [de Lorgeril et al. 1994]. Part of α-linolenic acid's effect might be due to its ability to act as a precursor to the longer chain, more highly unsaturated n-3 fatty acids EPA and DHA.

Fish oil fatty acids appear to protect against colorectal, breast and prostate cancer [Bartsch et al. 1999]. Dietary modification to include oily fish, PUFA supplements or functional foods might promote apoptosis of cancer cells or their precursors and prevent tumour development at an early stage. Moreover raising intake of fish oil fatty acids appears beneficial, not only against heart disease and cancer, but also against inflammatory bowel disease and rheumatoid arthritis, with little evidence of adverse side-effects [Connor 2000]. In dietary oils and fats, PUFAs are present predominantly in the form of triglycerides, also termed triacylglycerols. In vivo, PUFAs are found in many forms, including phospholipids, triacylglycerols (and to a lesser extent di- and mono- acylglycerols), cholesterol esters, and non-esterified fatty acids (NEFA), also termed free fatty acids (FFA).

PUFAs (n-3 and n-6) in human plasma and tissues are derived from diet, as mammals cannot synthesise them de novo. In mammals, linoleic acid (LIN; 18:2, n-6) comes from diet, and arachidonic acid (AA; 20:4, n-6) is synthesised by elongation and desaturation of linoleic acid. EPA (20:5, n-3) and DHA (22:6, n-3) can be synthesised from dietary α-linolenic acid (18:3, n-3), and they can also come directly from diet (e.g. oily fish). Plasma fatty acid concentrations are rather variable, depending on diet and the individual fatty acid species in question. For example, in a group of apparently healthy postmenopausal women in the USA, the average plasma level (free plus esterified) of EPA was 110 μM and that of DHA was 283 μM [Wander and Du 2000]. However, in a group of patients in the UK (male and female, average age 69 y) awaiting carotid endarterectomy, the average plasma level of DHA was only a quarter of that of the above-mentioned "healthy" group of USA women (K.L.H. Carpenter and I.R. Challis, unpublished observation). On dietary supplementation with fish oil, at a level equivalent to consumption of ca. 400 g salmon per day (for the particular type of fish oil used in this study, EPA > DHA), the EPA and DHA concentrations (free plus esterified) in plasma of the USA women after 5 weeks rose to 734 μM and 515 μM respectively [Wander and Du 2000].

Understanding the mechanisms by which PUFAs and their products and metabolites induce apoptosis may provide important information relevant to optimising their beneficial effects, and to minimising any adverse effects, in vivo within the general population and possibly also in high-risk subjects and patients.

CELL DEATH AND ATHEROSCLEROTIC PLAQUE DESTABILISATION

Atherosclerosis is a chronic inflammatory disease. Early lesions, termed fatty streaks, consist of clusters of lipid-filled macrophage "foam cells" directly beneath the endothelial surface of the artery wall. In the intermediate stage a fibrous cap consisting of smooth muscle cells and connective tissue starts to develop under the endothelium and over the macrophage foam cells, and some extracellular lipid starts to appear in the core of the lesion. By the advanced stage (plaque) the lesion has a distinct fibrous cap and an acellular lipid core (gruel). Macrophage foam cells at the shoulders of the lesion appear to be dying and spilling their contents into the core. The relative proportions of cap and core vary. Fatty streaks and intermediate lesions are asymptomatic. Advanced lesions are often "silent" also, but in some cases they can be sufficiently large to impede blood flow. Moreover, some advanced plaques are prone to rupture, with serious clinical consequences. Advanced lesions are mostly found at sites of branches (e.g. carotid artery; abdominal aorta) or bends (e.g. coronary arteries) suggesting that haemodynamic stress plays an important role in lesion development.

A major cause of heart attacks and strokes is thrombo-embolism from ruptured atherosclerotic plaques, which exposes highly thrombogenic contents. Plaques with proportionally large lipid cores and thin fibrous caps are unstable and prone to rupture. Conversely, plaques with relatively thick fibrous caps and small lipid cores are more stable. Rupture-prone, unstable plaques contain large lipid deposits within a macrophage infiltrate, which enters from the bloodstream (monocytes) and accumulates at the plaque "shoulder." Macrophages accumulate lipid, forming "foam cells" which die spilling their contents into the core of the lesion, enlarging the lipid pool of the core, and predisposing to haemorrhage and an increase in intra-plaque pressure. Death of smooth muscle cells (SMC) attenuates the fibrous cap, which also contributes to plaque destabilisation. Moreover macrophages can secrete enzymes such as matrix metalloproteinases that can degrade the fibrous cap. Plaques tend to rupture at the shoulder. In cases of sudden coronary death, apoptotic macrophages were found localised at the site of plaque rupture [Kolodgie et al. 2000].

Among the evidence implicating oxidative stress and cell death in atherosclerosis is that oxidised LDL (oxLDL) and lipid oxidation products occur in atherosclerotic lesions [Yla-Herttuala et al. 1989 and 1990; Carpenter et al. 1995; Waddington et al. 2001], and that some of these substances induce death, including apoptosis, in macrophages and SMC [Guyton et al. 1995; Marchant et al. 1995; Hardwick et al. 1996; Siow et al. 1999; Müller et al. 1998; Carpenter et al. 2001 and 2003; Clare et al. 1995; Müller et al. 1996].

PUFAs and Atherosclerosis

Recently, fish-oil (rich in EPA and DHA) supplementation of patients awaiting carotid endarterectomy lowered the number of macrophages within the excised advanced atherosclerotic plaques, relative to plaques from patients supplemented with sunflower oil (rich in LIN) or with control oil (rich in OA and palmitic acid) [Thies et al. 2003]. Also, more of the patients in the fish-oil supplemented group had plaques with thick fibrous caps, and fewer had thin fibrous caps, than the patients in the sunflower and control oil groups. Since macrophages appear to be major contributors to plaque instability, by degrading the fibrous cap, Thies and colleagues [2003] suggested that macrophage death induced by EPA and DHA might be responsible for the lowering in number of macrophages in plaques and hence to a lower proportion of patients with plaques possessing thin fibrous caps. However they also acknowledged that actual mechanisms by which EPA and DHA supplementation might lead to the suggested rise in plaque stability need to be established. Fish-oil supplementation of mildly hypertriacylglycerolaemic men increased the susceptibility of their LDL to ex vivo oxidation [Leigh-Firbank et al. 2002], whilst lowering their plasma concentrations of triacylglycerol (fasting and postprandial) and NEFA (postprandial), raising platelet EPA and DHA content, and decreasing platelet AA content. Whether the effect of EPA and DHA on LDL oxidisability would translate into increased cell-death in atherosclerotic lesions is unknown. Within this context, the balance between PUFAs and natural antioxidants such as tocopherols is likely to be important.

The idea of Thies and colleagues [2003] that macrophage death might be beneficial in advanced lesions is debatable. Above, we have mentioned that apoptotic macrophages have been found at the shoulders of "culprit" ruptured plaques in cases of sudden coronary death [Kolodgie et al. 2000]. Macrophages that die in advanced plaques are incompletely scavenged, evidenced by the detection of apoptotic bodies, which are highly condensed remnants of apoptotic cells [Hegyi et al. 2001]. Moreover the lipid contents of macrophages appear to be spilled to contribute to the acellular "lipid core" (gruel) of the plaque. The unscavenged apoptotic bodies and the extracellular lipid in plaques may constitute inflammatory stimuli that help propagate the chronic inflammatory state of lesions, by activating live macrophages that are in lesions and causing recruitment of monocytes from the bloodstream that once inside the lesion mature into macrophages, accumulate lipid and die, in a vicious cycle.

An alternative explanation for the macrophage-lowering effect of EPA and DHA in lesions is monocyte recruitment to the plaque. 4-Hydroxyhexenal (HHE), produced by peroxidation of n-3 PUFAs, is a weaker chemoattractant for monocytes than is HNE, a peroxidation product of n-6 PUFAs [Müller et al. 1996]. Therefore, although being more peroxidisable, oxidation of EPA-/DHA-rich LDL may produce less chemotactic degradation products than LDL rich in n-6 PUFAs, resulting in decreased monocyte infiltration.

LIPOPROTEIN-ASSOCIATED PHOSPHOLIPASE A₂ AND DEATH OF MONOCYTE-MACROPHAGES

A major source of PUFAs in atherosclerosis is plasma low-density lipoprotein (LDL). Much evidence implicates oxidation of LDL in atherogenesis, including the apoptosis-inducing effect of oxidised LDL (oxLDL) on HMM in vitro. LDL oxidation involves peroxidation of the PUFA chains of LDL lipids, which are predominantly esters. Various LDL oxidation products such as 4-hydroxynonenal (HNE) [Müller et al. 1996], oxysterols [Clare et al. 1995], and lipid hydroperoxides [Muralidhar et al. 2004] can induce death in HMM in vitro. Radical scavengers such as alpha-tocopherol and BO-653 can prevent both LDL oxidation and the ensuing HMM death [Marchant et al. 1995; Müller et al. 1999]. Lipoprotein-associated phospholipase A_2 (Lp-PLA$_2$) is a naturally present LDL-borne enzyme that hydrolyses oxidised phospholipids (but not non-oxidised phospholipids) forming lysophosphatidylcholine and oxidised, non-esterified fatty acids (oxNEFA).

Treatment of LDL with inhibitors of Lp-PLA$_2$ diminished the ensuing toxicity when the LDL was oxidised and added to HMM in vitro, even though the Lp-PLA$_2$ inhibitors did not diminish LDL oxidation [Carpenter et al. 2001]. The inhibitors of Lp-PLA$_2$ were the highly specific SB222657 and the broad-spectrum serine esterase/protease inhibitors Pefabloc and diisopropyl fluorophosphate (DFP), and all of them inhibited the rise in lysophosphatidylcholine levels that occurred when LDL was oxidised in the inhibitors' absence. SB222657 treatment of LDL also diminished oxLDL-induced apoptosis in HMM. In the same study, we also compared the toxicities of lysophosphatidylcholine and a phosphatidylcholine that we chemically synthesised to contain an oxidatively fragmented chain (1-palmitoyl-2-(9-oxononanoyl)-*sn*-glycero-3-phosphocholine), and found that lysophosphatidylcholine was appreciably the more toxic of the two species for HMM. Thus all the evidence suggests that by preserving oxidised phospholipids from hydrolysis, the death-inducing effect of oxidised LDL can be diminished.

We found that a mildly oxidised form of LDL was a stronger death inducer in HMM than a moderately oxidised form of LDL [Carpenter et al. 2003]. This was true for toxicity, measured by lactate dehydrogenase (LDH) release, and also true for apoptosis induction (nucleosome ELISA). The mildly oxidised LDL had a higher hydroperoxide content (FOX assay) than the moderately oxidised LDL, whilst the latter had higher levels of later-stage lipid oxidation products (malondialdehyde and 7-oxysterols) and more negative charge (indicating modification of LDL protein by aldehydes). Inhibition of Lp-PLA$_2$ by the specific inhibitor SB222657 diminished both the LDH release and apoptosis for both the mildly and moderately oxidised LDLs. This observation was consistent with evidence from different experiments [Macphee et al. 1999] that Lp-PLA$_2$ can hydrolyse phospholipids with full-length PUFA-hydroperoxide chains as well as those with oxidatively fragmented PUFA chains. The oxidised non-esterified fatty acid (oxNEFA) fraction arising from Lp-PLA$_2$-mediated hydrolysis of oxLDL has been shown to possess chemoattractant activity for human monocytes, and pretreatment of LDL with SB222657 before oxidation inhibited the subsequent chemoattractant production [Macphee et al. 1999]. The same study established that the oxNEFA fraction was the main chemoattractant (for monocytes) within oxLDL lipids.

Lp-PLA$_2$ has rather permissive substrate requirements [Min et al. 1999 and 2001], so besides hydrolysing oxidised phosphatidylcholine it might also hydrolyse oxidised forms of the less abundant LDL phospholipid classes, and maybe also hydrolyse oxidised tri- and di-acylglycerols.

Experiments with the PPARγ antagonist GW9662, the PPARγ agonist ciglitazone and the Lp-PLA$_2$ inhibitor SB222657 suggested non-hydrolysed, oxidised phospholipids in oxLDL activate PPARγ as a cellular defence mechanism in HMM [Carpenter et al. 2003]. The significance of PPARγ is discussed in more detail below, in the section entitled "PUFAs and activation of peroxisome proliferator activated receptors".

Elevation of plasma Lp-PLA$_2$ has emerged as a novel inflammatory marker for cardiovascular risk, independent of various established risk factors and other markers of inflammation, in several recent studies, reviewed by Macphee et al. [2005]. Also reviewed were some apparent exceptions to this, notably a genetic variant with reduced Lp-PLA$_2$ activity, which may or may not be associated with increased atherosclerosis within the Japanese population. Mature macrophages and to a lesser degree freshly isolated monocytes secrete Lp-PLA$_2$ identical to LDL associated Lp-PLA$_2$ found in plasma [Stafforini et al. 1990; Tjoelker et al. 1995; Hakkinen et al. 1999]. Lp-PLA$_2$ mRNA and protein occur in macrophages in rabbit and human atherosclerotic lesions [Hakkinen et al. 1999]. Moreover, Lp-PLA$_2$ is highly expressed in rupture-prone lesions [Macphee et al. 2005]. Administration of Lp-PLA$_2$ inhibitors to healthy volunteers dose-dependently reduced plasma Lp-PLA$_2$ activity by up to 95 %. Initial clinical studies in patients undergoing carotid endarterectomy suggest that Lp-PLA$_2$ inhibitors (administered for 14 d prior to surgery) can inhibit activity of this enzyme in atherosclerotic lesions and in plasma [Macphee et al. 2005]. Whether Lp-PLA$_2$ inhibitors can confer clinical benefit on cardiovascular outcomes will require further studies, of longer duration.

PUFAs AND DEATH OF MONOCYTE-MACROPHAGES

The pro-apoptotic activity of PUFAs cannot entirely be explained in all cases by peroxidation, formation of reactive oxygen species (ROS) and degradation products. In vitro, HMM treated with PUFAs showed a general trend for increasing apoptosis with increasing degree of fatty acid unsaturation. However, arachidonic acid (AA; 20:4, n-6) stood out above the trend (in contrast to its behaviour in cancer cell lines, see below) as it induced apoptosis more strongly than both the more highly unsaturated (and more peroxidisable) EPA and DHA [Muralidhar et al. 2004], suggesting that other mechanisms for apoptosis-induction by PUFAs were at work. In vivo, PUFAs are also substrates of enzyme complexes, such as cyclooxygenase (COX) and lipoxygenase (LOX). For example, AA is metabolised to prostaglandins, leukotrienes etc. In our study [Muralidhar et al. 2004], AA-induced apoptosis was diminished by the COX inhibitor indomethacin and by the LOX inhibitor nordihydroguaiaretic acid, suggesting roles for these enzymes in the induction of apoptosis by AA. Moreover 15(S)-hydroperoxy-5,8,11,13-eicosatetraenoic acid (15-HPETE) was a very strong inducer of apoptosis in HMM, whereas 15(S)-hydroxy-5,8,11,13-eicosatetraenoic acid (15-HETE) was innocuous. The failure of sulindac (another COX inhibitor) to diminish AA-induced apoptosis might be due to lack of metabolism in vitro to its sulphide form, which is a more active COX inhibitor [Roberts and Morrow 2001].

Indomethacin can inhibit both COX-1 and COX-2, though is reportedly more active against the former [Mitchell et al. 1993]. Interestingly indomethacin was more strongly apoptosis-inducing (for HMM) when added without AA than when AA and indomethacin were added together. Also AA (no indomethacin) was less strongly apoptosis-inducing than indomethacin (no AA). Indomethacin is reported to be an agonist for PPARγ and PPARα [Lehmann et al. 1997] and the COX-2 gene possesses a PPAR response element so is under PPAR control [Pontsler et al. 2002]. Cross-talk between AA, indomethacin, COX-2 and PPAR might thus occur. Since we found that AA was a PPARγ activator in HMM (discussed in the section on PPARγ below), it is thus conceivable that competition between AA and indomethacin might explain the lower apoptosis induction for AA plus indomethacin than for indomethacin alone.

Another possible explanation for indomethacin's inhibitory effect on AA-induced apoptosis could be as follows. COX enzymes (strictly termed prostaglandin endoperoxide H synthases) possess 2 active sites per protein molecule, the cyclooxygenase site (that oxidises AA to PGG_2) and the peroxidase site (that reduces PGG_2 to PGH_2), and NSAIDs such as indomethacin inhibit the cyclooxygenase site but not the peroxidase site [Smith et al. 2000]. The latter site would thus remain capable of reducing, for example, toxic 15-HPETE to innocuous 15-HETE.

Recently, 4-hydroxynonenal (HNE) has been shown to induce COX-2 in a murine macrophage cell line (RAW264.7) [Kumagai et al. 2004]. HNE is a peroxidation product of n-6 PUFAs. Major n-6 PUFAs are linoleic (18:2) and arachidonic (20:4) acids; the latter is the more susceptible to peroxidation. Several other lipid oxidation products, including hydroxy- and hydroperoxy- octadecadienoic acids (peroxidation products of linoleic acid) and 7-ketocholesterol were ineffective at COX-2 induction [Kumagai et al. 2004]. The same study found COX-2 colocalised with HNE in human atherosclerotic lesions. The study thus suggests that lipid peroxidation can promote an inflammatory response, and that in this context HNE may be a significant pro-inflammatory molecule in atherosclerosis.

Various anti-inflammatory agents including indomethacin, and also a selective 15-lipoxygenase inhibitor, were anti-atherogenic in animal models of atherosclerosis [Bailey and Butler 1973; Pratico et al. 2001; Sendobry et al. 1997]. Recently, indomethacin phenethylamide, a highly selective inhibitor for COX-2 in vitro and which also partially inhibited COX-1 in vivo, significantly reduced early and intermediate-stage atherosclerotic lesions in apoE-deficient mice [Burleigh et al. 2005]. COX-1 is found in most tissues and mediates normal function requiring prostaglandin synthesis. COX-2 is induced in inflammation and is expressed in atherosclerotic lesions in humans [Baker et al. 1999; Schonbeck et al. 1999] and mice [Burleigh et al. 2002], in macrophages, smooth muscle cells and endothelial cells. However COX-2 inhibitors to date do not appear to have any clear beneficial effect on atherosclerosis in the advanced stages. Moreover, in patients taking the COX-2 inhibitor Vioxx (rofecoxib), there were increased cardiovascular events, in the Adenomatous Polyp Prevention on Vioxx (APPROVe) trial [Bresalier et al. 2005]. As a consequence, Vioxx was removed from the market. The relationships of COX-1 and COX-2 to atherosclerosis appear complex and incompletely understood.

PUFA-INDUCED APOPTOSIS IN COLORECTAL CANCER CELLS

Consumption of dietary fish-oil, rich in n-3 PUFAs correlates inversely with risk of human colorectal cancer, and this protective relationship has been confirmed in animal models, reviewed by Bartsch et al. [1999]. However the mechanisms are not clear. One possible explanation might be that the fish oil promotes apoptosis (programmed cell death) of colorectal cancer cells or their precursors. Fish-oil is rich in the highly polyunsaturated fatty acids (PUFAs) eicosapentaenoic acid (EPA, 20:5, n-3) and docosahexaenoic acid (DHA, 22:6, n-3).

DHA and EPA are more potent than other less highly unsaturated PUFAs at inducing DNA fragmentation, indicative of apoptosis, in human colorectal cancer cells in culture (M.J. Arends and K. Müller, unpublished data). Oleic acid, a monounsaturate, was innocuous. This structure-activity relationship suggests a peroxidative mechanism of apoptosis induction, as there is a well-known rise in the susceptibility of lipids to peroxidation with increasing degree of unsaturation (i.e. with greater numbers of carbon-carbon double bonds per molecule). Our data for human colorectal cancer cells follow the same pattern of increasing induction of apoptosis in pancreatic cancer and leukaemic cells with increasing degree of unsaturation of PUFAs shown in previous work [Hawkins et al. 1998]. Hence, modulation of the threshold of susceptibility to apoptosis in normal or premalignant colonic cells or induction of apoptosis in colorectal cancer cells via manipulation of fatty acid composition may be a useful chemo-preventative strategy.

Increasing evidence from the literature suggests mitochondria have a co-ordinating role in a common pathway leading to cell death, reviewed by Ferri and Kroemer [2001]. Mitochondria appear capable of acting as responders to changes emanating from the nucleus and from extra-nuclear components of the cell, as well as to changes within the mitochondria themselves. Mitochondrial release of cytochrome c into the cytosol activates a cascade of caspases, including caspase-9 initially and caspase-3 in the execution stages, culminating in apoptosis with caspase-activated DNase bringing about internucleosomal DNA cleavage. The p53 protein acts as a guardian of genomic integrity, which normally responds to DNA damage or oxidative stress by triggering either apoptosis or growth arrest, but which is often mutated in cancer, thereby rendering the cells more resistant to therapy. PUFA-induced peroxidative DNA damage may induce responses by p53-dependent and p53-independent mechanisms, and DNA mismatch repair pathways.

The human colorectal cancer cell lines that we studied were characterised for status of p53 and also for that of mismatch repair (MMR) and chromosomal instability [Abdel-Rahman et al. 2001]. The MMR system, which can respond to oxidative DNA damage [DeWeese et al. 1998] is a complex, multi-enzyme pathway for proof-reading newly-synthesised DNA. The MMR system can become defective as a result of inactivation of any of its components, leading to an inability to repair DNA mismatches and slippage errors leading to changes in length of repetitive sequences that can be detected as microsatellite instability. MMR mutations can be somatic or germ-line, the latter as in Hereditary Non-Polyposis Colorectal Cancer syndrome [Toft and Arends 1998]. The MMR system is capable of acting, at least in part, via p53 to induce apoptosis after DNA damage [Toft et al. 1998 and 1999]. Wild type p53 induces apoptosis via transcriptional activation of a number of genes involved in apoptotic pathways, including members of the Bcl family, such as Bax, which acts through mitochondria. A notable feature of mitochondria is that they possess a characteristic lipid, cardiolipin, which has a naturally high content of PUFA. Peroxidation of cardiolipin appears to promote apoptosis, discussed in more detail in the section entitled "Cardiolipin and apoptosis" below.

In the human colorectal cancer cell lines, the presence of wild-type p53 (p53-wt) promoted PUFA-induced apoptosis, in comparison to mutant p53 (p53-mut). Even so, apoptosis in the p53-mut cell lines incubated with the most highly unsaturated PUFA (DHA; 22:6, n-3) was clearly elevated above background (i.e. the same cell-lines cultured with no additions, or with vehicle control, or with the innocuous monounsaturate oleic acid) indicating p53-independent induction of apoptosis in the p53-mut cell lines. The influence on apoptosis of MMR status appeared subordinate to p53 status. Levels of DNA oxidative damage in PUFA-treated colorectal cancer cell lines, measured as 8-hydroxy-2'-deoxyguanosine (8OHdG) in DNA were consistent with this apoptosis pattern (K.L.H. Carpenter, M.T. O'Connell and M.J. Arends, unpublished data). We also measured 8OHdG in DNA from 17 human colorectal tumours, which had been characterised for MMR status. For the 9 tumours with 8OHdG levels greater than or equal to the median level, incidence of MMR deficiency (evidenced by microsatellite instability in 7 out of 9 tumours) was greater than for the 8 tumours with 8OHdG levels below the median (microsatellite instability in 3 out of 8 tumours).

For all of the human colorectal cancer cell lines tested, the monounsaturate oleic acid (18:1, n-9) was innocuous, and DHA (22:6, n-3) was the most apoptosis-inducing of all the fatty acids tested. The combination of p53-wt with MMR-deficiency (LoVo cell line) appeared to sensitise cells to apoptosis induction by the less potent PUFAs with 2 or 3 carbon-carbon double bonds, i.e. linoleic acid (18:2, n-6) and α-linolenic acid (18:3, n-3), so that apoptosis increased in a linear fashion, when % apoptotic cells (% sub-G_0/G_1 cells) were plotted against number of carbon-carbon double bonds per fatty acid molecule. For the other cell lines, with the combinations p53-wt plus MMR-proficiency (C70), p53-mut plus MMR-deficiency (HCT116), and p53-mut plus MMR-proficiency (HT29), linoleic and α-linolenic acids were, like oleic acid, innocuous, whilst apoptosis was elevated with arachidonic acid (20:4, n-6), eicosapentaenoic acid (20:5, n-3) and docosahexaenoic acid (22:6, n-3), which was the most apoptosis-inducing. The combination of p53-wt with MMR-deficiency thus appears to be overall most susceptible to PUFA-induced apoptosis, and accordingly these cells (LoVo) developed relatively high levels of 8OHdG in response to DHA. Although cell death was not measured directly in parallel to 8OHdG accumulation, these studies suggest that DNA oxidation precedes cell death. These colorectal cancer cell lines are habitually adherent; dead or dying cells tend to detach. The 8OHdG measurements were for adherent cells at 24 or 48 h, times chosen to minimise loss of cells, whereas the cell death measurements were for combined adherent and non-adherent cells after 72 h. Fatty acid concentrations were 200 μM for the apoptosis experiments and 100 or 200 μM for the 8OHdG experiments.

The results for colorectal cancer cells were thus consistent with the idea that lipid peroxidation can promote DNA oxidative damage leading to apoptosis, especially in the presence of p53-wt. The combination of MMR-deficiency with p53-wt permitted accumulation of high levels of 8OHdG in response to polyunsaturated fatty acid and conferred a partial sensitisation to apoptosis. α-Tocopherol (100 μM) inhibited polyunsaturated fatty acid (PUFA)-induced 8OHdG accumulation in colorectal cancer cells (tested in HT29 and HCT116); its effect on cell death was not tested.

The maintenance of normal integrity of colonic crypts involves a balance between proliferation and apoptosis. Proliferation of colorectal crypt cells is elevated in colorectal cancer compared with non-cancer controls [Mills et al. 2001]. Cancer cells have an avid appetite for lipid. Dietary supplementation with DHA and EPA appeared to diminish proliferative activity of crypts in a group of colorectal cancer patients [Huang et al. 1996].

PUFAS AND ACTIVATION OF PEROXISOME PROLIFERATOR ACTIVATED RECEPTORS

Various PUFAs and their oxidation products are able to activate peroxisome proliferator activated receptors (PPARs) [Forman et al. 1997; Kliewer et al. 1997; Nagy et al. 1998]. Three isoforms are known: PPARα, PPARγ and PPARδ (also termed PPARβ). PPARs are ligand-dependent transcription factors belonging to the nuclear hormone gene superfamily, and have many regulatory activities, especially those involving lipid handling. Activation of PPARγ plays an important role in differentiation of adipocytes and of other cell types as well as in glucose utilisation, whilst PPARα target genes are involved in fatty acid catabolism and utilisation. PPARγ activation can also be involved in apoptosis induction, at least partly by negatively interfering with the anti-apoptotic NFκB signalling pathway. NFκB activation appears to play a role in oncogenesis [Baldwin 2001]. The inhibitory effect of PPARγ on NFκB appears to be due to direct interaction between PPARγ and NFκB forming a transcriptionally inactive complex [Chung et al. 2000]. PPARγ may be able to exert an anticancer effect by promoting differentiation and apoptosis. Recently the PPARγ ligand troglitazone was shown to induce apoptosis in liver cancer cells [Toyoda et al. 2002]. Treatment of HT-29 colon cancer cells with ciglitazone, a PPARγ-activator, down-regulated COX-2 expression [Yang and Frucht 2001], which could constitute an anti-cancer mechanism. Although incompletely understood, PPARγ is considered to be a tumour suppressor and anti-inflammatory [Patel et al. 2001], although some exceptions exist in certain animal models [Saez et al. 1998]. PPARδ appears to function mainly as a tumour promotor [Park et al. 2001]. PPARγ is expressed in human colon tumours and appears predominantly non-mutated (51/55 sporadic cases) [Sarraf et al. 1999]. PPARγ has been suggested to be a potential therapeutic target for colon cancer [Yang and Frucht 2001].

In our study of PUFA-induced HMM apoptosis, we tested the effect of the 2 most potent apoptosis inducers (AA and DHA) and the 2 least potent apoptosis inducers (LIN and OA) on PPARγ expression [Muralidhar et al. 2004]. We measured PPARγ at 24 h (an early time point in apoptosis induction preceding execution phase), whereas our apoptosis measurements were at 48 h. We found that AA and DHA significantly increased PPARγ expression in both cytoplasm and nuclei, suggestive of activation, whereas LIN and OA did not increase PPARγ expression, relative to control HMM. We used a well-known PPARγ activator 15-deoxy-delta^{12,14}-prostaglandin J$_2$ (15d-PGJ$_2$) as a positive control, giving increased PPARγ expression in HMM. 15d-PGJ$_2$ is a COX product of AA, and is formed naturally in the resolution phase of inflammation. Whether significant amounts of 15d-PGJ$_2$ arise from AA incubated with HMM in vitro is unknown. We found that 15d-PGJ$_2$ at 1-10 μM for 24 h induced death of HMM [Muralidhar et al. 2004]; our PPARγ measurements were therefore done with 1 μM 15d-PGJ$_2$ at 8 h to minimise loss of cells. Our findings for 15d-PGJ$_2$ were consistent with those of other researchers, who reported that 15d-PGJ$_2$ activated PPARγ and induced apoptosis in HMM at 1 μM for 24 h [Chinetti et al. 1998] and in an endothelial cell line at 10 μM for 20 h [Bishop-Bailey and Hla 1999]. Apoptosis induction by 15d-PGJ$_2$ might not necessarily involve PPARγ. For example, 15d-PGJ$_2$ was reported to induce apoptosis by intracellular ROS production and activation of caspase 3 cascade in HL-60 human leukaemic cells [Chen et al. 2005].

PPARγ activation is, as discussed above, widely regarded as apoptosis-promoting. However, it may in some cases protect against cell death. Ciglitazone and rosiglitazone, both PPARγ activators, had biphasic effects on T-cell death [Wang et al. 2002]. In HMM, ciglitazone was innocuous when tested at 3 μM [Carpenter et al. 2003], its reported EC$_{50}$ for PPARγ activation in CV-1 cells [Willson et al. 1996]. As mentioned earlier, (in the section on Lp-PLA$_2$ and apoptosis) evidence from experiments with appropriate inhibitors of PPARγ and of Lp-PLA$_2$, and activator of PPARγ, suggested that non-hydrolysed oxidised phospholipids in oxLDL appeared to activate PPARγ in a defence mechanism against cell death [Carpenter et al. 2003]. Oxidised alkyl phosphatidylcholine (the *O*-alkyl linkage in the *sn*-1 position, and the oxidised chain ester-linked in the *sn*-2 position), a sub-class of oxidised phosphatidylcholine in oxLDL, can specifically bind to and activate PPARγ [Davies et al. 2001]. The binding appeared a characteristic of the intact (non-hydrolysed) form since oxNEFAs were inefficient competitors. Oxidised phosphatidylcholine can activate PPARα [Lee et al. 2000], but this requires phospholipase A$_2$ activity [Delerive et al. 2000], suggesting that the oxNEFA thereby liberated were the actual PPARα ligands. In our own study [Carpenter et al. 2003] PPARγ thus appears likely to be more important than PPARα in the putative defence mechanism triggered by non-hydrolysed oxidised phosphatidylcholine in HMM.

Atherosclerosis is a chronic inflammatory disease. PPARγ activation in macrophages in vitro has mixed consequences which if true in vivo could be pro- or anti-inflammatory and pro- or anti-atherogenic. These include reduction of inflammatory cytokines [Jiang et al. 1998], inhibition of MMP-9 gelatinolytic activity [Marx et al. 1998], and stimulation of cholesterol efflux via the ABCA1 pathway [Chinetti et al. 2001]. Activation of PPARγ by oxLDL upregulates CD36 (scavenger receptor B), of which oxLDL is a ligand, leading to enhanced uptake [Tontonoz et al. 1998]. This might promote foam cell formation, but appears to be offset by enhanced cholesterol efflux (see above).

PPARγ occurs in macrophages in atherosclerotic lesions, in a pattern highly correlated with oxidation-specific epitopes [Ricote et al. 1998; Marx et al. 1998]. PPARγ activation leading to macrophage apoptosis might be anti-inflammatory and hence anti-atherogenic, particularly as macrophages are able to kill SMC [Boyle et al. 2001] and thereby erode the fibrous cap. However, if apoptotic macrophages are inefficiently scavenged and contribute to the lipid core debris, together with necrotic macrophages, then death induction by peroxidised PUFAs, especially AA, could exert a pro-atherogenic influence. Evidence for the lack of phagocytosis of a proportion of apoptotic bodies is provided by the presence of free, intact, apoptotic bodies within the acellular lipid core of human advanced atherosclerotic lesions [Hegyi et al. 2001]. If, on the other hand, PPARγ activation promotes macrophage survival, then this might result in smaller lipid cores within lesions, and perhaps also less plaque rupture, particularly as macrophage apoptosis at the vulnerable shoulders of plaques was found associated with rupture of "culprit" plaques in sudden coronary death [Kolodgie et al. 2000].

CARDIOLIPIN AND APOPTOSIS

An important component of mitochondria is the phospholipid cardiolipin, which in mammals is virtually unique to mitochondria. It is most abundant in the inner mitochondrial membrane. The fatty acid chains of cardiolipin have a naturally high PUFA content, e.g. bovine heart cardiolipin contains > 80 % linoleic acid. Moreover cardiolipin composition is more responsive than other phospholipids to dietary PUFA in vivo, or supplementation of culture medium with PUFA in vitro. Cardiolipin was enriched to 48 % DHA by dietary fatty acid manipulation in mammals [Berger et al. 1992], and to 50 % DHA in HT-29 colon cancer cells by culturing with 50 μM DHA for 36 h [Watkins et al. 1998]. Cardiolipin fatty acid composition affects electron transport complex activity [Daum 1985], which will affect electron leakage and hence mitochondrial ROS production. HT-29 colorectal cancer cells produced elevated intracellular ROS as a result of DHA enrichment [Watkins et al. 1998]. Raising the degree of unsaturation of the cardiolipin will also increase its susceptibility to peroxidation.

Cytochrome c in the inter-membrane space of mitochondria is bound to native cardiolipin on that face of the inner membrane [Ott et al. 2002]. Peroxidation of cardiolipin releases cytochrome c from the bound state to the free state within the intermembrane space [Ott et al. 2002]. Cardiolipin is a major constituent of contact sites where the inner and outer mitochondrial membranes meet [Lutter et al. 2000 and 2001]. Increasing the PUFA content of cardiolipin appears to favour the formation of contact sites [Gasnier et al. 1998]. Truncated Bid or tBid (a Bcl family member that links the death receptor pathways to the mitochondrial effector mechanisms of apoptosis) appears targeted to cardiolipin at the contact sites, where pores form [Lutter et al. 2000]. It is plausible that cardiolipin might also play a role in permeabilisation of mitochondria by Bax in a similar fashion, since Bax appears to act at contact sites [Doran and Halestrap 2000]. Recently, caspase 2 has been shown to permeabilise the outer mitochondrial membrane and disrupt the binding of cytochrome c to anionic phospholipids, notably cardiolipin [Enoksson et al. 2004].

An interesting paper that supports the pro-apoptotic role of cardiolipin peroxidation is Nomura et al. [2000], entitled: "Mitochondrial phospholipid hydroperoxide glutathione peroxidase inhibits the release of cytochrome c from mitochondria by suppressing the peroxidation of cardiolipin in hypoglycaemia-induced apoptosis". Mitochondria-targeted antioxidants MitoQ and MitoVit E added in vitro were more effective than their untargeted counterparts at protecting Friedreich Ataxia fibroblasts against death induced by intracellular oxidative stress [Jauslin et al. 2003].

Interestingly, palmitic (16:0) and stearic (18:0) fatty acids induced apoptosis in myocytes in vitro, whereas the effect was counteracted by oleic acid (18:1) [de Vries et al. 1997]. These effects could be attributed to alteration of phospholipid membranes, including in mitochondria, though analysis of fatty acid chains was done for total cellular phospholipid, rather than a specific mitochondrial fraction. A complex dynamic mechanism seems to exist linking dietary fatty acid species with mitochondrial structure-function changes and energy metabolism, illustrated by studies in animals by Innis and Clandinin in the 70's and 80's [Renner et al. 1979; Innis and Clandinin 1981a,b,c; Clandinin and Innis 1983]. Interestingly, dietary fatty acid composition seems to influence not only the fatty acid composition of the cardiolipin (the most diet-responsive lipid) and other phospholipids in mitochondria, but also the phospholipid class distribution, e.g. the ratio of cardiolipin to phosphatidylcholine in mitochondria, without affecting the total phospholipid level in mitochondria (micrograms/mg protein).

The issue of variation in cardiolipin relative to phosphatidylcholine is interesting bearing in mind Barth Syndrome, an X-linked cardiomyopathy with abnormal mitochondria. In Barth Syndrome there is a four-fold reduction, compared to normal, in cardiolipin pool size (% of total cellular phospholipids), shown in fibroblasts. This reduction in cardiolipin is due to defective remodelling, i.e. diminished ability to incorporate linoleic acid into phosphatidyl glycerol and cardiolipin after de novo cardiolipin biosynthesis, followed by degradation of the abnormally acetylated cardiolipin [Vreken et al. 2000]. Apart from cardiolipin, there were no other differences between Barth Syndrome and normal, for pool size of any of the other classes of phospholipids (% of total cellular phospholipids).

The defects of Barth Syndrome highlight the requirement for incorporation into cardiolipin of PUFA, principally linoleic acid (18:2, n-6), for normal function of mitochondria. Linoleic acid cannot be biosynthesised by mammals so has to come from diet.

We have already mentioned that cardiolipin is susceptible to auto-oxidation. Notably, the preparation (coating) of plates for testing serum for "anti-phospholipid" and "anti-cardiolipin" antibodies, which are inflammatory markers, involves the drying (overnight at $4^{\circ}C$) of an ethanol solution of cardiolipin, during which time auto-oxidation of the cardiolipin occurs [Horkko et al. 1996]. Monoclonal antibodies to oxLDL also bound to oxidised cardiolipin. Probably this is because anti-phospholipid/anti-cardiolipin and anti-oxLDL antibodies all recognise epitopes of oxidised phospholipid. Possibly, oxidised cardiolipin might constitute an epitope on apoptotic bodies, if leftovers of mitochondria are exposed, which might be pro-inflammatory. Although the vast majority of the literature regards cardiolipin as an exclusively mitochondrial lipid, it has been reported as a minor phospholipid in plasma, where it is carried mostly in LDL [Deguchi et al. 2000]. These authors established that plasma cardiolipin was not due to cell remnants in their samples, and suggested that circulating anti-cardiolipin antibodies might arise as a response to oxidised cardiolipin within LDL. Cardiolipin is susceptible to hydrolysis, at least under some conditions. For example, in kidney homogenates, deacylation of endogenous cardiolipin, by endogenous phospholipases, was described as "the most prevalent lipolytic event" [Helmy et al. 2004]. However, hydrolysis of cardiolipin by endogenous mitochondrial phospholipase A_2 was quoted as being relatively slow compared to hydrolysis of phosphatidylethanolamine [de Winter et al. 1987]. Storage of cardiolipin in solution in chloroform (a solvent that usually contains traces of HCl due to decomposition) resulted in auto-oxidation and hydrolysis [Parinandi et al. 1988]. Whether oxidised cardiolipin is less or more susceptible to hydrolysis than non-oxidised cardiolipin is not known. It cannot be ruled out that oxidised cardiolipin might be susceptible to some kind of phospholipase that hydrolyses oxidised chains but not non-oxidised, like Lp-PLA$_2$, also known as. platelet-activating factor acetylhydrolase (PAF-AH). As mentioned earlier, this enzyme is secreted by monocytes and macrophages, and is carried predominantly on LDL. Moreover, intracellular isoforms of PAF-AH have been reported in the literature, but the area is not well explored, discussed in Carpenter et al. [2001].

TOXICITY OF SATURATED FATTY ACIDS

So far we have focussed on the toxicity of polyunsaturated fatty acids, as a consequence of their susceptibility to peroxidation, as contrasted with the innocuousness of the monounsaturate oleic acid, which is relatively insusceptible to peroxidation. Saturated fatty acids might thus be expected to be innocuous also, as they are not prone to peroxidation. However, perhaps surprisingly, saturated fatty acids are not necessarily innocuous but appear to be involved in the phenomenon of lipoapoptosis as a consequence of inappropriate over-accumulation of saturated fatty acids in non-adipose tissues. In some cases, it appears that over-accumulation of saturates gives rise to increased cellular production of ROS and reactive nitrogen species, as described below. So, paradoxically, abnormal accumulation of non-peroxidisable saturated fatty acids can give rise to increased oxidative stress, which might conceivably in turn damage cellular polyunsaturated fatty acids.

Elevated plasma levels of free fatty acids (FFA; also termed non-esterified fatty acids, NEFA) have been implicated in obesity-associated health risks, such as hyperlipidemia, cardiomyopathy, kidney failure, reproductive disorders, insulin resistance and diabetes. All of these may be caused by the failure of leptin-mediated liporegulation and ensuing lipotoxicity/lipoapoptosis [Unger 2002; Unger and Orici 2002].

Leptin, a hormone produced by adipocytes, is now thought to act by promoting lipid-storage in adipocytes in order to prevent ectopic fat deposition in non-adipose tissues. Genetic disorders can lead to leptin deficiency or tissue non-responsiveness to leptin resulting in intracellular lipid accumulation (steatosis) and ultimately lipotoxicity in non-adipose tissues, associated with dysfunction of pancreatic β-cells, myocardium, kidney and skeletal muscle. In diet-induced obesity, leptin levels initially increase, allowing fat storage in adipose tissues without ectopic fat deposition or adverse effects. However, resistance to leptin activity develops eventually, resulting in ectopic fat storage in non-adipose tissues, lipotoxicity/lipoapoptosis and ultimately organ failure. Several studies suggest that lipoapoptosis results mainly from the accumulation of long-chain fatty acids, particularly saturated fatty acids [Eitel et al. 2002; Maestre et al. 2003; Listenberger et al. 2003; Okuyama et al. 2003; El-Assaad et al. 2003; Welters et al. 2004; Mishra and Simonson 2005].

The loss of pancreatic β-cells is a characteristic of both type 1- and type 2-diabetes. In type 1-diabetes, an autoimmune reaction leads to infiltration of pancreatic islets by macrophages and T-cells, which secrete cytokines, such as IFN-β, IL-1β and TNF-α. This leads to increased nitric oxide production (NO) in pancreatic islets cells and apoptosis. In type 2-diabetes, β-cell death is thought to be mainly due to lipoapoptosis, possibly aggravated by increased plasma glucose levels [Welters et al. 2004]. Saturated fatty acids, mainly palmitate or stearate, have been shown to induce apoptosis in rat INS 832/13 cells and human islet β-cells [Eitel et al. 2002; El-Assaad et al. 2003; Maestre et al. 2003], in the β-cell line HIT-T15 [Okuyama et al. 2003], but also in human mesangial cells [Mishra and Simonson 2005], in human ovarian granuloma cells [Mu et al. 2001], rat testicular Leydig cells [Lu et al. 2003], human breast cancer cells [Hardy et al. 2003] and in CHO cells [Listenberger et al. 2003].

The mechanisms by which saturated fatty acids induce apoptosis are still debated. In β-cells inhibition of FA β-oxidation was shown to aggravate palmitate-induced apoptosis [El-Assaad et al. 2003]. NO synthase inhibitors prevented palmitate-induced toxicity, indicating that nitric oxide production is involved in apoptosis induction [Okuyama et al. 2003]. In INS-1 cells incubation with palmitate led to increased superoxide production, cytochrome c and AIF release into the cytosol and increased bax expression [Maestre et al. 2003]. FFAs induced apoptosis in β-cells also by the induction of an ER-stress response independent of NFκB and nitric oxide formation [Kharroubi et al. 2004]. In CHO cells, palmitate-induced apoptosis was associated with an increase in the generation of ROS and ceramide [Listenberger et al. 2003]. In cardiomyocytes and breast cancer cells palmitate is thought to induce apoptosis by reducing cardiolipin synthesis, [El-Assaad et al. 2003 and refs therein; Hardy et al. 2003]. In human mesangial cells, palmitate and stearate induced apoptosis via caspase-9/3-dependent and -independent pathways. The caspase-9/3-independent pathway was probably mediated by the release of endonuclease G from mitochondria. [Mishra and Simonson 2005]. Palmitate-induced apoptosis *in vitro* can be aggravated by the simultaneous presence of high glucose concentrations [El-Assaad et al. 2003; Okuyama et al. 2003]. Okuyama et al. suggested that palmitate toxicity via increased NO production was aggravated by glucose-induced superoxide production through enhanced cellular formation of toxic peroxynitrite [Okuyama et al. 2003].

In contrast to the toxicity of saturated fatty acids, monounsaturated fatty acids, such as oleate or linoleate, were mostly found to be innocuous or even protected against saturated FA toxicity [Eitel et al. 2002; El-Assaad et al. 2003; Listenberger et al. 2003; Hardy et al. 2003; Welters et al. 2004; Mishra and Simonson 2005].

One possible mechanism for the protective effect of monounsaturated FFA is their stabilizing effect on mitochondria. In the rat β-cell line BRIN-BD11 inhibitor studies showed that the protective effect of palmitoleate could be due to attenuation of cytochrome c release from mitochondria via increases in cardiolipin synthesis [Welters et al. 2004]. In CHO cells, oleate protection was associated with an increased ability of the cells to store FA in the form of neutral lipid, i.e. oleate channels palmitate away from apoptosis-inducing pathways to non-toxic lipid storage pathways. Studies on genetically manipulated cells suggest that endogenous unsaturated FA promote neutral lipid storage. Furthermore, cells with increased neutral lipid storage are resistant to palmitate-induced apoptosis. Alternatively, cells with decreased capacity for triglyceride synthesis are more sensitive to palmitate-induced cell death [Listenberger et al. 2003]. In MDA-MB-231 breast cancer cells treated with palmitate, cardiolipin levels decreased significantly after 4 h, but remained unchanged in oleate-treated cells. Cardiolipin decrease was responsible for the release of cytochrome c and induction of apoptosis. The data indicate that cell survival depends on an adequate pool of unsaturated phospholipids necessary for cardiolipin synthesis. Oleate inhibits palmitate-induced apoptosis, probably by channelling palmitate to inert triglyceride stores and by sustaining CL synthesis [Hardy et al. 2003].

Diabetes therapy aiming at maintaining or restoring the existing β-cell mass could be achieved by β-cell transplantation, β-cell neogenesis, or prevention of β-cell apoptosis. GLP-1 (glucagon-like peptide) and liraglutide (a GLP-1 analogue) blocked the pro-apoptotic activities of both cytokines and fatty acids in rat islet cells. This anti-apoptotic activity of liraglutide was mediated via the GLP-1 receptor. Liraglutide inhibition of apoptosis was not mediated by inhibition of ceramide synthase or by inhibition NO production. Rather, the anti-apoptotic effect of liraglutide was mediated by intracellular cAMP and PI3 kinase activity [Bregenholt et al. 2005]. In the β-cell line RIN m5F, palmitate-induced apoptosis was also inhibited by elevating intracellular cAMP-levels. However, anti-apoptotic activity of cAMP was mediated via protein kinase A at low concentrations and through the cAMP-GEF pathway (cAMP – guanine nucleotide exchange factor) at high concentrations [Kwon et al. 2004]. These results indicate that GLP-1 agonist treatment may be a rational regimen for retaining/restoring pancreatic β-cell mass critical for both type 1 and type 2 diabetes.

Long-term treatment with TZDs (thiazolidinediones) has been shown to result in lowering of FFA levels in plasma, prevention of lipid deposition in β-cells, skeletal muscle, cardiac muscle and liver and in a redistribution of intracellular lipid from insulin-responsive organs to peripheral adipocytes. This also has a positive effect on cardiovascular risk factors, such as endothelial dysfunction, VSMC proliferation, and lipoprotein profile [Wyne 2003].

CONCLUSION

Epidemiological evidence suggests that diets rich in PUFAs, especially EPA and DHA, are beneficial against atherosclerosis and cancer. In vitro work has shown that PUFAs can induce apoptosis by many mechanisms: peroxidation with production of reactive oxygen species and toxic degradation products, formation of pro-apoptotic metabolites via COX and LOX, activation of PPARgamma, or effects on cardiolipin synthesis and oxidisability. Similarly, high levels of saturated fatty acids have been shown to be detrimental to pancreatic beta-cells and can lead to diabetes etc., and in turn to cardiovascular complications. This article highlights the need to tie together in vitro research and in vivo effects, with the view to the development of improved dietary or drug-based strategies for preventing and combating these diseases.

ACKNOWLEDGEMENTS

We thank the British Heart Foundation (KLHC, MJA, KM, IRC), Cancer Research UK (MJA), the Research Advisory Group and Charities Committee of Addenbrooke's Hospital (KLHC, MJA) and the Wellcome Trust (JNS) for financial support.

REFERENCES

Abdel-Rahman WM, Katsura K, Rens W, Gorman PA, Sheer D, Bicknell D, Bodmer WF, Arends MJ, Wyllie AH, Edwards PA. (2001) Spectral karyotyping suggests additional subsets of colorectal cancers characterized by pattern of chromosome rearrangement. *Proc Natl Acad Sci USA* 98:2538-2543.

Bailey JM, Butler J. (1973) Anti-inflammatory drugs in experimental atherosclerosis. I. Relative potencies for inhibiting plaque formation. *Atherosclerosis* 17:515-522.

Baker CS, Hall RJ, Evans TJ, Pomerance A, Maclouf J, Creminon C, Yacoub MH, Polak JM. (1999) Cyclooxygenase-2 is widely expressed in atherosclerotic lesions affecting native and transplanted human coronary arteries and colocalizes with inducible nitric oxide synthase and nitrotyrosine particularly in macrophages. *Arterioscler Thromb Vasc Biol.* 19:646-55.

Baldwin AS. (2001) Control of oncogenesis and cancer therapy resistance by the transcription factor NF-kappaB. *J Clin Invest* 10:241-246.

Bartsch H, Nair J, Owen RW. (1999) Dietary polyunsaturated fatty acids and cancers of the breast and colorectum: emerging evidence for their role as risk modifiers. *Carcinogenesis* 20:2209-18.

Berger A, Gershwin ME, German JB. (1992) Effects of various dietary fats on cardiolipin acyl composition during ontogeny of mice. *Lipids* 27:605-612.

Bishop-Bailey D and Hla T. (1999) Endothelial cell apoptosis induced by the peroxisome proliferator- activated receptor (PPAR) ligand 15-deoxy-delta12, 14-prostaglandin J2. *J Biol Chem* 274: 17042-17048.

Boyle JJ, Bowyer DE, Weissberg PL and Bennett MR. (2001) Human blood-derived macrophages induce apoptosis in human plaque- derived vascular smooth muscle cells by Fas-ligand/Fas interactions. *Arterioscler Thromb Vasc Biol* 21: 1402-1407.

Bregenholt S, Moldrup A, Blume N, Karlsen AE, Friedrichsen BN, Tornhave D, Knudsen LB, Petersen JS. (2005) The long-acting glucagons-like peptide-1 analogue, liraglutide, inhibits β-cell apoptosis in vitro. *Biochem Biophys Res Commun* 330: 577-584.

Bresalier RS, Sandler RS, Quan H, Bolognese JA, Oxenius B, Horgan K, Lines C, Riddell R, Morton D, Lanas A, Konstam MA, Baron JA; Adenomatous Polyp Prevention on Vioxx (APPROVe) Trial Investigators. (2005) Cardiovascular events associated with rofecoxib in a colorectal adenoma chemoprevention trial. *N Engl J Med* 352:1092-102.

Burleigh ME, Babaev VR, Oates JA, Harris RC, Gautam S, Riendeau D, Marnett LJ, Morrow JD, Fazio S, Linton MF. (2002) Cyclooxygenase-2 promotes early atherosclerotic lesion formation in LDL receptor-deficient mice. *Circulation* 105:1816-1823.

Burleigh ME, Babaev VR, Patel MB, Crews BC, Remmel RP, Morrow JD, Oates JA, Marnett LJ, Fazio S, Linton MF. (2005) Inhibition of cyclooxygenase with indomethacin phenethylamide reduces atherosclerosis in apoE-null mice. *Biochem Pharmacol* 70:334-342.

Carpenter KL, Challis IR, Arends MJ. (2003) Mildly oxidised LDL induces more macrophage death than moderately oxidised LDL: roles of peroxidation, lipoprotein-associated phospholipase A_2 and PPARgamma. *FEBS Lett* 553:145-150.

Carpenter KL, Dennis IF, Challis IR, Osborn DP, Macphee CH, Leake DS, Arends MJ, Mitchinson MJ. (2001) Inhibition of lipoprotein-associated phospholipase A_2 diminishes the death-inducing effects of oxidised LDL on human monocyte macrophages. *FEBS Lett* 505:357-363.

Carpenter KL, Taylor SE, van der Veen C, Williamson BK, Ballantine JA, Mitchinson MJ. (1995) Lipids and oxidised lipids in human atherosclerotic lesions at different stages of development. *Biochim Biophys Acta* 1256:141-150.

Chen YC, Shen SC, Tsai SH. (2005) Prostaglandin D(2) and J(2) induce apoptosis in human leukemia cells via activation of the caspase 3 cascade and production of reactive oxygen species. *Biochim Biophys Acta* 1743:291-304.

Chinetti G, Griglio S, Antonucci M, Torra IP, Delerive P, Majd Z, Fruchart JC, Chapman J, Najib J, Staels B. (1998) Activation of proliferator-activated receptors alpha and gamma induces apoptosis of human monocyte-derived macrophages. *J Biol Chem* 273:25573-25580.

Chinetti G, Lestavel S, Bocher V, Remaley AT, Neve B, Torra IP, Teissier E, Minnich A, Jaye M, Duverger N, Brewer HB, Fruchart JC, Clavey V and Staels B. (2001) PPAR-alpha and PPAR-gamma activators induce cholesterol removal from human macrophage foam cells through stimulation of the ABCA1 pathway. *Nat Med* 7: 53-58.

Chung SW, Kang BY, Kim SH, Pak YK, Cho D, Trinchieri G and Kim TS. (2000) Oxidized low density lipoprotein inhibits interleukin-12 production in lipopolysaccharide-activated mouse macrophages via direct interactions between peroxisome proliferator-activated receptor-gamma and nuclear factor-kappa B. *J Biol Chem* 275: 32681-32687.

Clandinin MT, Innis SM. (1983) Does mitochondrial ATP synthesis decline as a function of change in the membrane environment with ageing. *Mech Ageing Dev.* 22:205-8.

Clare K, Hardwick SJ, Carpenter KL, Weeratunge N, Mitchinson MJ. (1995) Toxicity of oxysterols to human monocyte-macrophages. *Atherosclerosis* 118:67-75.

Connor WE. (2000) Importance of n-3 fatty acids in health and disease. *Am J Clin Nutr* 71(suppl) 171S-175S.

Daum G. (1985) Lipids of mitochondria. *Biochim Biophys Acta* 822:1-42.

Davies SS, Pontsler AV, Marathe GK, Harrison KA, Murphy RC, Hinshaw JC, Prestwich GD, Hilaire AS, Prescott SM, Zimmerman GA, McIntyre TM. (2001) Oxidized alkyl phospholipids are specific, high affinity peroxisome proliferator-activated receptor gamma ligands and agonists. *J Biol Chem* 276:16015-23.

Davies SS, Pontsler AV, Marathe GK, Harrison KA, Murphy RC, Hinshaw JC, Prestwich GD, Hilaire AS, Prescott SM, Zimmerman GA, McIntyre TM. (2001) Oxidized alkyl phospholipids are specific, high affinity peroxisome proliferator-activated receptor gamma ligands and agonists. *J Biol Chem* 276: 16015-23.

de Lorgeril M, Renaud S, Mamelle N, Salen P, Martin JL, Monjaud I, Guidollet J, Touboul P, Delaye J. (1994) Mediterranean alpha-linolenic acid-rich diet in secondary prevention of coronary heart disease. *Lancet* 343:1454-9.

de Vries JE, Vork MM, Roemen TH, de Jong YF, Cleutjens JP, van der Vusse GJ, van Bilsen M. (1997) Saturated but not mono-unsaturated fatty acids induce apoptotic cell death in neonatal rat ventricular myocytes. *J Lipid Res.* 38:1384-94.

de Winter JM, Lenting HB, Neys FW, van den Bosch H. (1987) Hydrolysis of membrane-associated phosphoglycerides by mitochondrial phospholipase A$_2$. *Biochim Biophys Acta.* 917:169 -77.

Deguchi H, Fernandez JA, Hackeng TM, Banka CL, Griffin JH. (2000) Cardiolipin is a normal component of human plasma lipoproteins. *Proc Natl Acad Sci USA.* 97:1743-8.

Delerive P, Furman C, Teissier E, Fruchart J, Duriez P, Staels B. (2000) Oxidized phospholipids activate PPARalpha in a phospholipase A$_2$-dependent manner. *FEBS Lett.* 471:34-8.

DeWeese TL, Shipman JM, Larrier NA, Buckley NM, Kidd LR, Groopman JD, Cutler RG, te Riele H, Nelson WG. (1998) Mouse embryonic stem cells carrying one or two defective Msh2 alleles respond abnormally to oxidative stress inflicted by low-level radiation. *Proc Natl Acad Sci USA* 95:11915-20.

Doran E, Halestrap AP. (2000) Cytochrome c release from isolated rat liver mitochondria can occur independently of outer-membrane rupture: possible role of contact sites. *Biochem J* 348 Pt 2:343-50.

Eitel K, Staiger H, Brendel MD, Brandhorst D, Bretzel RG, Häring H-U, Kellerer M. (2002) Different role of saturated and unsaturated fatty acids in β-cell apoptosis. *Biochem Biophys Res Comm* 299: 853-856.

El-Assaad W, Buteau J, Peyot M-L, Nolan C, Roduit R, Hardy S, Joly E, Dbaibo G, Rosenberg L, Prentki M. (2003) Saturated fatty acids synergize with elevated glucose to cause pancreatic β-cell death. *Endocrinology* 144: 4154-4163.

Enoksson M, Robertson JD, Gogvadze V, Bu P, Kropotov A, Zhivotovsky B, Orrenius S. (2004) Caspase-2 permeabilizes the outer mitochondrial membrane and disrupts the binding of cytochrome c to anionic phospholipids. *J Biol Chem.* 279:49575-8.

Ferri KF and Kroemer G. (2001) Organelle-specific initiation of cell death pathways. *Nature Cell Biology* 3: E255-E263.

Forman BM, Chen J and Evans RM. (1997) Hypolipidemic drugs, polyunsaturated fatty acids, and eicosanoids are ligands for peroxisome proliferator-activated receptors alpha and delta. *Proc Natl Acad Sci USA* 94: 4312-4317.

Gasnier F, Rey C, Hellio Le Graverand MP, Benahmed M, Louisot P. (1998) Hormone-induced changes in cardiolipin from Leydig cells: possible involvement in intramitochondrial cholesterol translocation. *Biochem Mol Biol Int* 45:93-100.

GISSI-Prevenzione Investigators. (1999) Dietary supplementation with n-3 polyunsaturated fatty acids and vitamin E after myocardial infarction: results of the GISSI-Prevenzione trial. *Lancet* 354: 447-455.

Guyton JR, Lenz ML, Mathews B, Hughes H, Karsan D, Selinger E, Smith CV. (1995) Toxicity of oxidized low density lipoproteins for vascular smooth muscle cells and partial protection by antioxidants. *Atherosclerosis* 118:237-249.

Hakkinen T, Luoma JS, Hiltunen MO, Macphee CH, Milliner KJ, Patel L, Rice SQ, Tew DG, Karkola K, Yla-Herttuala S. (1999) Lipoprotein-associated phospholipase A_2, platelet-activating factor acetylhydrolase, is expressed by macrophages in human and rabbit atherosclerotic lesions. *Arterioscler Thromb Vasc Biol* 19: 2909-17.

Hardwick SJ, Hegyi L, Clare K, Law NS, Carpenter KL, Mitchinson MJ, Skepper JN. (1996) Apoptosis in human monocyte-macrophages exposed to oxidized low density lipoprotein. *J Pathol* 179:294-302.

Hardy S, El-Assaad W, Przybytkowski E, Joly E, Prentki M, Langelier Y. (2003) Saturated fatty acid-induced apoptosis in MDA-MB-231 breast cancer cells. A role for cardiolipin. *J. Biol. Chem* 278: 31861-31870.

Hawkins RA, Sangster K, Arends MJ. (1998) Apoptotic death of pancreatic cancer cells induced by polyunsaturated fatty acids varies with double bond number and involves an oxidative mechanism. *J Pathol* 185:61-70.

Hegyi L, Hardwick SJ, Siow RC and Skepper JN. (2001) Macrophage death and the role of apoptosis in human atherosclerosis. *J Hematother Stem Cell Res* 10: 27-42.

Helmy FM, Hassanein M, Juracka A. (2004) Studies on the endogenous phospholipids of mammalian kidney and their in vitro hydrolysis by endogenous phospholipases: a thin layer chromatographic and densitometric study. *Cell Biochem Funct* 22:379-87.

Horkko S, Miller E, Dudl E, Reaven P, Curtiss LK, Zvaifler NJ, Terkeltaub R, Pierangeli SS, Branch DW, Palinski W, Witztum JL. (1996) Antiphospholipid antibodies are directed against epitopes of oxidized phospholipids. Recognition of cardiolipin by monoclonal antibodies to epitopes of oxidized low density lipoprotein. *J Clin Invest* 98:815-25.

Huang Y-C, Jessup JM, Forse RA, Flickner S, Pleskow D, Anastopoulos HT, Ritter V, Blackburn GL. (1996) n-3 Fatty acids decrease colonic epithelial cell proliferation in high-risk bowel mucosa. *Lipids 31* Suppl: S313-S317.

Innis SM, Clandinin MT. (1981a) Dynamic modulation of mitochondrial inner-membrane lipids in rat heart by dietary fat. *Biochem J* 193:155-67.

Innis SM, Clandinin MT. (1981b) Dynamic modulation of mitochondrial membrane physical properties and ATPase activity by diet lipid. *Biochem J* 198:167-75.

Innis SM, Clandinin MT. (1981c) Mitochondrial-membrane polar-head-group composition is influenced by diet fat. *Biochem J* 198:231-4.

Jauslin ML, Meier T, Smith RA, Murphy MP. (2003) Mitochondria-targeted antioxidants protect Friedreich Ataxia fibroblasts from endogenous oxidative stress more effectively than untargeted antioxidants. *FASEB J* 17:1972-4.

Jiang C, Ting AT and Seed B. (1998) PPAR-gamma agonists inhibit production of monocyte inflammatory cytokines. *Nature* 391: 82-86.

Kharroubi I, Ladriere L, Cardozo AK, Dogusan Z, Cnop M, Eizirik DL. (2004) Free fatty acids and cytokines induce pancreatic β-cell apoptosis by different mechanisms: role of nuclear factor-κB and endoplasmic reticulum stress. *Endocrinology* 145: 5087-5096.

Kliewer SA, Sundseth SS, Jones SA, Brown PJ, Wisely GB, Koble CS, Devchand P, Wahli W, Willson TM, Lenhard JM and Lehmann JM. (1997) Fatty acids and eicosanoids regulate gene expression through direct interactions with peroxisome proliferator-activated receptors alpha and gamma. *Proc Natl Acad Sci USA* 94: 4318-4323.

Kolodgie FD, Narula J, Burke AP, Haider N, Farb A, Hui-Liang Y, Smialek J, Virmani R. (2000) Localization of apoptotic macrophages at the site of plaque rupture in sudden coronary death. *Am J Pathol* 157:1259-1268.

Kumagai T, Matsukawa N, Kaneko Y, Kusumi Y, Mitsumata M, Uchida K. (2004) A lipid peroxidation derived inflammatory mediator: identification of 4-hydroxy-2-nonenal as a potential inducer of cyclooxygenase-2 in macrophages. *J Biol Chem* 279:48389-96.

Kwon G, Pappan KL, Marshall CA, Schaffer JE, McDaniel ML. (2004) cAMP dose-dependently prevents palmitate-induced apoptosis by both protein kinase A- and cAMP-guanine nucleotide exchange factor-dependent pathways in β-cells. *J Biol Chem* 279: 8938-8945.

Lee H, Shi W, Tontonoz P, Wang S, Subbanagounder G, Hedrick CC, Hama S, Borromeo C, Evans RM, Berliner JA, Nagy L. (2000) Role for peroxisome proliferator-activated receptor alpha in oxidized phospholipid induced synthesis of monocyte chemotactic protein-1 and interleukin-8 by endothelial cells. *Circ Res* 87:516-21.

Lee H, Shi W, Tontonoz P, Wang S, Subbanagounder G, Hedrick CC, Hama S, Borromeo C, Evans RM, Berliner JA, Nagy L. (2000) Role for peroxisome proliferator-activated receptor alpha in oxidized phospholipid-induced synthesis of monocyte chemotactic protein-1 and interleukin-8 by endothelial cells. *Circ Res* 87: 516-21.

Lehmann JM, Lenhard JM, Oliver BB, Ringold GM, Kliewer SA (1997) Peroxisome proliferator-activated receptors alpha and gamma are activated by indomethacin and other non-steroidal anti-inflammatory drugs. *J Biol Chem* 272:3406-3410.

Leigh-Firbank EC, Minihane AM, Leake DS, Wright JW, Murphy MC, Griffin BA and Williams CM (2002) Eicosapentaenoic acid and docosahexaenoic acid from fish oils: differential associations with lipid responses. *Br J Nutr* 87: 435-45.

Listenberger L., Han X, Lewis SE, Cases S, Farese RV, Ory DS, Schaffer JE. (2003) Triglyceride accumulation protects against fatty acid-induced lipotoxicity. Proc Natl *Acad Sci* USA 100: 3077-3082.

Lu Z-H, Mu Y-M, Wang B-A, Li X-L, Lu J-M, Li J-Y, Pan C-Y, Yanase T, Nawata H. (2003) Saturated free fatty acids, palmitic acid and stearic acid, induce apoptosis by stimulation of ceramide generation in rat testicular Leydig cell. *Biochem Biophys Res Commun* 303: 1002-1007.

Lutter M, Fang M, Luo X, Nishijima M, Xie X, Wang X. (2000) Cardiolipin provides specificity for targeting of tBid to mitochondria. *Nat Cell Biol* 2:754-61.

Lutter M, Perkins GA, Wang X. (2001) The pro-apoptotic Bcl-2 family member tBid localizes to mitochondrial contact sites. *BMC Cell Biol* 2:22.

Macphee C, Benson GM, Shi Y, Zalewski A. (2005) Lipoprotein-associated phospholipase A$_2$: a novel marker of cardiovascular risk and potential therapeutic target. *Expert Opin Investig Drugs* 14: 671-679.

MacPhee CH, Moores KE, Boyd HF, Dhanak D, Ife RJ, Leach CA, Leake DS, Milliner KJ, Patterson RA, Suckling KE, Tew DG, Hickey DM. (1999) Lipoprotein-associated phospholipase A$_2$, platelet-activating factor acetylhydrolase, generates two bioactive products during the oxidation of low-density lipoprotein: use of a novel inhibitor. *Biochem J* 338:479-87.

Maestre I, Jordan J, Calvo S, Reig JA, Cena V, Soria B, Prentki M, Roche E. (2003) Mitochondrial dysfunction is involved in apoptosis induced by serum withdrawal and fatty acids in the beta-cell line Ins-1. *Endocrinology* 144: 335-345.

Marchant CE, Law NS, van der Veen C, Hardwick SJ, Carpenter KL, Mitchinson MJ. (1995) Oxidized low-density lipoprotein is cytotoxic to human monocyte macrophages: protection with lipophilic antioxidants. *FEBS Lett* 358:175-178.

Marx N, Sukhova G, Murphy C, Libby P and Plutzky J. (1998) Macrophages in human atheroma contain PPARgamma: differentiation- dependent peroxisomal proliferator-activated receptor gamma(PPARgamma) expression and reduction of MMP-9 activity through PPARgamma activation in mononuclear phagocytes in vitro. *Am J Pathol* 153: 17-23.

Mills AJ, Mathers JC, Chapman PD, Burn J, Gunn A. (2001) Colonic crypt proliferation state assessed by whole crypt microdissection in sporadic neoplasia and familial adenomatous polyposis. *Gut* 48: 41-46.

Min JH, Jain M., Wilder C, Paul L, Apitz-Castro R, Aspleaf DC, Gelb MH. (1999) Membrane-bound plasma platelet activating factor acetylhydrolase acts on substrate in the aqueous phase. *Biochemistry* 38: 12935-42.

Min JH, Wilder C, Aoki J, Arai H, Inoue K, Paul L, Gelb MH. (2001) Platelet-activating factor acetylhydrolases: broad substrate specificity and lipoprotein binding does not modulate the catalytic properties of the plasma enzyme. *Biochemistry* 40: 4539-49.

Mishra R, Simonson MS. (2005) Saturated free fatty acids and apoptosis in microvascular mesangial cells: palmitate activates pro-apoptotic signalling involving caspase 9 and mitochondrial release of endonuclease G. *Cardiovascular Diabetology* 4: 2.

Mitchell JA, Akarasereenont P, Thiemermann C, Flower RJ, Vane JR. (1993) Selectivity of nonsteroidal antiinflammatory drugs as inhibitors of constitutive and inducible cyclooxygenase. *Proc Natl Acad Sci U S A* 90:11693-11697.

Mu Y-M, Yanase T, Nishi Y, Tanaka A, Saito M, Jin CH, Mukasa C, Okabe T, Nomura M, Goto K, Nawata H. (2001) Saturated FFAs, palmitic acid and stearic acid, induce apoptosis in human granulosa cells. *Endocrinology* 142:3590-3597.

Müller K, Carpenter KL, Mitchinson MJ. (1998) Cell-mediated oxidation of LDL: comparison of different cell types of the atherosclerotic lesion. *Free Radic Res* 29:207-220.

Müller K, Carpenter KL, Freeman MA, Mitchinson MJ. (1999) Antioxidant BO-653 and human macrophage-mediated LDL oxidation. *Free Radic Res* 30:59-71.

Müller K, Hardwick SJ, Marchant CE, Law NS, Waeg G, Esterbauer H, Carpenter KL, Mitchinson MJ. (1996) Cytotoxic and chemotactic potencies of several aldehydic components of oxidised low density lipoprotein for human monocyte-macrophages. *FEBS Lett* 388:165-168

Muralidhar B, Carpenter KL, Müller K, Skepper JN, Arends MJ. (2004) Potency of arachidonic acid in polyunsaturated fatty acid-induced death of human monocyte-macrophages: implications for atherosclerosis. *Prostaglandins Leukot Essent Fatty Acids* 71:251-262.

Nagy L, Tontonoz P, Alvarez JG, Chen H, Evans RM. (1998) Oxidized LDL regulates macrophage gene expression through ligand activation of PPARgamma. *Cell* 93: 229-240.

Nomura K, Imai H, Koumura T, Kobayashi T, Nakagawa Y. (2000) Mitochondrial phospholipid hydroperoxide glutathione peroxidase inhibits the release of cytochrome c from mitochondria by suppressing the peroxidation of cardiolipin in hypoglycaemia-induced apoptosis. *Biochem J* 351:183-93.

Okuyama R, Fujiwara T, Ohsumi J. (2003) High glucose potentiates palmitate-induced NO-mediated cytotoxicity through generation of superoxide in clonal β-cell HIT-T15. *FEBS Lett* 545: 219-223.

Ott M, Robertson JD, Gogvadze V, Zhivotovsky B, Orrenius S. (2002) Cytochrome c release from mitochondria proceeds by a two-step process. *Proc Natl Acad Sci U S A* 99:1259-1263.

Parinandi NL, Weis BK, Schmid HH. (1988) Assay of cardiolipin peroxidation by high-performance liquid chromatography. *Chem Phys Lipids* 49:215-20.

Park BH, Vogelstein B, Kinzler KW. (2001) Genetic disruption of PPARdelta decreases the tumorigenicity of human colon cancer cells. *Proc Natl Acad Sci U S A* 98:2598-2603.

Patel L, Pass I, Coxon P, Downes CP, Smith SA, Macphee CH. (2001) Tumor suppressor and anti-inflammatory actions of PPARgamma agonists are mediated via upregulation of PTEN. *Curr Biol* 11:764-768.

Pontsler AV, St Hilaire A, Marathe GK, Zimmerman GA, McIntyre TM. (2002) Cyclooxygenase-2 is induced in monocytes by peroxisome proliferator activated receptor gamma and oxidized alkyl phospholipids from oxidized low density lipoprotein. *J Biol Chem* 277:13029-13036.

Pratico D, Tillmann C, Zhang ZB, Li H, FitzGerald GA. (2001) Acceleration of atherogenesis by COX-1-dependent prostanoid formation in low density lipoprotein receptor knockout mice. *Proc Natl Acad Sci U S A* 98:3358-3363.

Renner R, Innis SM, Clandinin MT. (1979) Effects of high and low erucic acid rapeseed oils on energy metabolism and mitochondrial function of the chick. *J Nutr* 109:378-87.

Ricote M, Huang J, Fajas L, Li A, Welch J, Najib J, Witztum JL, Auwerx J, Palinski W and Glass CK. (1998) Expression of the peroxisome proliferator-activated receptor gamma (PPARgamma) in human atherosclerosis and regulation in macrophages by colony stimulating factors and oxidized low density lipoprotein. *Proc Natl Acad Sci U S A* 95: 7614-7619.

Roberts LJ and Morrow JD. (2001) Analgesic-antipyretic and antiinflammatory agents and drugs used in the treatment of gout. In: *Goodman and Gilman's The Pharmacological Basis of Therapeutics*, pp. 687-731 [JG Hardman, LE Limbird and AG Gilman, editors]: 10th Edn., McGraw-Hill, New York.

Saez E, Tontonoz P, Nelson MC, Alvarez JG, Ming UT, Baird SM, Thomazy VA, Evans RM. (1998) Activators of the nuclear receptor PPARgamma enhance colon polyp formation. *Nat Med* 4:1058-1061.

Sarraf P, Mueller E, Smith WM, Wright HM, Kum JB, Aaltonen LA, de la Chapelle A, Spiegelman BM, Eng C. (1999) Loss-of-function mutations in PPARgamma associated with human colon cancer. *Mol Cell* 3: 799-804.

Schonbeck U, Sukhova GK, Graber P, Coulter S, Libby P. (1999) Augmented expression of cyclooxygenase-2 in human atherosclerotic lesions. *Am J Pathol* 155:1281-91.

Sendobry SM, Cornicelli JA, Welch K, Bocan T, Tait B, Trivedi BK, Colbry N, Dyer RD, Feinmark SJ, Daugherty A. (1997) Attenuation of diet-induced atherosclerosis in rabbits with a highly selective 15-lipoxygenase inhibitor lacking significant antioxidant properties. *Br J Pharmacol* 120:1199-1206.

Siow RC, Richards JP, Pedley KC, Leake DS, Mann GE. (1999) Vitamin C protects human vascular smooth muscle cells against apoptosis induced by moderately oxidized LDL containing high levels of lipid hydroperoxides. *Arterioscler Thromb Vasc Biol* 19:2387-2394.

Smith WL, DeWitt DL, Garavito RM. (2000) Cyclooxygenases: structural, cellular, and molecular biology. *Annu Rev Biochem* 69:145-182.

Stafforini DM, Elstad MR, McIntyre TM, Zimmerman GA, Prescott SM. (1990) Human macrophages secret platelet-activating factor acetylhydrolase. *J Biol Chem* 265: 9682-7.

Thies F, Garry JM, Yaqoob P, Rerkasem K, Williams J, Shearman CP, Gallagher PJ, Calder PC and Grimble RF (2003) Association of n-3 polyunsaturated fatty acids with stability of atherosclerotic plaques: a randomised controlled trial. *Lancet* 361: 477-85.

Tjoelker LW, Wilder C, Eberhardt C, Stafforini DM, Dietsch G, Schimpf B, Hooper S, Le Trong H, Cousens LS, Zimmerman GA, et al. (1995) Anti-inflammatory properties of a platelet-activating factor acetylhydrolase. *Nature* 374: 549-53.

Toft NJ, Arends MJ, Wyllie AH, te Riele H, Clarke AR. (1998) No evidence of female embryonic lethality in mice nullizygous for both *Msh2* and *p53*. *Nature Genetics* 18:17-18.

Toft NJ, Arends MJ. (1998) DNA mismatch repair and colorectal cancer. *Journal of Pathology* 185:123-129.

Toft NJ, Winton DJ, Kelly J, Howard LA, Dekker M, te Riele H, Arends MJ, Wyllie AH, Margison GP, Clarke AR. (1999) *Msh2* status modulates both apoptosis and mutation frequency in the murine small intestine. *Proc Natl Acad Sci USA* 96:3911-3915.

Tontonoz P, Nagy L, Alvarez JG, Thomazy VA, Evans RM. (1998) PPARgamma promotes monocyte/macrophage differentiation and uptake of oxidized LDL. *Cell* 93: 241-252.

Toyoda M, Takagi H, Horiguchi N, Kakizaki S, Sato K, Takayama H, Mori M. (2002) A ligand for peroxisome proliferator activated receptor gamma inhibits cell growth and induces apoptosis in human liver cancer cells. *Gut* 50: 563-567.

Unger RH. (2002) Lipotoxic diseases. *Annu Rev Med* 53: 319-336.

Unger RH, Orci L. (2002) Lipoapoptosis: its mechanism and its diseases. *Biochim Biophys Acta* 1585: 202-212.

Vreken P, Valianpour F, Nijtmans LG, Grivell LA, Plecko B, Wanders RJ, Barth PG. (2000) Defective remodeling of cardiolipin and phosphatidylglycerol in Barth syndrome. *Biochem Biophys Res Commun* 279:378-82.

Waddington E, Sienuarine K, Puddey I, Croft K. (2001) Identification and quantitation of unique fatty acid oxidation products in human atherosclerotic plaque using high performance liquid chromatography. *Analytical Biochemistry* 292:234-244.

Wander RC and Du S-H. (2000) Oxidation of plasma proteins is not increased after supplementation with eicosapentaenoic and docosahexaenoic acids. *Am J Clin Nutr* 72: 731-737.

Wang YL, Frauwirth KA, Rangwala SM, Lazar MA and Thompson CB. (2002) Thiazolidinedione activation of peroxisome proliferator-activated receptor gamma can enhance mitochondrial potential and promote cell survival. *J Biol Chem* 277: 31781-31788.

Watkins SM, Carter LC, German JB. (1998) Docosahexaenoic acid accumulates in cardiolipin and enhances HT-29 cell oxidant production. *J Lipid Res* 39:1583-1588.

Welters HJ, Tadayyon M, Scarpello JHB, Smith SA, Morgan NG. (2004) Mono-unsaturated fatty acids protect against β-cell apoptosis induced by saturated fatty acids, serum withdrawal or cytokine exposure. *FEBS Lett* 560: 103-108.

Willson TM, Cobb JE, Cowan DJ, Wiethe RW, Correa ID, Prakash SR, Beck KD, Moore LB, Kliewer SA, Lehmann JM. (1996) The structure-activity relationship between peroxisome proliferator- activated receptor gamma agonism and the antihyperglycemic activity of thiazolidinediones. *J Med Chem* 39: 665-668.

Wyne KL. (2003) Free fatty acids and type 2 diabetes mellitus. *Am J Med* 115:29S-36S.

Yang WL and Frucht H. (2001) Activation of the PPAR pathway induces apoptosis and COX-2 inhibition in HT-29 human colon cancer cells. *Carcinogenesis* 22: 1379-1383.

Yla-Herttuala S, Palinski W, Rosenfeld ME, Parthasarathy S, Carew TE, Butler S, Witztum JL, Steinberg D. (1989) Evidence for the presence of oxidatively modified low density lipoprotein in atherosclerotic lesions of rabbit and man. *J Clin Invest* 84:1086-1095.

Yla-Herttuala S, Rosenfeld ME, Parthasarathy S, Glass CK, Sigal E, Witztum JL, Steinberg D. (1990) Colocalization of 15-lipoxygenase mRNA and protein with epitopes of oxidized low density lipoprotein in macrophage-rich areas of atherosclerotic lesions. *Proc Natl Acad Sci U S A* 87:6959-6963.

In: Leading Topics in Cancer Research
Editor: Lee P. Jeffrie, pp. 219-233

ISBN 1-60021-332-4
© 2007 Nova Science Publishers, Inc.

Chapter 8

PROMISING NEWCASTLE DISEASE VIRUS (NDV) THERAPY IN HUMAN HIGH GRADE GLIOMAS

Laszlo K. Csatary, Christina Csatary,
Gyorgy Gosztonyi and Bela Bodey[*]

[1]United Cancer Research Institute, Alexandria, VA,
[2]Childrens Center for Cancer and Blood Diseases, Childrens Hospital Los Angeles,
Los Angeles, and Department of Pathology, Keck School of Medicine,
University of Southern California, Los Angeles, CA

ABSTRACT

The employment of virus therapy to treat human neoplasms has a three decade history. One such virus that has been explored is the Newcastle Disease Virus (NDV) Vaccine (MTH-68/N). MTH-68/N vaccine therapy has been employed in a number of different neoplasms with success. This success has also been demonstrated in glioblastomas and high grade gliomas. Glioblastoma multiforme (GBM) is the most common primary brain tumor and by far it is the most aggressive form of glial tumors. This neoplasm has a poor prognosis, averaging six months to a year. Nine cases of advanced GBM and high grade glioma were treated with the NDV vaccine (MTH-68/N) after the classical modalities of anti-neoplastic therapy failed. Our results included survival rates of ten years, nine years, eight years, six years, five years, three years, nine months, and six months post-diagnosis for the eight surviving patients. Against all odds, these surviving patients have also returned to a lifestyle that resembles their pre-morbid daily routines. They enjoy good clinical health. These patients have regularly received the MTH-68/N vaccine for a number of years without interruption as a form of monotherapy once the classical modalities failed. The MRI and CT results have revealed an objective decrease in size of the tumors, in some cases the near total disappearance of the mass. There has also been documented decrease in mass effect following administration of the

---

[*] *Corresponding Author: Bela Bodey, M.D., D. Sc.;* 8000-1 Canby Avenue, Reseda, CA 91335, USA; E-mail:
Bodey18@aol.com;

MTH-68/N vaccine. Although one of our patients did succumb to complications of his malignancy, the results are nonetheless extremely promising in that there is not only a decrease in tumor burden but also a return of pre-morbid functioning. It should be stressed that the positive results may be due to the long-term employment of the vaccine. This chapter seeks to shed light on the background of NDV with a focus on the possible mechanism of action. There is also a detailed description of the clinical course of each of the cases, the revealing and convincing clinical findings, as well as of the functional improvement that the patients experienced with the use of the MTH-68/N and MTH-68/H vaccine after all classical modalities failed and hope was nearly lost.

Keywords: Glial cell precursors (astrocytes, oligodendrocytes, ependymocytes); Astrocytoma; (ASTR); Glioblastoma (GBM); Neoplasm associated marker (NAM); Neoplasm associated antigen (NAA); Monoclonal antibody (MoAB); Cellular Immunophenotype (CIP); Newcastle Disease Virus (NDV) Vaccine (MTH-68/N); Spontaneous Regression (SR); Monoclonal Antibodies (MoABs).

INTRODUCTION

"This peculiarity of the membrane, namely, that it becomes continuous with the interstitial matter, the real cement, which binds the nervous elements together and that in all its properties it constitutes a tissue different from the other forms of connective tissue, has induced me to give it a new name, that of neuro-glia (nerve cement)."

Rudolf Virchow, April 3, 1858 [1]

HUMAN GLIAL TUMORS

The most common brain tumors develop from glial cell precursors (astrocytes, oligodendrocytes, ependymocytes). Glial tumors [mainly astrocytomas (ASTRs)], especially glioblastomas, are characterized by hypercellularity, pleomorphism, a number of cell mitoses, CIP heterogeneity, various grades of necrosis, and multiple endothelial cell proliferations related to newly generated, tumor-related capillaries. Furthermore, glial tumors are characterized by high grade local invasiveness and a relatively low metastatic tendency. [2-4]

Malignant childhood ASTRs appear within the neuro-glial or macroglial central nervous system (CNS) [5]; they account for over 50% of all intracranial tumors. [3,4,6] Cairncross [7] interpreted the histogenesis of ASTRs in the light of parallel concepts emerging from investigations in myeloproliferative disorders. [8,9] According to the stem cell hypothesis, ASTRs originate from a common pluripotent, neuro-ectodermally derived precursor cell, whose progeny retain the ability to differentiate and do so along astrocytic lines. [10] The majority of malignant glial tumors are incurable with the current classical therapeutical modalities, including surgical resection, radiotherapy, and chemotherapy. [11] This may well be the direct result of the biological variability of these tumors (*e.g.* multiple stem cell lines, intrinsic and acquired multidrug resistance).

The molecular pathogenesis of human brain tumors has been intensely studied during the past few years. Genetic alterations of chromosome 17p are associated with pilocytic ASTRs

(World Health Organization (WHO) grade I), mutations at 17p and 19q are common in anaplastic ASTRs (WHO grade III) and abnormal chromosomes 17p, 19q and 10 are associated with the most malignant glioblastoma multiforme (WHO grade IV). [3,12] It is well established that low-grade ASTRs have an intrinsic tendency for progressive IP dedifferentiation toward higher-grade, more malignant ASTRs. [13]

Glioblastoma multiforme (GBM), the most malignant neoplasm of the human CNS, develops rapidly *de novo* (primary glioblastoma) or through malignant cellular IP progression from low-grade or anaplastic ASTR (so-called secondary glioblastoma). [14] It was recently reported that mutations of the p53 gene are present in more than two-thirds of secondary glioblastomas, but rarely occur in primary GBMs, suggesting the presence of divergent genetic pathways. [15]

The majority of malignant glial tumors are incurable with the current classical therapeutical modalities. Still the prognosis of high grade gliomas remains somewhat unpredictable because histologic features alone provide an imperfect assessment of the biologic behavior of a given lesion. [16] Whereas some patients experience prolonged disease control after surgery and adjuvant therapy, others with lesions that appear comparable exhibit rapid disease progression and death. Proliferative activity provide a potential correlate of tumorbiologic aggressiveness. [17]

In recent years, there is increasing recognition of polyphenotypic high-grade malignancies in CNS tumor literature. Some of these tumors have been regarded as variants of PNET or as extrarenal malignant rhabdoid tumors (MRTs). Jay and co-workers [18] have described two posterior fossa neoplasms, both of which displayed a "polyphenotypic" expression of neural, epithelial, myogenic, and glial markers. The histological and ultrastructural appearances were inconsistent with glioma, PNET, meningioma, ependymoma, choroid plexus carcinoma, sarcoma, germ cell tumor, and other tumors in the WHO classification. Although the polyphenotype raises the issue that these may represent variants of MRT or the atypical teratoid-rhabdoid tumor, the morphologic findings in the two cases were very dissimilar. The two cases presented by the authors underscore the problems in nosology and classification of polyphenotypic tumors of the CNS. This is particularly significant, as therapeutic protocols for PNET, MRT, and non-CNS polyphenotypic tumors are quite different.

Concurrent viral infections which induce a virus interference phenomenon can significantly modify the outcome of hypothetical viral diseases. [19,20] Participation of one or more viral infections during the intimate steps of the oncogenetic changes was shown in 33% of human cancer. Attenuated (non-pathogenic) avian viruses have been used as a form of non-specific immunobiological, fourth modality treatment of advanced human cancer. The mechanism of viral interference requires the presence of suitable interfering virus, which is apathogenic to the host and is capable of eliminating the harmful effects of the pathogenic virus. [21,22] We also propose an enhancement of the host tumor-directed immune response induced by the superinfecting apathogenic virus. [23] Detection of *de novo* synthesis of new neoplastic cell associated surface antigens after viral superinfection could also benefit the understanding of this complex immunobiological phenomenon. [24]

IMMUNOSUPPRESSION WITHIN THE CELLULAR MICROENVIRONMENT OF CHILDHOOD BRAIN TUMORS

Important immunological parameter changes have been determined in children suffering from brain tumors: 1) low numbers of circulating T lymphocytes; 2) impaired cytotoxicity of T lymphocyte (CD8$^+$, tumor infiltrating and TAA directed lymphocytes express a defective high affinity interleukin-2 receptor (IL-2R); 3) poor mitogenic responsiveness of tumor infiltrating T lymphocytes in vitro; 4) decreased antibody responsiveness (result of defective CD4$^+$ T helper lymphocyte functions); 5) abnormal delayed hypersensitivity responses; and 6) CD4$^+$ and CD8$^+$ lymphocytes derived from TIL are killed by autologous glioma cells in vitro. [25,26]

Soluble factors, secreted by brain tumor cells are responsible for the impaired anti-neoplastic cellular immune responses. In vitro experiments have revealed that T lymphocytes from normal individuals cultured in the presence of brain tumor cell supernatants exhibit the very same immunological abnormalities mentioned above.

A dominant suppressor growth factor involved in the intratumoral defense mechanisms of neoplastically transformed cells is the transforming growth factor-β2 (TGF-β2). TGF-β2 is derived from primary brain tumors (autocrine secretion), and has been shown to suppress the in vitro generation of cytotoxic T lymphocytes (CTL) from TIL derived from peripheral blood lymphocytes [27], and thus its in vivo secretion at the tumor site may well be responsible for the intense suppression of CD8$^+$ CTL. [28,29] Brain tumors have been shown to express predominantly low levels of MHC class I molecules, as well as ICAM-1 and to produce TGF-β2, all of which serve as explanations of the inability to effectively isolate and expand infiltrating immunological effectors (CTL) from these neoplasias. [32] This combination of factors probably represents a common tumor biological phenomenon and apparently renders the infiltrating cells incapable of proliferation and considerably lowers their immunological (cytotoxic) efficacy, and may be crucial in the inability of the infiltrating immunological effector cells to overcome tumor progression. [30,31]

Other tumor derived soluble factors, such as prostaglandin E$_2$ (PGE$_2$), interleukin-1 receptor (IL-1R) antagonist, and interleukin-10 (IL-10) may also contribute to the observed immunosuppression in childhood brain tumors. [2]

NEWCASTLE DISEASE VIRUS (NDV) VACCINE (MTH-68/N)

> A miracle cannot prove what is impossible,
> It is helpful only as confirmation of what is possible.
> *Maimonides (1135-1204)*

The antineoplastic effect of NDV was first published in 1965. [22] In the last three decades, Csatary and co-workers have employed chicken Newcastle Disease Virus (NDV), which is harmless to humans, as a live vaccine named MTH-68/N. [19,23,24,32] Similar clinically favorable results were also achieved when other attenuated veterinary virus vaccines were employed on several human viral infections. Since the early 1970s, all together 38 viruses have been reported as having had antineoplastic effects on mammalian neoplasms. [21]

Newcastle disease virus (NDV) infects a wide variety of birds and it can also infect humans, but, in humans it causes only mild flu-like symptoms or conjunctivitis and/or laryngitis. MTH68/H is a unique mesogenic NDV strain. NDV is classified as avian paramyxovirus-1 (APMV1), in the Rubulavirus genus of the family Paramyxoviridae in the order Mononegavirales. Members of this family have a single stranded, linear, RNA, with an elliptical symmetry. The total genome is roughly 16,000 nucleotides long and contains six genes encoding six major polypeptides: nucleocapsid protein, phosphoprotein, matrix protein, fusion (F) protein, hemagglutinin-neuraminidase (HN), and large RNA-dependent polymerase protein. Replication of the virus takes place in the cytoplasm of the host cell.

Based on their pathogenicity on birds, NDV strains are classified into highly velogenic, intermediate (mesogenic) or lentogenic strains. Mesogenic strains are avirulent for chickens older than 6 weeks of age but retain their virulence for day-old chickens (intracerebral pathogenicity index: $\sim$ 1.0-1.5). F protein, which is synthesized as non-functional precursor F_0 and proteolytically cleaved to yield polypeptides F_1 and F_2 by host proteases, is an important determinant of NDV pathogenicity. Different pathotypes are characterized by differences in the amino acid sequences surrounding the F_0 cleavage site, which hosts the molecular marker for virulence.

Restriction enzyme site mapping of the F protein gene and sequence analysis can be employed to classify the NDV isolates into different genotypes. By this analysis our another vaccine, the mesogenic MTH68/H strain was proven to belong to genotype III group as well as the strain Mukteswar while the other NDV vaccine strains (La Sota, B1) were different and classified as genotype II. The believed parent of MTH68/H, the velogenic virus Herts '33 strain belongs to genotype IV and no close relations to MTH68/H can be proven. (In the same study a remarkable genetic stability of MTH68/H, even after prolonged passage was proven.)

The perception is that some NDV strain can replicate up to 10,000 times better in human neoplastically transformed cells than in most normal human cells (and the widely believed fact that the virus is non-toxic) aroused the interest in the cancer therapy.

The NDV strains believed to be suitable for antineoplastic therapy can be further classified as either lytic or nonlytic for human cells. Lytic strains and nonlytic strains both appear to replicate much more efficiently in human neoplastic cells than they do in most normal human cells and viruses of both strain types have been investigated as potential anticancer agents. One major difference between lytic strains and nonlytic strains is that lytic strains are able to make infectious progeny virus particles in human cells, whereas nonlytic strains are not. The progeny virus particles made by nonlytic strains contain inactive versions of these molecules. The production of infectious progeny virus particles by lytic strains gives them the ability to kill host cells fairly quickly.

The NDV strains that have been evaluated most widely for the treatment of human neoplasms are MTH-68, PV-701, 73-T and Ulster. The first three are lytic while Ulster is nonlytic.

Among the few real potentially effective NDV strains evaluated for the treatment of cancer MTH68/H is unique. The medicinal product containing the highly purified unique live MTH68/H strain is freeze dried with specific innocuous stabilisers assuring the long stability of the finished product.

The other specificity of MTH-68/H that these viruses can destroy their host cells: (1) by inducing necrosis or lysis by their excessive replication; (2) by inducing programmed cell death, apoptosis. The replication competent MTH-68/H virus selectively target neoplastically transformed cells and destroy their host tumour cells while leave the normal cells uninfected. The MTH-68/H strain's safety is extensively proven as well as the excellent tolerability by patients with minimal, if any, side effects.

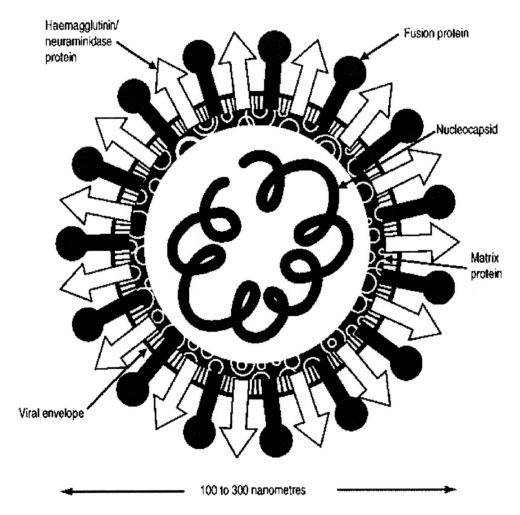

Significant changes appear in the clinical laboratory parameters (liver transaminases and other enzymes, blood cells) following the treatment with NDV vaccine MTH-68/N, demonstrating a stop or slow down in the progression of the primary cancer disease. [33] A majority of the cases of primary and metastatic tumors had a partial or total regression after the NDV vaccine was employed. Patients classified in the stage of advanced neoplastic disease ended up in the tumor free clinical condition. During the long time of survival a malignization (immunophenotype changes) of glial tumors cannot be ascertained. There is no immunophenotypic change in the rhombencephalic manifestation, both tumors are WHO grade III, anaplastic astrocytomas. There is no dedifferentiation in the expression of GFAP, as shown by immunostaining.

CASE STUDIES

Case 1

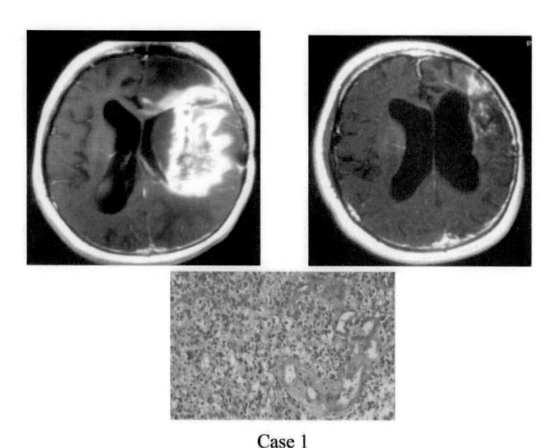

Case 1

Case 1 is that of a 14-year old male (now approximately 22) who was diagnosed with a large left fronto-temporal mass seen on a computed tomogaphic scan (CT) in September of 1994. The tumor was grossly debulked followed by a course of 56 Gray radiation to the tumor bed. Pathology showed the mass to be gliobastoma multiforme (grade IV glioma). In March 1995, he was started on adjuvant Tamoxifen therapy at 100 mg daily, which proved to be unsuccessful when an MRI in November 1995 showed a local recurrence of the tumor. The patient was then started on Cyclophosphamide at $3600mg/m^2$ with Vincristine at 1.5 mg. After a single course of therapy, another MRI showed clear-cut progression of the tumor. The chemotherapy regimen was changed to Carboplation at a dose of 500 mg/m^2 with VP16 100 mg/m^2 daily for two days, cycled with Cisplatin 100 mg/m^2. Another MRI performed in March of 1996 showed continued tumor enlargement, with the patient's functional and neurological states deteriorating and increasing right-sided weakness and aphasia. The patient became wheel chair bound with a Karnovsky core of 40 and received Phenytoin for frequent seizures. In April 1996, MTH-68 (NDV vaccine) was intravenously initiated at one vial per day ($10^{7.4}$ electroimmunodiffusion (EID) [egg infective dose] 50 per vial). The dose was increased to two vials daily for two months, to three vials daily until December 1997, and then to four vials daily, which he continued to receive. The patient also continued with Tamoxifen. A borderline increase in tumor size was observed on MRIs completed between May and November 1996 despite the patient's neurological and functional improvement. However, from November 1996 to September 1998, MRIs revealed progressive shrinkage of the tumor by approximately 95%. The patient also remained on Dexamethasone, which was tapered off from a dosage of 20 mg daily in April 1996 to 0 mg/day by January of 1997, at which time Phenytoin and Tamoxifen were also discontinued.

The patient has had no seizures since July 1996. Since January 1997, he has only received MTH-68 and in the year 2000, the patient's dosage was slowly decreased. After having been treated with MTH-68 for five and a half years, the patient walks with a mild hemi-paresis and attends regular college where he receives above average grades. He has also just recently received his driver's license.

Case 2

Case 2 is that of an 18-year-old girl who was first presented with a month of severe headaches and vomiting. An MRI and CT showed a large frontal mass, which was revealed to be a high-grade glioma, malignant astrocytoma by biopsy after a surgical resection in July 1995. The surgery removed about 70% of the tumor mass, with the patient then receiving 6000cGY of radiation and undergoing four cycles of chemotherapy. The chemotherapy consisted of BCNV, Carboplatin, and VP16. The patient also had bilateral shunts placed. In September 1996, an MRI showed a recurrence of the tumor in the same location. The patient then underwent a gross surgical resection of the entire mass, after which she received no further treatment. Surgical pathology findings were unable to determine if her cytology revealed a low grade of high grade glioma. In November of 1996, a small local recurrence was discovered and by March 1997, a large "butterfly" mass in the frontal region extended to the contralateral side and deep into the brain tissue. The patient was no longer considered for any of the conventional modalities and was at this point bedridden and ashasic, with right-sided hemiplagia and right facial palsy. The patient's neurological and functional status was dismal. She was also Cushinoid and obese because of the ongoing Dexamethason treatment at 30 mg daily. In July of 1997, the patient began MTH-68 therapy intranasally and was changed to IV MTH-68 in September 1997. MTH-68 has been her only therapy since then, receiving a daily dose of one vial until January 2001 at which time it was decreased to four times a week. In April 2001, her dosage was even furthered decreased to two times a week. An MRI in March 2000 revealed an almost complete disappearance of the tumor mass, with residual scarring and changes secondary to surgery and radiation.

The patient's neurological and functional status has improved dramatically over this period. Her right-side facial palsy gradually improved and her speech is now back to normal. Her right-sided hemiparesis also improved, with the patient being able to walk with two-sided assistance or a walker. She has now finished the tenth grade and is functioning at a Karnovsky level of 70. She has also undergone a Dexamethasone taper to 0 mg/day and no longer has Cushinoid appearance, allowing her to maintain a total weight of 50 kilos. The patient is still alive and continues to receive MTH-68 as her sole therapy.

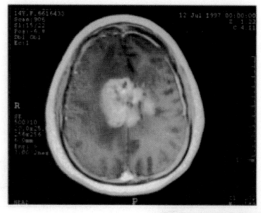
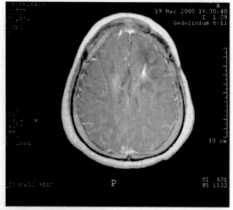

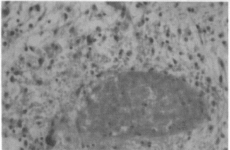

Case 2

Case 3

The patient is a seven year old male, born on October 11, 1994, who was first diagnosed with glioblastoma multiforme in February 1996. At that time, the patient underwent a partial resection of the tumor in the temporo-parietal region. Surgical pathology confirmed that the mass was a glial tumor with moderate cellular differentiation, disorganized architecture, and moderate atypia of nuclei, with infiltrate into the surrounding tissue. Post-surgically, the patient underwent a year of intense chemotherapy and significant progression of the tumor was noted during this time. The patient was advised to seek some alternative therapy and further operative resection when chemotherapy was discontinued. A VP shunt was placed for the treatment of hydrocephalus. In August of 1997, the patient began MTH-68 treatment, which he has continued until the present time. Since that time, the patient has had tumor recurrence and has had two partial resections. The patient has, nonetheless, had good neuro-cognitive and physical development. An MRI in June 2002 revealed six small lesions, two unchanged in the right uncus and in the left occipital region, an extremely small new hypophysical lesion and in the third ventricle and in the right sub-frontal region. The cystic lesion previously operated on shows slow insidious progression. The patient has since had a repeat sterotactic resection of the cystic lesion. Currently, the patient is alive with his glioblastoma being under control through surgical resection and ongoing MTH-68 therapy. The patient remains neuro-cognitively intact.

Case 4

The patient is a 44-year old American female who after collapsing in September of 1998 was diagnosed with bifrontal glioblastoma multiforme. She underwent two major craniotomies for resection of two large tangerine sized frontal tumors. Afterwards, she underwent experimental ultrapheresis and a course of Thalidomie and chemotherapy. In March 1999, a shunt was placed for treatment of hydrocephalus. The patient also received radiation therapy in the summer of 1999, before starting MTH-68 therapy in September of that year. The treatment was administered intravenously daily and then orally and nasally with a nebulizer. She has not received any other therapy since then. MRIs in the year 2000 (February, May, August, and December) showed a residual cystic structure in the left frontal lobe, with enhancement surrounding the cystic space extending caudally into the brain parenchyma as well as diffuse dural enhancement. Yet, these findings remained stable and showed no significant progression throughout the year. In January 2001, the patient began suffering from seizures and developed partial complex epilepsy. She received Depakote and Neurontin for seizure control, with her seizures diminishing in frequency and severity. In April 2001, her MRI showed residual or recurrent neoplasm in the left frontal lobe peri-cystically and diffuse dural enhancement once again. However, no progression was noted in the MRI (no change from December 2000 findings).

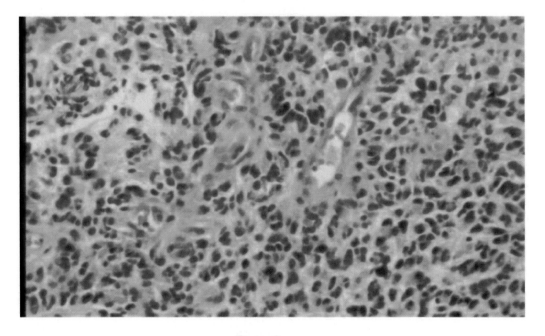

Case 4

Presently, the patient remains independent in most of her activities and is able to partake in family affairs and play Scrabble. Although she can no longer work as a magazine editor since January 2002, she is increasingly able to read and write. Her short-term memory, concentration, and neuro-cognitive status is improving. The patient has no problems with gait or movement and has been seizure free for some time now. For the last two years, MTH-68 has been her sole therapy.

It is quite obvious from the above case studies that the MTH-68/N virus vaccine therapy is successful. The normal survival time for patients diagnosed with glioblastoma multiforme rarely exceeds more than one year; this diagnosis often spells a death sentence. However, with the MTH-68/N virus vaccine therapy, patients diagnosed with glioblastoma are far exceeding these limited time frames, with all of them still living today. A great majority of patients with glioblastomas live a very limited, bed-ridden life that is far from their daily routine. Because of the MTH-68/N virus vaccine therapy, these patients have in fact returned to living a far more normal life, resuming many of their usual daily activities and way of living. From the case studies, it should also be duly noted that Csatary and co-workers have maintained use of the virus vaccine over a long period of time, with some of the patients taking the therapy for years at a time. The possible secret behind the success of the therapy is that the vaccine is relentlessly administered over a long period of time.

Since 1996, MTH-69/H viral treatment has also been extended to high-grade gliomas, during which time 15 patients suffering from such tumors have been treated. In 6 patients the treatment did not arrest tumor growth, they died of the progression of their neoplasm. Two patients died of causes unrelated to their brain tumor. Seven patients are alive, they reacted favorably to the treatment. In 3 of them, the therapeutic results are promising with survival times of 16 to 30 months, but these survival periods are still not long enough to allow trustworthy evaluation. The remaining 4 patients exhibit survival times of 6 to 10 years and offer reliable grounds to demonstrate the efficacy of oncolytic viral treatment. All four patients exhausted the potentials of conventional therapeutic modalities and were in the phase of relentless progression of their tumor.

Below, we provide a description of four cases treated with MTH-68/H.

Case 1

This is a 23-year-old male with a left fronto-temporal GBM. Conventional therapy could not prevent recurrence. MTH-68/H therapy resulted in continuous regression of his tumor. In 2002 only residual changes could be shown. Since 1998 the patient drives a car and could attend college.

Case 2

This is a 22-year-old female, operated on because of a left fronto-temporal glioma, WHO Grade III/IV. Severe progression despite radio- and chemotherapy and reoperation. Institution of MTH-68/H therapy was followed by a dramatic improvement, with almost complete disappearance of the tumor. In 2000, only residual changes could be displayed.

Case 3

This case is that of an 11-year-old boy. In 1996, a left temporo-parietal GBM was partially resected. In spite of intense chemotherapy, there was severe tumor progression. In 1997 i.v. MTH-68/H therapy was started, leading to significant clinical improvement. In 1998 two stereotactic resections were performed because of focal recurrences. Since 2002, there has been a stable clinical condition with ongoing MTH-68/H therapy. From histology and MRI studies only written reports are available.

Case 4

This case is that of a 49-year-old woman. In 1998, there was a partial resection of a bifrontal GBM, followed by intense chemotherapy and radiation. MTH-68-H therapy was started in1999. From 2000, there was gradual improvement concomitant with reduction of the tumor mass.

Summing up the data of these 4 cases we can conclude that these patients have survived and improved under continuous MTH-68/H therapy as a monotherapy for 5 to 9 years. The overall survival – from the establishment of the diagnosis – amounts to 7 to 11 years.

Coming back to the original survey of all treated patients, the question arises, why does roughly half of the patients respond well to oncolytic viral treatment, and why is the other half of the patients unresponsive, when all of them had the same type of tumor, and the conditions of the treatment were identical in both groups.

The most perplexing case is that of a young boy, who developed two tumor manifestations, which responded in a very opposite way to oncolytic viral treatment. This boy, 12 years old at the beginning of his illness, presented with a left thalamic glioma, which proved to be an anaplastic astrocytoma (WHO Grade III). Following partial resection he underwent intense radiation and chemotherapy, but his tumor progressed powerfully. At this time i.v. MTH-68/H therapy was started, combined with oral valproic acid (VPA), an antiepileptic drug, which recently was noted to have antineoplastic effects in gliomas. Within 4 months a dramatic reduction of tumor extension and improvement of the clinical condition could be registered. At this time, however, a new tumor manifestation appeared in the roof of the IVth ventricle. The boy underwent surgery again; at histological examination this tumor manifestation corresponded also to an anaplastic astrocytoma. Despite continuing oncolytic viral, VPA and dexamethasone treatment his condition deteriorated rapidly and he died four months after the second operation.

DISCUSSION

In the four cases of GBM and high grade glioma reported by us in this case study, each of the four patients had the MTH-68/N virus vaccine therapy administered after the three anti-neoplastic classical modalities had been exhausted. This vaccine was given to them for a longer period of time, much longer than other researchers have done with other vaccine therapies. In fact, all four patients are still alive and continue to receive the vaccine. Employing the MTH-68/N virus vaccine therapy as a form of monotherapy, the survival times of Case 1 has been eight years, seven years for Case 2, six years for Case 3, and four years for Case 4, which far exceeds expected times of survival. Moreover, our definition of survival differs from others and is not simply living, but rather incorporates the idea that these patients return to their previous daily routines, to a more normal way of living. These patients have truly shown great clinical improvement.

Similiar results have also been found in other human neoplasms and have been published. [32,33]

It is quite possible that some authors would attempt to interpret our results as a form of spontaneous regression (SR). Spontaneous regression is defined as an occurrence when the malignant neoplastic mass partially or completely disappears without any treatment or as a result of therapy considered inadequate to influence systemic neoplastic disease. [34,35] This definition is accepted, but it should be noted that the true existence of SR of neoplasms is often questioned and some simply do not accept this pathophysiological phenomenon. SR was reported in a case of pilocytic astrocytoma in a patient without neurofibromatosis type 1, but never in high grade glial tumors and GBM. [36] The employment of a virus vaccine therapy is a very specific alternative/immunotherapeutic anti-neoplastic treatment.

Neoplasm associated markers (NAMs) are the biochemical and immunological counterparts of the morphology of neoplasms. [37,38] The expression of an immunocytochemically defined CAM is also related to the tissue of origin and is not a random event.

During the past two decades, the use of monoclonal antibodies (MoABs) against oncofetal, neoplasm associated, cell lineage specific, differentiation, cancer/testis, endothelial, and cell proliferation related antigens in the diagnosis, biological assessment of prognosis, and in the immunotherapy of systematic neoplastic disease has gained increased importance. [39] A sensitive direct correlation exists between the expression of certain molecules and the development of an invasive, highly malignant CIP of neoplastic cells, allowing for the occurrence of angiogenesis and metastasis. The development of molecular biological neoplasm detection has led to the development of different NAAs. NAAs have been used in the immuno-diagnostic of human malignancies and in various neoplasms as immunotherapy through monoclonal antibodies. In the case of brain tumors, however, such protocols of using MoABs has never been established and has, thus far, proven to be unsuccessful.

The MTH-68/N virus vaccine therapy is three decades in the making, with Dr. Csatary beginning his initial work on this therapy three decades ago. Nowadays, there are numerous groups of physcians and scientists all over the world employing the MTH-68/N virus vaccine therapy. This vaccine tends to be only employed once the other classical anti-neoplastic treatments have failed and it has, nonetheless, achieved great success. How many more decades of results are needed for this therapy to accepted as a permanent modality of human neoplasms, especially since this therapy does not interfere with the three classical modalities and will actually only enhance the therapeutic effects of these already accepted treatments?

REFERENCES

[1]   Virchow, R. Cellular pathology. (RM de Witt, New York, 1860).

[2]   Bodey B., Bodey B. Jr., and Siegel S.E. Immunophenotypical (IP) differential diagnosis and immunobiology of childhood primary brain tumors. A decade of experience. *Int J Pediatric Hematol/Oncol 6*, 65-84 (1998).

[3]   von Deimling, A., Louis, D.N., and Wiestler, O.D. Molecular pathways in the formation of gliomas. *Glia 15*, 328-338 (1995).

[4]   Kleihues, P., Soylemezoglu, F., Schauble, B., Scheithauer, B.W., and Burger, P.C. Histopathology, classification, and grading of gliomas. *Glia 15*, 211-221 (1995).

[5]   Williams, B.P., Abney, E.R., and Raff, M.C. Macroglial cell development in embryonic rat brain: studies using monoclonal antibodies, flourescence-activated cell sorting and cell culture. *Dev Biol 112*, 126-134 (1985)

[6]   Katsura, S., Suzuki, J., and Wada, T. Statistical study of brain tumours in the neurosurgical clinics in Japan. *J Neurosurg 16*, 570-580 (1959).

[7]   Cairncross, J.G. The biology of astrocytoma: lessons learned from chronic myelogenous leukemia-hypothesis. *J Neuro-Oncol 5*, 99-104 (1987).

[8]   Greaves, M., Janossy, G., Francis, G., and Minowada, J. Membrane phenotypes of human leukemic cells and leukemic cell lines: Clinical correlates and biological implications. In: Differentiation of normal and neoplastic hemopoietic cells. Vol. 5 (Clarkson B, Marks PL, and Till J, eds) 823-841 (Cold Spring Harbor Conferences on Cell Proliferation, Cold Spring Harbor Laboratory, New York, 1977).

[9]   Burns, B.F. Molecular genetic markers in lymphoproliferative disorders. *Clin Biochem 22*, 33-39 (1989).

[10]   Bodey, B., Zeltzer, P.M., Saldivar, V., and Kemshead, J.: Immunophenotyping of childhood astrocytomas with a library of monoclonal antibodies. *Int J Cancer 45*, 1079-1087 (1990).

[11]   Bullard, D.E., Gillespie, Y., Mahaley, M.S., and Bigner, D.D. Immunobiology of human gliomas. *Semin Oncol 13*, 94-109 (1986).

[12]   Ohgaki, K., Schäuble, B., zur Hausen, A., von Ammon, K., and Kleihues, P. Genetic alterations associated with the evolution and progression of astrocytic brain tumors. *Virchows Arch 427*, 113-118 (1995).

[13]   Bodey, B., Gröger, A.M., Bodey, B. Jr., Siegel, S.E., and Kaiser, H.E. Immunocytochemical detection of p53 protein expression in various childhood astrocytoma subtypes: Significance in tumor progression. *Anticancer Research 17*, 1187-1194 (1997).

[14]   Biernat, W., Kleihues, P., Yonekawa, Y., and Ohgaki, H. Amplification and overexpression of MDM2 in primary (de novo) glioblastomas. *J Neuropathol Exp Neurol 56*, 180-185 (1997).

[15]   Watanabe, K. *et al.* Overexpression of the EGF receptor and p53 mutations are mutually exclusive in the evolution of primary and secondary glioblastomas. *Brain Pathol 6*, 217-223 (1996).

[16]   Watanabe, K., Tachibana, O., Yonekawa, Y., Kleihues, P., and Ohgaki, H. Role of gemistocytes in astrocytoma progression. *Lab Invest 76*, 277-284 (1997).

[17]   Pollack, I.F., Campbell, J.W., Hamilton, R.L., Martinez, A.J., and Bozik, M.E: Proliferation index as a predictor of prognosis in malignant gliomas of childhood. *Cancer 79*, 849-856 (1997).

[18]   Jay, V., Edwards, V., Halliday, W., Rutka, J., and Lau, R. "Polyphenotypic" tumors in the central nervous system: problems in nosology and classification. *Pediatr Pathol Lab Med 17*, 369-389 (1997).

[19]   Csatary, L.K. Viruses in the treatment of cancer. *Lancet 2*, 825 (1971).

[20]   Csatary, L.K., Romvary, J., Kasza, L., Schaff, S., and Massey, R.J. *In vivo* interference between pathogenic and non-pathogenic viruses. *J Med 16*, 563-573 (1985).

[21]   Webb, H.E., and Gordon-Smith, C.E. Viruses in the treatment of cancer. *Lancet 1*, 1206-1208 (1970).

[22]   Cassell, W., and Garrett, R.E.: Newcastle disease virus as an antineoplastic agent. *Cancer 18*, 863-868 (1965).

[23]   Csatary, L.K. *et al.* Attenuated vetenary virus vaccine for the treatment of cancer. *Cancer Detection and Prevention 17*, 619-627 (1993).

[24] Csatary, L.K., Csatary, E., and Moss, R.W. Re: Scientific interest in newcastle disease virus is reviving. *J Natl Cancer Inst 92*, 493-494 (2000).

[25] Walker, P.R., and Sikorska, M.: New aspects of the mechanism of DNA fragmentation in apoptosis. Biochem Cell Biol *75:* 287-299, 1997.

[26] Walker, P.R., Saas, P., and Dietrich, P-Y. Role of Fas ligand (CD95L) in immune escape: the tumor cells strikes back. *J Immunol 158*, 4521-4524 (1997).

[27] Mule, J.J., Schwarz, S.L., Roberts, A.B., Sporn, M.B., and Rosenberg, S.A. Transforming growth factor-beta inhibits the *in vitro* generation of lymphokine-activated killer cells and cytotoxic T cells. *Cancer Immunol Immunother 26*, 95-100 (1988).

[28] Sporn, M.B., Roberts, A.B., Wakefield, L.M., and Assoian, R.K. Transforming growth factor-beta: biological function and chemical structure. *Science 233*, 532-534 (1986).

[29] Rivoltini, L., *et al.* Phenotypic and functional analysis of lymphocytes infiltrating paediatric tumours, with a characterization of the tumour phenotype. *Cancer Immunol Immunother 34*, 241-251 (1992).

[30] Bodey B., Bodey B. Jr., and Siegel S.E. Immunophenotypic characterization of infiltrating poly- and mononuclear cells in childhood brain tumors. *Modern Pathology 8*, 333-338 (1995).

[31] Bodey B., Bodey B. Jr., Siegel S.E., and Kaiser H.E. Immunocytochemical detection of leukocyte-associated and apoptosis-related antigen expression in childhood brain tumors. *Critical Reviews Oncology/Hematology 39*, 3-16 (2001).

[32] Csatary, L.K., *et al.*: Beneficial treatment of patients with advanced cancer using a Newcastle disease virus vaccine (MTH-68/H). *Anticancer Res 19*, 635-638 (1999).

[33] Fábián, Zs., *et al.* Induction of apoptosis by a newcastle disease virus vaccine (MTH-68/H) in PC12 rat phaeochromocytoma cells. *Anticancer Research 21*, 125-135 (2001).

[34] Bodey B., Bodey B. Jr., Siegel S.E., and Kaiser H.E. Spontaneous regression of neoplasms in mammals. Review of the cases published between 1988 and 1997. *IN VIVO 12*, 107-122 (1998).

[35] Bodey B. Spontaneous Regression of Neoplasms: New Possibilities for Immunotherapy. *EOBT*, in print (2002).

[36] Gallucci, M., Catalucci, A., Scheithauer, B.W., and Forbes G.S. Spontaneous involution of pilocytic astrocytoma in a patient without neurofibromatosis type 1: case report. *Radiology 214*, 223-226 (2000).

[37] Bodey, B. The significance of immunocytochemistry in the diagnosis and therapy of neoplasms. *EOBT 2*, 371-393 (2002).

[38] Bodey B., Bodey B. Jr, Siegel S.E., and Kaiser H.E. Fas (APO-1, CD95) receptor expression in childhood astrocytomas. Is it a marker of the major apoptotic pathway or a signaling receptor for immune escape of neoplastic cells? *IN VIVO 13*, 357-373 (1999).

[39] Bodey B. Genetically Engineered Antibodies for Direct Anti-Neoplastic Treatment and Neoplactic Cells Directed Delivery of Various Therapeutic Agents. *EOBT 1*, 603-617 (2001).

In: Leading Topics in Cancer Research
Editor: Lee P. Jeffries, pp. 235-251

ISBN 1-60021-332-4
© 2007 Nova Science Publishers, Inc.

Chapter 9

PROTECTIVE EFFECT OF ALPHA-TOCOPHEROL (VITAMIN E) IN HEAD AND NECK CANCER RADIATION-INDUCED MUCOSITIS

Paulo Renato Ferreira and Marta Pereira-Lima

Department of Radiation Oncology, Hospital de Clinicas de Porto Alegre, Universidade Federal do Rio Grande do Sul, Porto Alegre, RS, Brazil

ABSTRACT

The fundamental principle of radiotherapy is to destroy malignant cells while minimizing damage to normal tissues. Almost all patients who receive radiotherapy to the head and neck area develop some grade of acute mucositis, which is not only painful, but may compromise tumor control by determining decrease in dose intensity and interruptions of the treatment. The term 'oral mucositis' describes the adverse effect of chemotherapy or radiation induced inflammation of the oral mucosa. Symptoms of mucositis vary from pain and discomfort to an inability to tolerate food or fluids. The degree and duration of mucositis in patients receiving radiotherapy are related to radiation source, cumulative dose, dose intensity, volume of irradiated mucosa, smoking/alcohol consumption and oral hygiene conditions. To our knowledge, there is no other controlled study which has evaluated vitamin E as a single radioprotective agent in patients with head and neck tumors treated with radiation therapy alone or post-operative. For this reason, we conducted a double-blind, randomized trial with the objective to investigate the potential mucosal protection of vitamin E in irradiated patients with head and neck cancer, motivated by its simplicity of administration, no severe toxicity in conventional doses, low cost and easy availability.

The fundamental principle of radiotherapy is to destroy malignant cells while minimizing damage to normal tissues. Almost all patients who receive radiotherapy to the head and neck area develop some grade of acute mucositis [1], which is not only painful, but may compromise tumor control by determining decrease in dose intensity and interruptions of the treatment [2]. The term 'oral mucositis' describes the adverse effect of chemotherapy or radiation induced inflammation of the oral mucosa [3]. Symptoms of mucositis vary from pain and discomfort to an inability to tolerate food or fluids. The degree and duration of mucositis in patients receiving radiotherapy are related to radiation source, cumulative dose, dose intensity, volume of irradiated mucosa, smoking/alcohol consumption and oral hygiene conditions [4, 5]. The pathogenesis of oral mucositis is thought to involve direct and indirect mechanisms. It is generally believed that oral mucositis is consequent to the direct inhibitory effects of therapy on DNA replication and mucosal cell proliferation [6]. Indirect effects result from release of inflammatory mediators, loss of protective salivary constituents, therapy-induced neutropenia, and the emergence of microorganisms on damaged mucosa [7]. Sonys et al [8] proposed a four phase hypothesis as to the mechanisms of the development of mucositis: 1) inflammatory or vascular phase, induced by toxic cytokines released from epithelial cells after chemotherapy or radiotherapy administration; 2) epithelial phase, characterized by atrophy and ulceration due to reduced renewal of the oral basal epithelium; 3) ulcerative or bacteriological phase, during which some areas of erosion become covered with a fibrinous pseudomembrane. Bacterial colonization occurs, producing endotoxins which contribute to further cytokines release; and 4) healing phase, with epithelial renewal and reestablishment of the local flora. Histopathologically, edema and vascular changes such as thickening of the tunica intima, reduction in the size of the lumen and destruction of the elastic and muscle fibers of the vessel walls are noted [9]. A number of agents with potentially mucosal protection capabilities and different mechanisms of action in radioinduced mucositis has been investigated in randomized trials. Most of them have reduced number of patients, and their efficacy and safety have not been clearly established [1,10,11]. Consequently, there is no standard intervention for oral radioinduced mucositis [7].

PREVENTION AND TREATMENT OF RADIOINDUCED MUCOSITIS

General Measures

Adequate mouth and dental hygiene during the radiotherapy period is one of the most effective measure to prevent mucositis [11,12]. Abrasive toothpastes, oral irritating solutions, smoking, alcohol, acid or excessively hot or cold foods should be avoided [13]. In a consensus conference, the National Institute of Health of the USA [14] recommended some previous measures for head and neck patients candidates to radiotherapy, such as patient and family counseling about side effects of therapy, treatment of preexisting dental cavities at least 14 days before treatment commencement, and intensive use of toothpaste, dental floss and frequent mouth washes with oral fluoride.

Oral Antiseptics, Antibiotics and Antiinflamatories

The oropharyngeal bacterial flora is composed mainly of anaerobics, streptococci and neisseria sp. Necrotic tumors are an adequate medium for many microorganisms, and radiotherapy may predispose to bacterial overgrowth by damaging dividing cells leading to colonization by abnormal bacteria and by reducing saliva. Oral antiseptics such as chlorhexidine, have been tested as mucosal protectants, but no significant effect has been observed [15,16,17]. By the other hand, iodine povidone was reported to decrease incidence, intensity and duration of oral mucositis when compared with placebo [18]. The antibiotic association of polimyxin E, tobramycin and anfotericin B was evaluated by three trials, which found different conclusions. Spijkervet *et al.* [15] conducted a three arm trial comparing polimixin E, tobramycin and anfotericin B versus chlorhexidine versus placebo in patients with head and neck tumors treated with radiotherapy alone. There was a significant reduction in mucositis intensity in the first arm. In a similar larger trial, Symonds *et al.* [19] confirmed these results. However, Okuno *et al.* [20] found no differences favouring these antibiotics association. In a trial conducted by Leborgne et al [21], prednisone reduced interruptions in radiotherapy necessary for recovering of oral toxicity, but it had no effect on intensity and duration of mucositis. Two additional pilot studies confirmed the efficacy of corticosteroids versus placebo [22,23].

Anti-Ulcer Agents

Because ulceration of the oral epithelium is part of the mucositis process, the preventive role of anti- peptic ulcer agents has been evaluated. Sucralfate has been the most investigated agent in randomized trials, but results are conflicting. Lievens *et al.* [24], Barker *et al.* [25], Epstein *et al.* [26], Makkonen *et al.* [27] and Ferreira [28] have found no significant differences between sucralfate and placebo, whereas Scherlacher *et al.* [29], Valls *et al.* [30] and Franzén *et al.* [31] found significant mucosal protection. In a literature review, Belka *et al.* [32] concluded that, except in pelvic tumors, sucralfate has limited benefit in radiation induced mucositis of the head and neck.

Prostaglandins and Antiprostaglandins

Prostaglandins are radioprotective drugs, especially of the gastrointestinal tract [11]. Some small trials found reduction in mucositis intensity with prostaglandin E (PGE_2) in irradiated patients with head and neck tumors [33,34,35]. The role of prostaglandins in the infammatory process envolved in mucositis was investigated by Pillsbury *et al.* [36]. Compared to placebo, indometacin, an anti-prostaglandin agent, reduced intensity and postponed the onset of mucositis in irradiated patients with head and neck tumors.

Colony Stimulating Factors

Granulocytes colony stimulating factor (G-CSF) and granulocytes and macrophages colony stimulating factor (GM-CSF) are glycoproteins related to neutrophille and monocytes/macrophages proliferation and differentiation [11]. GM-CSF may also stimulate proliferation and migration of oral mucosal cells [37,38]. Two phase II studies showed that GM-CSF reduced the incidence of mucositis in patiens undergoing total body irradiation (TBI) [39,40] and radiotherapy for head and neck cancer [41,42,43]. Keratinocyte growth factor-2 (KGF-2) is an new class of agent that has no in vitro or in vivo proliferative effects on human epithelial-like tumor, but it selectively induces epithelial cell proliferation, differentiation and migration. This failure to stimulate tumor cell growth characterizes the ability of this drug to specifficaly target normal epithelial cells [44,45]

Amifostine

Amifostine, an aminothyol with radioprotective capabilities in normal tissues, was tested in some trials with patients with head and neck tumors. Büntzel et al. [46] evaluated 39 patients treated with radiotherapy and chemotherapy and found that amifostine reduced significantly the frequency of grade 3 and 4 mucositis, with apparently no interference on the therapeutic effect of therapy. Similar results were observed in a small trial conducted by Wagner et al. [47], where amifostine reduced both intensity and duration of oral mucositis. However, data for protection of mucositis are considered marginal and insufficient to recommend amifostine at this time [48].

Other Agents

Other agents with different mechanisms of action have been used as potential radioprotectants. Capsaicin, an agent which has been used in neuropathic syndroms, was topically employed in the oral mucosa of 11 patients with head and neck tumors undergoing chemoradiotherapy [49]. There was a significant reduction in pain intensity. Silver nitrate at 2% was investigated in 16 patients with head and neck tumors submitted to a split- course hiperfractionated radiotherapy. In the 5 days before and the 2 days after the onset of radiotherapy, left oral mucosa was topically treated with silver nitrate 3 times a day. The right size was kept as control without medication. Duration and intesity of mucositis were significantly reduced.

Vitamins

Several vitamins have shown radioprotective activity in animal and human models. Ascorbic acid (vitamin C) protected mouse spermatogonies against irradiation of ^{125}I [50]. In a randomized clinical trial, β-caroten, a vitamin A precursor, significantly reduced grades 3 and 4 oral mucositis in patients with head and neck tumors treated by radiotherapy and chemotherapy [51]. Although one study reported no radioprotective effect of vitamin E in rats by the criteria of chromosomal aberrations [52], many authors found significant evidence of intestinal [53,54,55,56] and oral mucosal protection [57] in irradiated rodents receiving systemic or topic vitamin E. Some phase III clinical trials also found significant oral mucosal protection when vitamin E was used alone in chemotherapy studies or combined to other protective agents in a chemoradiation study. In a randomized, double-blind trial with 18 evaluable patients treated with chemotherapy alone for several malignancies, Wadleigh et al [58] found that daily doses of 400 mg of vitamin E topically applied significantly speeded the healing of oral mucositis. The duration of mucositis (median of 3 days) was significantly shorter in the vitamin E group comparing to placebo group (only 1 among 9 patients had healing of mucosal lesions on the five days of observation). No toxicity was observed. The authors concluded that topical use of vitamin E is safe in preventing oral mucositis induced by chemotherapy.

One trial evaluated vitamin E and other similar drugs as radioprotective agents, in which vitamin E was not the experimental drug. Osaki et al. [59] randomized 63 patients with head and neck tumors treated with radiotherapy and concomitant chemotherapy. The experimental group received daily doses of azelastine, a histamin H1 antagonist with antioxidant activity, vitamin C, vitamin E and gluthation. The control group received identical treatment, but no azelastine. The study showed that 21 patients of the experimental group had grades 1 and 2 oral mucositis, and 16 had lesions grades 3 and 4. In the control group, only 5 patients had grades 1 and 2 oral mucositis, but 21 had lesions grades 3 and 4. The authors conclude that azelastine may be useful in the prevention of grades 3 and 4 oral mucositis induced by chemoradiotherapy.

In another randomized trial, Lopez et al [60] evaluated 19 patients with acute myelogenous leukemia treated with either induction or intensive chemotherapy followed by autologous bone marrow transplant. The duration of grades 3-4 of oral mucositis was significantly shorter in patients receiving 2 ml of topical vitamin E over the oral mucosa in the arm treated with induction chemotherapy. The plasmatic concentration of vitamin E was unexpectedly lower in patients receiving vitamin E than in patients receiving placebo. Their data suggested that the intestinal absorption of vitamin E does not seem significant, and that the mucosal protective action is mainly due to a local effect.

RATIONAL FOR THE PREVENTIVE EFFECT OF VITAMIN E IN RADIOINDUCED MUCOSITIS

As experimentally demonstrated in the intestinal mucosa of rodents, there is substantial data to support that radiation induced oxygen free radicals act as mediators of cell injury following ionizing irradiation [53,54,61]. Free radicals induce DNA structural modifications which are incompatible with cell survival, if not repaired [62]. They also remove hydrogen atoms from cell membrane fatty acids, a reaction called lipidic peroxidation, which results in alterations of membrane permeability and, ultimately, in cell death [63].

Under physiological conditions, some protective mechanisms are important natural defensive agents against the oxidative action caused by free radicals, such as cytoprotective enzymes (superoxide dismutase, catalase, glutathione peroxidase) and antioxidants (tocopherols, carotenes, ascorbic acid, reduced glutathione) [64]. Providing ionizing radiation and many cytotoxic drugs are known to produce free radicals, and because they are implicated in the process of cell killing, mutagenesis, transformation and carcinogenesis, it is reasonable to assume that scavenging free radicals agents would play a significant role in modulating these processes [55].

Alpha-tocopherol, the main constituent of vitamin E, is the most important natural antioxidant present in the human blood [63]. Its main biological function is to scavenge peroxil free radicals (HO_2) in the cell membrane. Vitamin E has been reported as capable to stabilize cellular membranes and to improve herpetic gengivitis, possibly through its antioxidant activity [65,66,67]. According to Köstler et al [68], the rational for the topical use of vitamin E as a mucosal protective agent is based upon its antioxidant and membrane stabilizing action, which interferes with the inflammatory damage caused by reactive oxygen free radicals created in the course of chemotherapy or radiotherapy. Consequently, because vitamin E is inexpensive, readily available and well tolerated, confirmatory and prophylactic trials would be of great interest.

A DOUBLE-BLIND, RANDOMIZED TRIAL ON THE PROTECTIVE EFFECT OF VITAMIN E ON RADIOINDUCED MUCOSITIS IN HEAD AND NECK CANCER

To our knowledge, there is no other controlled study which has evaluated vitamin E as a single radioprotective agent in patients with head and neck tumors treated with radiation therapy alone or post-operative. For this reason, we conducted a double-blind, randomized trial with the objective to investigate the potential mucosal protection of vitamin E in irradiated patients with head and neck cancer, motivated by its simplicity of administration, no severe toxicity in conventional doses, low cost and easy availability [69,70]. Our study admitted patients with confirmed histological diagnosis of cancer of the oral cavity and oropharynx referred to radiotherapy. They were evaluated at Hospital de Clinicas de Porto Alegre – Universidade Federal do Rio Grande do Sul (UFRGS) and received irradiation alone or post-operative at Hospital Sao Lucas da PUCRS - Pontificia Universidade Catolica do Rio Grande do Sul (HSL-PUCRS) in Porto Alegre, Southern Brazil. The trial was approved by the Scientific and Bioethics Committees of both institutions in accordance with the precepts established by the Helsinki Declaration. An informed consent was obtained from all patients. Admission requirements consisted of: 1) a minimal irradiated buccal mucosal area $\geq$ 12,2 cm^2. The limits of this area, measured on verification films, were the hard palate (superior), the floor of the mouth (inferior), the anterior border of the vertical portion of the mandible (posterior) and the distal border of the irradiation field (anterior); 2) age $\geq$ 21; 3) Zubrod [71] performance status grade 2 or lower, 4) tolerance of solid food at study entry, and 5) no trismus, concomitant use of oral anticoagulants, previous or current history of other cancers, previous history of radiotherapy in the head and neck area nor previous or concomitant chemotherapy. The initial evaluation consisted in history, physical/ otolaryngological/dental examination, computed tomography of the head and neck, chest x-ray study and complete blood count. Patients were staged according to the UICC (International Union Against Cancer) -TNM classification [72].

Randomization process was conducted by coworkers not directly involved in this study. Patient's names were picked out by lot and allocated in a grid with 5 blanks per line, according to the group of treatment: vitamin E or placebo. Intermittently, the line sequences were changed in order to improve the randomization. Neither the authors nor patients were aware of the identification of the prescribed drugs. Patients were given either 400 mg of vitamin E (Ephynal©, Produtos Roche Quimicos e Farmaceuticos, Sao Paulo, SP, Brazil) or 500 mg of placebo (Efamol Pure Evening Primrose Oil©, Kentville, NS, Canada). The drugs were available as an oil solution enclosed in capsules. Patients were taught to dissolve it in saliva, rinse it all over the oral cavity during 5 minutes, and then swallow it immediately before every session of irradiation, Monday through Friday, from the first to the last day of radiotherapy. A second capsule was similarly administered at patient's home after 8-12 hours. Both vitamin E and placebo capsules had the same size, shape, color and texture and were given to the patients in vials supplied weekly. The drug used as placebo is a combination of fatty acids (oleic, linoleic, gama-linoleic, palmitic, stearic and others), but also contains 2.5 % of vitamin E in its formula (13 I.U. per capsule of 500 mg). Prescribed analgesics were paracetamol/codeine or dipyrone whenever necessary.

Radiotherapy was provided by a Cobalt 60 unit (Theratron Phoenix) operating at 80 cm target-skin distance. Two parallel opposed fields were designed with customized alloy shielding blocks to include the tumor within a 2 cm safe margin and the upper cervical lymph nodes bilaterally. Anterior supraclavicular fields were added whether metastatic cervical lymph nodes were present or the primary tumor was located in tonsils or tongue. A daily dose of 2 Gy/section/5 days a week was calculated at the midline up to a cumulative dose of 44 Gy/4.5 weeks. A first field reduction was made for spinal cord sparing up to the dose of 60 Gy/6 weeks. A second reduction was made to encompass only the tumor within 1 cm margins up to the final dose of 70 Gy/7 weeks. Patients previously treated with complete or incomplete resections were planned to receive total doses of 50 or 60 Gy in 5 and 6 weeks, respectively, with a similar technique. Check films were obtained during patient set up and weekly for subsequent quality control, throughout radiotherapy. Protocol violations were established when patients: 1) did not receive the prescribed dose of irradiation, 2) interrupted radiotherapy more than 3 consecutive fractions, or 3) did not take the protocol medications adequately.

A comprehensive dentistry evaluation was made in order to assure adequate balancing of pre-treatment conditions related to secondary factors associated with mucositis severity. Patients had their weight recorded and oral mucositis evaluated and graded by the same investigator on the first day of radiotherapy, and then subsequently once a week until the last fraction. The RTOG/EORTC [73] (Radiation Therapy Oncology Group/European Organization for Research and Treatment of Cancer) objective grading system was used: grade 0- no changes over baseline; grade 1- Injection. May experience mild pain. No analgesics required; grade 2- patchy mucositis may produce inflammatory serosanguinous discharge. May experience moderate pain requiring analgesia; grade 3- confluent fibrinous mucositis. May experience severe pain requiring narcotic; grade 4-ulceration, hemorrhage or necrosis. For the purposes of this study, symptomatic mucositis was considered as grade ≥ 2. To evaluate the impact on quality of life, at the end of the treatment patients filled out a questionnaire based on the World Health Organization Grading of Mucositis/Stomatitis [7], where they informed the occurrence of pain and oral intake difficulty during radiotherapy. This subjective grading system consisted in the following scale: grade 0- no pain; grade 1- painful mucositis did not require modifications in oral intake; grade 2- painful mucositis, can eat but did require decrease in liquids intake any time during radiotherapy; grade 3- painful mucositis prevented oral intake; 4-painful mucositis required parenteral or enteral support any time during radiotherapy.

The main endpoint was the severity of oral mucositis. All randomized patients were counted for the analysis, according to the intention to treat principle. Not all the patients completed 7 weeks of radiotherapy because some had been submitted to previous surgery and required lower doses of irradiation. "Patients-week" were defined as the number of patients at

risk who were in the study in every week of radiotherapy. For every patient-week, each
record of symptomatic buccal mucositis was considered as a single event. The number of
events of symptomatic mucositis was correlated with the number of patients-week, aiming to
take into account the duration of time the patient suffered the toxicity. A density of incidences
of symptomatic mucositis was calculated as a coefficient obtained by the number of
symptomatic mucositis events divided by the number of patients-week in every week of
radiotherapy. The study was designed to test a moderate to large effect. The expected sample
size was estimated based on a 15% difference in the scores of symptomatic mucositis between
vitamin E and placebo groups from a previous pilot study carried out with 28 patients
reported elsewhere [74]. One hundred fifty-one patients-week were estimated as necessary in
each arm. A significant level of 5% and a statistical power of 80% were adopted in order to
test a minimal incidence difference of at least 15 events for every 100 patients-week.
Secondary endpoints were duration of mucositis and weight loss. For the same significance
level, statistical power and sample size, the estimated differences required for the duration of
symptomatic mucositis and weight loss between both groups were at least 10 days and 11 kg,
respectively.

Pre-treatment characteristics, as well as differences in the intensity of mucositis and
complications, were analyzed by the Pearson's Chi-square test with a confidence interval of
95% (CI95%). Student's t test and Mann-Whitney test were utilized to compare differences
between means and medians, respectively. Survival estimates were obtained by the Kaplan-
Meier test [75], and the differences between survival curves by the Log Rank Test. All P
values were two-tailed.

From December 1997 to December 1999, fifty-four patients were randomized. Twenty-
eight were accrued to vitamin E group and 26 to the placebo group. Frequencies of gender,
age, histological type, tumor location, stage, previous surgery, oral and dental evaluation,
smoking and alcohol consumption were similar in both arms (table 1). Most of the patients
were male. The mean age was 55.4 years (standard deviation [SD]=12.5). The most frequent
histology and anatomical site were squamous cell carcinoma and oral cavity, respectively.
Forty patients had stages III and IV disease: 24/28 (85.7%) belonged to the vitamin E group
and 16/26 (61.5%) to the placebo group (RR [relative risk]=1.39; CI95%=0.99-1.96;
P=0.086). Around 2/3 of the patients had been submitted to previous surgery. Most of them
had some type of oral or dental alteration (23/28 and 16/26 patients in vitamin E and placebo
groups, respectively), and history of cigarette and alcohol consumption. Three patients from
the vitamin E group did not receive the prescribed doses: two due to intense mucositis and
one due to death assigned to tumor progression. The median follow-up of the 54 patients was
12 months (range:2-24 months).

At twenty-four months, the estimated overall and median survivals for all patients were
44.8% and 9.5 months (range: 2-24) respectively. For patients of the vitamin E and placebo
groups, these figures were 32.2% and 8.5 months (range: 2-24) and 62.9% and 12.5 months
(range: 2-23) respectively (P=0.126).

All the patients developed varying degrees of mucositis during radiotherapy (table 2).
Symptomatic mucositis was more frequent in the placebo group than in the vitamin E group:
36 events of symptomatic mucositis were observed in 167 patients-week (21.6%) of the
vitamin E group, whereas 54 events of symptomatic mucositis were observed in 161 patients-
week (33.5%) of the placebo group. These data were computed in the calculation of a density

Table 1. Patient characteristics

Characteristics	Number of patients per treatment group (%)				P
	Vitamin E		Placebo		
Gender					0.999
Male	25	(89.3)	23	(88.5)	
Female	3	(10.7)	3	(11.5)	
AGE					0.268
Mean (standard deviation)	53.5 (9.1)		57.3 (15.3)		
Histology					0.347
Squamous cell carcinoma	26	(92.8)	21	(80.8)	
Undifferentiated Carcinoma	1	(3.6)	4	(15.4)	
Adenoid cystic carcinoma	0	(0)	1	(3.8)	
Fibrossarcoma	1	(3.6)	0	(0)	
Anatomical site					0.789
Tonsil	3	(10.7)	5	(19.2)	
Base of the tongue	4	(14.3)	2	(7.7)	
Retromolar trigone	3	(10.7)	2	(7.7)	
Soft palate	0	(0)	1	(3.8)	
Oral tongue	10	(35.7)	9	(34.6)	
Floor of the mouth	8	(28.6)	7	(26.9)	
Stage					0.142
I	0	(0)	3	(11.5)	
II	4	(14.3)	7	(26.9)	
III	5	(17.8)	4	(15.4)	
IV	19	(67.9)	12	(46.2)	
Previous Surgery					0.840
Yes	18	(64.3)	17	(65.4)	
No	10	(35.7)	9	(34.6)	
Oral and Dental Evaluation					0.610
Normal teeth and oral mucosa	5	(17.8)	10	(38.5)	
Single alterations					
Periodontal disease	5	(17.8)	4	(15.4)	
Increased coating of the tongue	3	(10.7)	1	(3.8)	
Fibrous hyperplasia	2	(7.1)	1	(3.8)	
Gingivitis	1	(3.6)	1	(3.8)	
Multiple alterations					
Periodontal disease, cavities, pericoronitis, fibrous hyperplasia, increased coating of the tongue	8	(28.6)	4	(15.4)	
No evaluation	4	(14.3)	5	(19.2)	
Cigarrette smoking history	27	(96.4)	24	(92.3)	0.603
Yes					
No	1	(3.6)	2	(7.7)	
Alcohol History					0.878
Yes	21	(75.0)	20	(77.0)	
No	7	(25.0)	6	(23.0)	

of incidences (RR= 0.643, 95CI%= 0.42-0.98, P= 0.038) (table 3). Accordingly, 8.3 patients-week were required for vitamin E avoiding one event of symptomatic mucositis. Maximum peaks of symptomatic mucositis occurred at the 6th week and 5th week for the vitamin E and placebo groups, respectively (figure 1). As shown in table 4, an analysis of the questionnaires answered by patients at the end of the treatment also revealed that vitamin E decreased pain and restriction in oral intake (grades 2-3) during radiotherapy (3/28 patients= 10.7% vs. 14/26 patients= 53.8%) (P=0.0001).

Table 2. Events of symptomatic mucositis according to the radiotherapy week and the number of patients-week

Week	Events of symptomatic mucositis					
	Vitamin E group (28 patients)			Placebo group (26 patients)		
	Patients-week	Number of events	(%)	Patients-week	Number of events	(%)
1	28	1	(3.6)	26	0	(0)
2	28	4	(14.3)	26	7	(27.0)
3	28	8	(28.6)	26	10	(38.5)
4	27	8	(29.6)	26	11	(42.3)
5	25	5	(20.0)	26	13	(50.0)
6	23	8	(34.8)	21	9	(42.9)
7	8	2	(25.0)	10	4	(40.0)
Total	167 (100)	36	(21.6)	161 (100)	54	(33.5)

Table 3. Density of incidences of symptomatic mucositis

Group	Number of events		Incidence per 100 patients-week
	Symptomatic mucositis	Patients-week	
Vitamin E	36	167	21.6
Placebo	54	161	33.5

[*] RR= 0.643, 95CI%= 0.42-0.98, P= 0.038

Table 4. Pain and oral intake restriction based on subjective data provided by patients at the end of the treatment[*]

Grade	Vitamin E Number of patients (%)		Placebo Number of patients (%)	
0	13	(46.4)	3	(11.5)
1	12	(42.8)	9	(34.6)
2	3	(10.7)	9	(34.6)
3	0	(0)	5	(19.2)
4	0	(0)	0	(0)
Total	28	(100)	26	(100)

[*] P= 0.0001

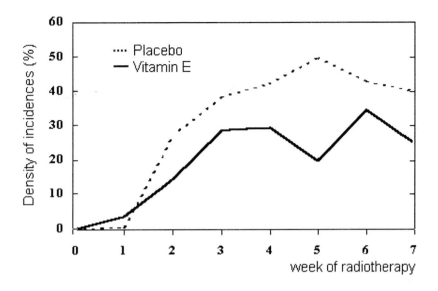

Figure 1. Density of incidences of symptomatic mucositis according to the week of radiotherapy.

Total doses of radiotherapy were similarly distributed in both arms (table 5). There was no dose-response relationship or mucosal area-dependence with the severity of mucositis. Mean doses at the primary site for the vitamin E and placebo groups were 61 Gy and 62 Gy (P=0.664) and mean durations of radiotherapy were 5.9 and 6.1 weeks, respectively (P=0.520). The median area of buccal mucosal irradiation for the vitamin E and placebo groups were 20.7 cm^2 (range:12.2-33.8) and 22.9 cm^2 (range:12.5-35.0), respectively (P=0.176).

Table 5. Frequency of the total doses of radiotherapy according to the treatment group[*]

Total dose (Gy)	Vitamin E	Placebo
	Number of patients (%)	Number of patients (%)
50	5 (17.8)	5 (19.2)
60	15 (53.5)	11 (42.3)
70	8 (28.6)	10 (38.4)
Total	28 (100)	26 (100)

[*] P=0.68

The median duration of symptomatic mucositis in patients of the vitamin E and placebo groups was one week (range: 0-5) and two weeks (range: 0-5), respectively (P=0.102). The initial mean weight in patients of the vitamin E and placebo groups (60.4 kg [SD= 10.4] and 66.2 kg [SD= 14.0], respectively) was compared to the mean weight during radiotherapy (55.5 kg [SD=20.8] and 60.7 kg [SD=22.1], respectively). The observed differences in weight were 4.9 kg and 5.5 kg, respectively (P=0.249).

Two thirds of the patients presented acute complications during the treatment (table 6). Mild nausea was the most frequent, but the majority of them may be related to the disease's natural history or to irradiation itself. Their frequencies in both treatment arms were similar (P=0.216). No late reactions were observed.

Table 6. Frequency of acute complications according to treatment group [*]

Complication	Treatment group [§]			
	Vitamin E 28 patients (%)		Placebo 26 patients (%)	
None	10	(35.7)	9	(34.6)
Mild nausea	12	(42.8)	10	(38.5)
Vomit	4	(14.3)	5	(19.2)
Fever	4	(14.3)	1	(3.8)
Candidiasis	2	(7.1)	4	(15.4)
Bleeding	2	(7.1)	9	(34.6)

[*] P=0.216.

[§] Some patients had more than one complication simultaneously.

In the vitamin E treated group, 6/9 patients had complete resolution of their mucositis within 4 days of initiating therapy, whereas in the placebo group only one patient had resolution of the lesions during the same time.

The proper assessment of the oral mucosa is of great importance before initiating therapy and throughout a treatment course. A variety of protocols and grading systems has been established and at least two of them incorporate both subjective and objective criteria: the RTOG/EORTC and the Wold Health Organization Grading of Mucositis/Stomatitis [7]. We used both scales based on their simplicity. Some studies define grade 3 and 4 as severe mucositis. No conventions for such reporting have been published. Many studies only report the incidence of severe reactions, whereas others combine "grade 2-3" reactions [76]. We considered RTOG grade 2 as symptomatic mucositis because it also expresses impairment in quality of life as consequence of inflammatory reaction, moderate to significant pain and necessity of analgesics. The frequency of symptomatic mucositis in the experimental arm was 64% of that observed in the placebo arm, which means that vitamin E reduced the risk of symptomatic mucositis development by 36%. By the other hand, since the differences in duration of mucositis and weight loss were lower than the minimal differences detectable by the sample size, our study had no sufficient statistical power to, conclusively, define whether vitamin E was capable or not to significantly influence these secondary endpoints.

The concentration of vitamin E in our placebo was considered acceptable for the purpose of this study because it corresponds to only 3.1% of drug concentration present in the active drug. The presence of vitamin E in placebo capsules has been reported in similar studies [58].

Although there was a trend of poorer survival in the experimental arm, it is unlikely that vitamin E has influenced short term survival, since the differences between both curves were non significant. We attribute this trend to the higher frequency of stages III and IV prevailing in the vitamin E arm, although these differences were also non significant. Mild nausea was more frequently reported by patients in the vitamin E group, whereas bleeding was more frequent in the placebo group. However, many of these symptoms may be attributable to radiotherapy and the tumor itself. Differences in complications between both groups were non significant, suggesting that vitamin E did not induce relevant toxicity.

We conclude that patients of the vitamin E group had lower frequencies of symptomatic mucositis than patients of the placebo group. On the other hand, our study had no sufficient statistical power to conclusively assess differences in the duration of symptomatic mucositis and weight loss. The administration of vitamin E was simple, side effects had low toxicity and no significant influence in survival was observed. We consider that vitamin E has a potential protective effect on the oral mucosa of irradiated patients with tumors of the oral cavity and oropharynx. The most effective dose, frequency of administration, and synergistic role of other natural antioxidants with vitamin E are issues still to be investigated. New studies are necessary to confirm our results and address further questions.

REFERENCES

[1]   Loprinzi CL, Gastineau DA, Foote RL: Oral complications. In: Abeloff M, Armitage JO, Lichter AS, Niederhuber JE, editors. *Clinical Oncology*. 2nd ed. New York: Churchill Livingstone; 2000. pp. 965-979.

[2]   Parsons J: the effect of radiation on normal tissues of the head and neck. In: Million R, Cassisi N, editors. *Management of the head and neck cancer: A multidisciplinary approach*. 2nd ed. Philadelphia: JB Lippincott; 1994, pp. 245-289.

[3]   Naidu MU, Ramana GV, Rani PU, Mohan IK et al: Chemotherapy-induced and/or radiation therapy-induced oral mucositis-complicating the treatment of cancer. *Neoplasia*. 2004;6:423-431.

[4]   Franzen L, Funegard U, Ericson T, and Henriksson R (1992). Parotid gland function during and following radiotherapy of malignancies in the head and neck. *Eur J Cancer* 1992:28, 457–462.

[5]   Verdi CJ: Cancer therapy and oral mucositis—an approval of drug prophylaxis. *Drug Saf* 1993:9: 185 – 195.

[6]   Lockhart PB, Sonis ST: Alterations in the oral mucosa caused by chemotherapeutic agents. *J Dermatol Surg* 1981;7:1019-1025.

[7]   Wilkes JD: Prevention and treatment of oral mucositis following cancer chemotherapy. *Semin Oncol* 1998;5:538-551.

[8]   Sonis ST: Mucositis as a biological process: a new hypothesis for the development of chemotherapy-induced stomatotoxicity. *Oral Oncol* 1998;34: 39-43.

[9]   Berger A, Kilroy T: Oral complications. In: De Vita VT, Hellman S, Rosenberg SA, editors. *Cancer, Principles and Practice of Oncology*. 5th ed. Philadelphia: JB Lippincott; 2001. pp. 2714-2725.

[10]   Berger A, Kilroy T: Oral complications. In: De Vita VT, Hellman S, Rosenberg SA, editors. *Cancer, Principles and Practice of Oncology*. 6th ed. Philadelphia: JB Lippincott; 2001. pp. 2881.

[11]   Symonds RP: Treatment-induced mucositis: An old problem with new remedies. *Br J Cancer* 1998;77:1689-1695.

[12]   Feber T. Management of mucositis in oral irradiation. *Clin. Oncol* (R. Coll. Radiol.) 1996;8: 106-111.

[13] Loprinzi CL.; Gastineau DA; Foote RL: Oral complications. In: Abeloff M., Armitage JO; Lichter AS; Niederhuber JE; (ed.) . *Clinical Oncology*. 2.ed. New York. Churchill Livingstone; 2000. p. 965-979.

[14] NIH Consens Statement Online - 1989 April 17-19. Oral complications of cancer therapy. *Diagnosis, prevention and treatment*. National Institutes of Health Consensus Development Conference Statement 1989;7: 1-11.

[15] Spijkervet FL; Van Saene HK; Panders AK et al:Effect of chlorhexidine rinsing on the oropharyngeal ecology in patients with head and neck cancer who have irradiation mucositis. *Oral Surg. Oral Med. Oral Path*1989;67: 154-158.

[16] Foote RL; Loprinzi CL; Frank R et al: Randomized trial of a chlorhexidine mouthwash for the alleviation of radiation induced mucositis. *J Clin. Oncol* 1994;12: 2630, 2633.

[17] Samaranayake LP; Robertson AG; Macfarlane TW et al: The effect of chlorhexidine and benzydamine on mucositis induced by therapeutic irradiation. *Clin. Radiat* 1988;39: 291-294.

[18] Adamietz I; Rahn R; Böttcher H et al: revention of radiochemotherapy-induced mucositis: Value of the prophylactic mouth rinsing with PVP-iodine solution. *Strahlenther Onkol* 1998; 174:149-155.

[19] Symonds RP, McIlroy P, Khorrami J et al: The reduction of radiation mucositis by selective decontamination antibiotic pastilles: a placebo-controlled double-blind trial. *Br J Cancer* 1996;74:312-317.

[20] Okuno S; Foote R; Loprinzi C et al: A randomized trial of nonabsorbable antibiotic lozenge given to alleviate radiation-induced mucositis. *Cancer* 1997;79: 2193-2199.

[21] Leborgne J; Leborgne F; Zubizarreta E et al:Corticosteroids and radiation mucositis in head and neck cancer. A double-bind placebo controlled randomized trial. Radiother. *Oncol* 1998; 47: 145-148.

[22] Rothwell BR; Speltor WS: Palliation of radiation-related mucositis. *Special Care Dentistry* 1990;10: 21-25.

[23] Abdelaal A; Barker D; Fergusson M. Treatment for irradiation-induced mucositis. *Lancet,* 1987;1:97-102.

[24] Lievens Y; Haustemans K; Van den Weyngaert D *et al:* Does sucralfate reduce the acute side effects in head and neck cancer treated with radiotherapy? A double-bind randomized trial. *Radiother Oncol* 1998;47: 149-153.

[25] Barker G; Loftus L; C et al: The effects of sucralfate suspension and diphenhydramine syrup plus kaolin-pectin on radiotherapy-induced mucositis. *Oral Surg. Oral Méd. Oral Pathol* 1991; 71:288-293.

[26] Epstein JB; Wong FL: The efficacy of sucralfate suspension in the prevention of oral mucositis due to radiation therapy. *Int J. Radiat Oncol Biol Phys* 1994;28: 693-698.

[27] Makkonen T; Böstrom P; Vilja P et al: Sucralfate mouth washing in the prevention of radiation-induced mucositis: a placebo-controlled double-bind randomized study. *Int J Radiat Oncol Biol. Phys* 1994;30:177-182,.

[28] Ferreira PR: Utilização de sucralfato para a prevenção de mucosite na radioterapia dos tumores da cabeça e pescoço: um estudo randomizado. *Radiol Bras* 1993; 26: 71-80.

[29] Scherlacher A; Beufort-Spontin E: Radiotherapy of head and neck neoplasms: prevention of the inflamation of the mucosa by sucralfate treatment. *HNO* 1990;38: 24-28.

[30] Valls A; Algara M; Domènech M et al: Efficacy of sucralfate in the prophylaxis of diarrhea secondary to acute radiation-induced enteritis. Preliminary results of a double-bind randomized trial. *Med Clin (Barc.)* 1991;96: 449-452.

[31] Franzén L; Henriksson R; Littbrand B et al: Effects of sucralfate on mucositis during and following radiotherapy of malignancies in the head and neck region. A double-blind placebo-controlled study. *Acta Oncol* 1995;34: 2, 219-223.

[32] Belka C; Hoffmann W; Paulsen F et al: The use of sucralfate in radiation oncology. *Strahlenter Onkol* 1997;173:247-2525 (abst).

[33] Matejka M; Nell A; Kment G et al: Local benefit of prostaglandin E2 in radiochemotherapy-induced oral mucositis. *Br J Oral Maxillofac Surg* 1990;28: 89-94.

[34] Sinzinger H; Porterder H; Matejka M et al: Prostaglandins in irradiation induced mucositis. *Lancet* 1989;1:556-558.

[35] Porteder H; Rausch E; Kment G et al: Local prostaglandin E$_2$ in patients with oral malignancies undergoing chemo and radiotherapy. *J . Craniomaxillo Surg* 1988;16: 371.

[36] Pillsbury H; Webster W; Rosenman J: Prostaglandin inhibitor and radiotherapy in advanced head and neck cancers. *Arch. Otolaryngol. Head Neck Surg* 1986;112:552-553.

[37] Dinarello C: Interleukin 1 and interleukin antagonism. *Blood* 1991;77:1627-1652.

[38] Zaghloul MS; DORIE M; KALLMAN RF: Interleukin 1 increases thymidine labeling index of normal tissues of mice but not the tumor. *Int J Radiat Oncol Biol Phys* 1994;29: 805-811.

[39] Troussard X; Macro M.; Vie B et al: Human recombinant granulocyte macrophage colony stimulating factor (hr GM-CSF) improves double hemibody irradiation (DHBI) tolerance in patients with stage III multiple myeloma. a pilot study. *Br J Hematol* 1995;89: 191-195.

[40] Taylor K; Jagannath S; Spitzer G et al: Recombinant human granulocyte colony stimulating factor hastens granulocyte recovery after high dose chemotherapy and autologous bone marrow transplantation in Hodgkin's disease. *J Clin Oncol* 1989;7: 791-1799.

[41] Kannan V; Bapsy P; Anantha N et al: Efficacy and safety of granulocyte macrophage colony stimulating factor (GM-CSF) on the frequency and severity of radiation mucositis in patients with head and neck carcinoma. *Int. J. Radiat. Biol. Phys* 1997;37:1005-1010.

[42] Rosso M; Blasi G; Gherlone E et al: Effect of of granulocyte macrophage colony stimulating factor (GM-CSF) on prevention of mucositis in head and neck cancer patients treated with chemo-radiotherapy. *J. Chemother* 1997;9:382-385.

[43] Throuvalas M; Antonadou D; Pulizzi M et al: Evaluation of the efficacy and safety of GM-CSF in the prophylaxis of patients with head and neck cancer treated by RT. *Apresentado na European Conference of Clinical Oncology* (ECCO), p. 593. Federation of European Cancer Societies, Paris, 1995 (abst 431).

[44] Meropol NJ, Somer RA, Gutheil J et al: Randomized phase I trial of recombinant keratinocyte growth factor plus chemotherapy: potential role as mucosal protectant. *J Clin Oncol* 2003;1452 – 1458.

[45] Alderson R, Gohari-Fritsch S, Olsen H et al: In vitro and in vivo effects of repifermin (keratinocyte growth factor-2, KGF-2) on human carcinoma cells. *Cancer Chemother Pharmacol* 2002;50,202 – 212.

[46] Büntzel J; Küttner K; Fröhlich D et al: Selective radioprotection with amifostine in concurrent radiochemotherapy for head and neck cancer. *Annals Onco* 1998;9: 505-509.

[47] Wagner W; Prott F; Schonekas K:. Amifostine: a radioprotector in locally advanced head and neck tumors. *Oncol. Rep* 1998;5:1255-1257.

[48] Wasserman T, Chapman J: Radiation response modulator. In: *Principles and practice of radiation oncology.* Perez C, Brady L, Halperin E, Schmidt-Ullrich R (eds.). Philadelphia: Lippincott Williams and Wilkins, 2004. P. 679.

[49] Berger A; Ederson M; Madoolman W et al: Oral capsaicin provides temporary relief for oral mucositis pain secondary to chemotherapy/radiation therapy. *J. Pain Symptom Manage* 1995;10: 243-248.

[50] Narra V Harpanhalli R; HOWELL R et al: Vitamins as radioprotectants in vivo. I. Protection by vitamin C against internal radionuclides in mouse testes: implications to the mechanisms of the Auger effect *Radiat Res* 1994137: 394-399.

[51] Mills E: The modifying effect of beta-carotene on radiation and chemotherapy induced oral mucositis. *Br J Cancer* 1988;57: 416-42.

[52] El-Nahas SM, Mattar FE, Mohamed AA: Radioprotective effect of vitamins C and E. *Mutat Res* 1993;301:143-147.

[53] Felemovicius I, Bonsak ME, Baptista ML: Intestinal radioprotection by vitamin E (alpha tocopherol). *Ann Surg* 1995;222: 4,504-508.

[54] Delaney JP, Bonsak M, Hall P: Intestinal radioprotection by two new agents applied topically. *Ann Surg* 1992;216: 417-421,

[55] Empey LR, Papp JD, Jewell LD, et al: Mucosal protective effects of vitamin E and misoprostol during acute radiation-induced enteritis in rats. *Dig Dis Sci* 1992;37:205-214.

[56] Blumenthal RD, Lew W, Reising A, et al: Anti-oxidant vitamins reduce normal tissue toxicity induced by radio-immunotherapy. *Int J Cancer* 2000;86:276-280.

[57] Shaheen AA, Hassan SM: Radioprotection of whole body gamma-irradiation-induced alteration in some haematological parameters by cysteine, vitamin E, and their combination in rats. *Strahlenther Onkol* 1991;167:498-501.

[58] Wadleigh RG, Redman RS, Graham ML, et al: Vitamin E in the treatment of chemotherapy-induced mucositis. *Am J Med* 1992;92: 481-484.

[59] Osaki T, Ueta E, Yoneda K, et al: Prophylaxis of oral mucositis associated with chemoradiotherapy for oral carcinoma by Azelastine hydrochloride (Azelastine) with other antioxidants. *Head Neck* 1994;16:331-339.

[60] Lopez I, Goudou C, Ribrag V, et al: Traitement des mucines par la vitamine E lors de l'administration d'anti-neoplastiques neutropéniants. *Ann Med Interne* 1994;145: 405-408.

[61] Schofield FF, Holden D, Carr HD: Bowel disease after radiotherapy. *J R Soc Med* 1983;76:463-466.

[62] Brock WA: Kinectis of micronucleus expression in synchronized irradiated Chinese hamster ovary cells. *Cell Tissue Kinet* 1985;18: 247-252.

[63] Van Acker SA, Hoyman L, Bast A: Molecular pharmacology of vitamin E: Structural aspects of antioxidant activity. *Free Radic Biol Med* 1993;15: 311-328.

[64] Ward R, Peters T: Free radicals. In: Marshal W, Bangert S, editors. *Clinical Biochemistry – Metabolic and Clinic Aspects*. London: Church Livingstone; 1995. pp. 765-777.

[65] Regan V.; Servinova E.; Packer L: Antioxidant effects of ubiquinones in microsomes and mitochondria are mediated by tocopherol recycling. *Biochem Biophys Res Commun* 1990;169: 851-856.

[66] Tampo Y, Yonaha M: Vitamin E and gluthatione are required for preservation of microsomal gluthatione S-transferase from oxidative stress in microsomes. *Pharmacology* 66:259, 1990.

[67] Starasoler S, Haber GS: Use of vitamin E oil in primary herpes gingivostomatitis in an adult. NY State Dentristy 1978;44:382.

[68] Köstler WJ, Hejna M, Wenzel C, et al: Oral Mucositis Complicating Chemotherapy and/or Radiotherapy: Options for Prevention and Treatment. *CA Cancer J Clin* 2001;51: 290-315.

[69] Ferreira PR, Fleck JF, Diehl A et al: Protective effect of vitamin E (VE) in head and neck cancer radiation induced mucositis: a double-blind randomized trial. *Presented in the annual meeting of American Society of clinical Oncology*, 2002 (abstr 909).

[70] Ferreira PR, Fleck JF, Diehl A et al: Protective effect of alpha-tocopherol in head and neck cancer radiation-induced mucositis: a double-blind randomized trial. *Head Neck* 2004;26:313-21.

[71] Zubrod CG, Scheiderman M: Appraisal of methods for the study of chemotherapy of cancer in man. *J Chronic Dis* 1960;11:7-33.

[72] UICC, *International Union Against Cancer. TNM Classification of Malignant Tumours.* 5th ed. Wiley-Liss Inc. 1997. p. 19.

[73] Cox JD, Stetz J, Pajak TF: Toxicity criteria of the Radiation Therapy Oncology Group (RTOG) and the European Organization for Research and Treatment of Cancer (EORTC). *Int J Radiat Oncol Biol Phys* 1995;31: 1341-1346.

[74] Ferreira PR, Fleck JF, Diehl AS, et al: Vitamin E preventing radiation-induced mucositis in head and neck cancer: Interim analysis of a randomized, double-blind clinical trial. Proceedings of the 29th Paulista Meeting of Radiology, Sao Paulo, Brazil. *Rev Imagem* 1999, p. 22 (suppl).

[75] Kaplan G, Meier P: Non-parametric estimation from incomplete observations. *J Am Stat* 1958;53: 457-481.

[76] Trotti A: Toxicity in head and neck cancer: A review of trends and issues. *Int J Radiat Oncol Biol Phys* 2000;47:1-12.

In: Leading Topics in Cancer Research
Editor: Lee P. Jeffries, pp. 253-292

ISBN 1-60021-332-4
© 2007 Nova Science Publishers, Inc.

Chapter 10

TRENDS IN CANCER VACCINE

*M. Hayden, S Schroter , N. Rehan, W. Ma and B. Minev**

Moores UCSD Cancer Center
La Jolla, CA 92093-0820 USA

ABSTRACT

Cancer vaccines are becoming a promising approach to the treatment of cancer. This chapter summarizes the scientific background for the design of therapeutic cancer vaccines, as well as the challenges in their development. The current approaches to the discovery of the tumor-associated antigens as a basis for the new cancer vaccines are reviewed. The most promising methods for cancer vaccine development are also discussed. In this chapter we categorize the therapeutic cancer vaccines as follows: peptide vaccines, recombinant viral vaccines, DNA vaccines, and dendritic cell-based immunotherapy. We focus on their advantages and disadvantages and their current uses in the treatment of cancer. An up-to-date description of the results of cancer vaccine clinical trials is provided. We also discuss the future prospects in the design and the utilization of the cancer vaccines.

Keywords: Cancer vaccines, antigen presentation, tumor-associated antigens, synthetic peptides, recombinant vaccines, DNA vaccines, dendritic cells

ABBREVIATIONS

CTL, cytotoxic T lymphocytes; DC, dendritic cells; ER, endoplasmic reticulum; IL-2, interleukin 2; MHC, major histocompatibility complex; rVV, recombinant vaccinia viruses;

---

* Correspondence: Boris R. Minev, M.D., Moores UCSD Cancer Center, Bldg. MCCT, Room 4313, 3855 Health Sciences Drive, #0820, La Jolla, CA 92093-0820. Tel: (858) 822-1327. Fax: (858) 534-7061

SRP, signal recognition particle; SSR, signal sequence receptor; TAA, tumor-associated antigens; TAP, transporter associated with antigen processing; TIL, tumor infiltrating lymphocytes

1. INTRODUCTION

The possibility for the development of cancer vaccines was first recognized in 1893 by the New York surgeon William Coley who reported the regression of several human sarcomas following immune stimulation with a bacterial toxin. Renewed interest in cancer vaccines today is based on two recent advances which have allowed the design of more specific vaccine approaches: improved molecular techniques for the identification of genes encoding tumor-associated antigens, and better understanding of the mechanisms involved in antigen processing, presentation, and T cell activation. T cells expressing CD4 molecules recognize peptides of 12-25 amino acids presented by MHC class II molecules (1). The cytotoxic T-lymphocytes (CTL) expressing CD8 molecules recognize class I restricted peptides of 8-10 residues which are the products of intracellularly processed proteins (2). Cytosolic peptides are transported across the endoplasmic reticulum (ER) membrane with the help of the ATP-dependent transporters associated with antigen processing (TAP) (3). Peptides complexed with class I molecules in the ER are then transported to the cell surface for recognition by CTL (2). The interaction between CTL and the target tumor cells begins with the binding of the peptide antigen associated with MHC class I molecule to the T cell antigen receptor. Lymphocyte-mediated cytolysis is further enhanced by accessory molecules such as lymphocyte function antigens LFA-1 and LFA-3, co-stimulatory molecules (CD28, B7), and intercellular adhesion molecule ICAM-1 (4).

T realization that MHC class I restricted tumor antigens can act as targets for cytotoxic T lymphocytes (CTL) (5) promoted the search for tumor antigen genes (6, 7). CTL appear to be among the most direct and effective elements of the immune system that are capable of generating antitumor immune responses (8). Tumor cells expressing the appropriate tumor-associated antigens can be effectively recognized and destroyed by these immune effector cells, which may result in dramatic clinical responses (9-11). Both the adoptive transfer of tumor-reactive CTL and active immunization designed to elicit CTL responses have been reported to lead to significant therapeutic antitumor responses in some patients (9-11). However, these promising approaches and their applicability to many tumor types are restricted because of the limited number of tumor-associated antigens or epitopes for CTL.

2. TUMOR-ASSOCIATED ANTIGENS

A variety of approaches have been used for the identification of tumor-associated antigens (TAA) recognized by CTL. Most of the melanoma antigens have been identified by screening cDNA expression libraries with CTL reactive against melanoma (8).

Another approach for the identification of TAA involves testing of known proteins for recognition by CTL. With this approach, Kawakami et al. found that the expression of tyrosinase and gp100 correlated with lysis by HLA-A2-restricted, melanoma-reactive CTL

(12). The same investigators demonstrated later that HLA-A2+ cell lines transfected with the gene encoding gp100 can be recognized by melanoma-reactive CTL (13). Tyrosinase gene product was also recognized by HLA-A2-restricted CTL (14).

Direct isolation and sequencing of peptides eluted from the tumor cells is another method of identifying tumor-associated peptide antigens. Several groups have used this approach to isolate peptides recognized by melanoma-specific CTL (15), as well as to sequence the peptides with a triple quadriple mass spectrometer (16). This technique is complementary to the genetic approach because it allows measurement of the abundance of the antigenic peptides derived from the gene sequence. This is very important for the recognition of tumor cells by CTL, because at least 200 molecules of a peptide must occupy MHC class I molecules in order for CTL to lyse cancer cells (17). Another advantage of this technique is the direct identification of peptides naturally processed and presented on the tumor cell surface.

More recently, computer programs have been used to identify peptide sequences of known proteins based on their binding affinity for selected HLA molecules (18). We analyzed the sequence of human telomerase reverse transcriptase (hTRT) (19) for peptide sequences containing known binding motifs for the HLA-A2.1 molecule (20). We also used the software of the Bioinformatics & Molecular Analysis Section (National Institutes of Health, Washington, DC), which ranks 8-10 mer peptides based on a prediction half-time dissociation coefficient from HLA class I molecules (21). We tested whether two of the highest-ranking peptides can generate *in vitro* CTL able to recognize peptide-pulsed targets and HLA-A2+ cancer cells. We demonstrated in this study that the hTRT-specific CTL of normal individuals and patients with cancer specifically lysed a variety of HLA-A2+ cancer cell lines, suggesting the existence of precursor CTL for hTRT in both normal individuals and in cancer patients (22). Since telomerase activity is increased in the vast majority of melanomas and most other human tumors, our findings could contribute to the generation of universal telomerase-based cancer vaccines.

Using different computer-based algorithms, we identified six epitopes recognized by human CTL within the sequence of the new tumor-associated antigen MG50, which we described previously (23). There are no obvious similarities in structure between MG50 and any of the melanoma antigens described previously. Thus, MG50 differs from published sequences of MAGE, BAGE, GAGE, PRAME, and NY-ESO-1 (the cancer/testis-specific antigens), gp100, tyrosinase, MART-1/Melan-A, TRP-1 and TRP-2 (the melanocyte differentiation antigens), and CDK4, β-catenin, and MUM-1 (mutated or aberrantly expressed antigens). MG50 protein is one of the few melanoma-associated antigens that is not a melanocyte differentiation antigen or a mutated protein. The MG50 gene may be important not only because of its novelty, but because it is a large gene encoding at least six HLA class I-restricted epitopes recognized by human CTL in the context of HLA-A2.1(23). Importantly, we found that all six peptides immunized CD8+ T cells to react against both long-term and short-term HLA-A2.1+ melanoma cell lines. These data indicated that the epitopes are naturally expressed on melanoma cells, and therefore MG50 may be an excellent target for immunotherapy of melanoma.

Serological analysis of recombinant cDNA expression library of human tumors with autologous serum (SEREX) is another approach used to isolate human tumor antigens (24). Examples are tyrosinase, MAGE, NY-ESO-1, SSX2, SCB-1, and CT7 (8). Some of these antigens are T-cell defined antigens, which emphasizes the usefulness of SEREX analysis in identifying new tumor antigens.

2.1 Melanoma Antigens

Human melanoma antigens can be classified into three groups: (i) antigens expressed in melanoma, normal melanocytes, and retina; (ii) antigens expressed in several cancers and testis; and (iii) antigens specific for individual tumors.

The first group consists of nonmutated shared tumor antigens. An interesting correlation between depigmentation of skin and hair and good clinical responses to chemotherapy and immunotherapy (25), suggests that the same population of CTL recognizes both melanoma antigens and nonmutated shared antigens on melanocytes. Rosenberg et al. observed tumor regression in patients who developed vitiligo after interleukin 2 (IL-2)-related immunotherapy, suggesting that autoreactive CTL may be involved in tumor regression (26). Tyrosinase, MART-1/Melan-A, gp100, TRP1/gp75, and TRP2 have been identified as shared melanoma antigens recognized by CTL (8). These antigens may form the basis for the development of effective vaccines, but their expression on normal tissues raises concerns about the possible development of immunological tolerance and autoimmunity associated with the immunotherapy.

The second group includes several families of antigens, specifically: MAGE, BAGE, GAGE, RAGE, and NY-ESO-1. The MAGE genes are silent in a large panel of healthy adult tissues, with the exception of testis and placenta (27). Recently, 5 MAGE-A1 epitopes recognized by CTL were identified by *in vitro* stimulation with dendritic cells transduced with a recombinant canarypoxvirus (ALVAC) containing the entire MAGE-A1 gene (28). Like the MAGE genes, BAGE (29) and GAGE (30) genes are predominantly expressed in melanomas. Another gene called RAGE (renal carcinoma antigen gene) (31) is also expressed in melanomas, sarcomas and bladder tumors. Another antigen in this group is NY-ESO-1. It is not expressed in normal human tissues except testis but is frequently expressed in melanoma, breast, prostate, bladder, lung carcinoma, and other types of cancers (32). Interestingly, both HLA-A2 and HLA-A31 restricted T-cell epitopes have been identified from its primary open reading frame (33). More recently, Jeager et al. identified 3 NY-ESO-1 epitopes presented by HLA class II molecules and recognized by CD4+ T lymphocytes of 2 melanoma patients (34). Since these antigens are expressed in a variety of cancers but not in healthy tissues, they may be appropriate targets for immunotherapy.

Finally, some antigens unique to individual tumors appear through tumor-specific mutations, deletions or recombination events. A point mutation might change a normal peptide unable to bind to MHC molecules into a peptide capable of binding to MHC and, therefore, presented to the immune system. Natural tolerance eliminates any CTL recognizing normal peptides capable of binding to MHC. In case of a point mutation however, the modified peptide may become a target detected by existing CTL. Several antigens generated by point mutations on a murine tumor were recognized by autologous CTL (35). Point mutations were also found to encode human tumor antigens recognized by CTL (36-38). This group of antigens should be recognized by melanoma-specific CTL because their precursors should not have been depleted by the process of natural self-tolerance. From the clinical perspective, however, these antigens may not be useful for development of cancer vaccines because of their restriction to very few individual tumors.

2.2 Other Tumor Associated Antigens

In breast cancer and other adenocarcinomas, a polymorphic epithelial mucin (PEM) has been characterized as a tumor antigen (39-42). Mucins are high molecular weight glycoproteins. The MUC-1 mucin consists of a heavily glycosylated tandemly repeating 20-amino acid sequence, specifically PDTRPAPGSTAPPAHGVTSA (39). Aberrant glycosylation of mucins on carcinomatous epithelial cells leads to the exposure of novel core epitopes that are recognized by cytotoxic T cells (40). Even though HLA-unrestricted recognition of MUC-1 has been reported (40, 41), the establishment of mucin-specific cytotoxic T cell lines (41, 42) was a very important achievement in the attempts to develop cancer vaccines targeting this antigen. More recently, MHC-restricted CTL epitopes from non-variable number of tandem repeat sequence of MUC-1 have been identified (43). Since PEM is much more highly expressed on carcinomas than on normal tissues, it could be a suitable target for immunotherapy.

The HER2/neu protooncogene, expressed in breast cancer and other human cancers, encodes a tyrosine kinase with homology to epidermal growth factor receptor, with a relative molecular mass of 185 kd (44). HER2/neu protein is a receptor-like transmembrane protein comprising a large cysteine-rich extracellular domain that functions in ligand binding, a short transmembrane domain, and a small cytoplasmic domain (44). HER2/neu is amplified and expressed in many human cancers, largely adenocarcinomas of breast, ovary, colon, and lung. In breast cancer, HER2/neu overexpression is associated with aggressive disease and is an independent predictor of poor prognosis (45). Several class I restricted HER2/neu-derived peptides which were recognized by breast and ovarian cancer-specific cytotoxic T lymphocytes have been described (46-48).

In contrast to classI TAA, little attention has been paid to the identification of class II TAA, mostly because of the difficulties in their identification. However, a growing number of studies confirm the important role of CD4+ T cells in controlling tumor growth (49). In addition to tyrosinase (50), MAGE-3 was also recognized by CD4+ T cells, which were generated by in vitro stimulation of peripheral blood mononuclear cells (PBMC) with dendritic cells (DC) pulsed with synthetic peptides or purified MAGE-3 protein (51). A genetic approach was developed for cloning genes encoding MHC class II restricted tumor antigens. This approach allows for the screening of an invariant chain-cDNA fusion library in a genetically engineered cell line expressing the essential components of the MHC class II processing pathways. The first antigen identified with this approach was CDC27, which is recognized by CD4+ HLA-DR4-restricted tumor infiltrating lymphocytes (52). It was recently reported that a MART-1-derived peptide presented by HLA-DR4 was able to induce the *in vitro* expansion of specific CD4+ T cells derived from normal DR4+ donors or from DR4+ patients with melanoma when pulsed onto autologous DC (53). This study found that CD4+ T cell immunoreactivity against this peptide coexisted with a high frequency of anti-MART-1$_{27-35}$-reactive CD8+ T cells in freshly isolated blood harvested from HLA-A2+/DR4+ patients with melanoma. Another recent study with cancer patients demonstrated the essential role of DC that are activated by CD4+ Th cells for optimal CTL induction (54).

These findings confirm that tumor-specific CD4+ T lymphocytes from cancer patients are required for optimal induction of CTL against the autologous tumors. Therefore, both class I and class II peptides could be used to optimize the therapeutic effect of the immunotherapy for melanoma.

3. NOVEL VACCINE APPROACHES

3.1 Peptide Vaccines

The identification of peptide sequences recognized by CTL has led to attempts to directly induce CTL-responses *in vivo* (55, 56). Successful immunization of mice has been accomplished with peptides formulated with immunostimulating complex (ISCOM) (57), entrapped in liposomes (58), encapsulated in microspheres (59), osmotically loaded into syngeneic splenocytes (60) or coated on their surface (61). Effective immune responses were also elicited in mice with a mutant p53 peptide in adjuvant (62), or with either mutant or wild type p53 peptides loaded on dendritic cells (63). We showed in two murine antigenic systems that fusion peptides with a synthetic ER-signal sequence at the NH$_2$-terminus of the minimal peptide were more effective than the minimal peptide alone in generating specific CTL-responses (64). Furthermore, we found that the CTL response was MHC Class II independent, could not be attributed to increased hydrophobicity of the fusion peptides and was very effective in prolonging the survival of tumor-challenged mice. More recently, we identified two HLA-A2.1 restricted peptides from telomerase reverse transcriptase (hTRT) and demonstrated that *in vivo* immunization of HLA-A2.1 transgenic mice generated a specific CTL response against both hTRT peptides (22). Based on the induction of CTL responses *in vitro* and *in vivo*, and the susceptibility to lysis of tumor cells of various origins by hTRT-specific CTL, we suggested that hTRT could serve as a universal cancer vaccine.

Increasing number of studies report peptide vaccination of cancer patients. Spontaneous CTL reactivity against the melanoma antigens Melan A/MART-1, tyrosinase and gp100 is frequently detected in melanoma patients and healthy individuals (65-67). These finding suggest that CTL responses against 'self' antigens are induced spontaneously in patients and healthy individuals and may be boosted by appropriate vaccination. Immunizations with a MAGE-3-derived peptide without any adjuvant induced limited tumor regressions in five out of 17 patients with melanoma (68). More recently the same group used an HLA-A1-restricted MAGE-3 peptide to immunize 39 patients with metastatic melanoma. Of the 25 patients who received the complete treatment, 7 displayed significant tumor regressions: three regressions were complete and 2 led to a disease-free state, which persisted for more than 2 years after the beginning of treatment (69). Salgaller et al. reported generation of CTL specific for one of three gp100-derived peptides in patients vaccinated with peptide in incomplete Freund's adjuvant (70). Immunization of three patients with advanced melanoma with peptide-pulsed autologous antigen presenting cells led to induction of peptide specific CTL (71). The peptide used in this study was derived from MAGE-1 and was restricted to HLA-A1.1. The lack of any therapeutic response observed in this trial might be explained by the advanced stage of the disease in these patients. In another study nine melanoma patients were vaccinated weekly for four weeks with a combination of peptides derived from the

MART-1, tyrosinase, and gp100 proteins (72). Successful immunization against peptides could be detected *in vitro* in two of six patients against the tyrosinase peptide, three of six patients against the MART-1 peptide, and none of six patients receiving the gp100 peptide. More recently, eighteen patients with melanoma were immunized with a peptide derived from MART-1, emulsified with incomplete Freund's adjuvant (56). An enhancement of cytotoxic activity against MART-1 was detected with minimal toxicity for the patients consisting of local irritation at the site of vaccination. Serial administrations of this peptide appeared to boost the level of cytotoxicity *in vitro*, although clinical regression of the tumor was not observed. Peptides derived from NY-ESO-1, one of the most immunogenic tumor antigens, were used to immunize 12 patients with metastatic NY-ESO-1 expressing cancers, including melanoma (73). This trial demonstrated induction of primary NY-ESO-1-specific CTL responses as well as stabilization of disease and regression of individual metastases in three patients. In another trial, patients with advanced pancreatic carcinoma were vaccinated with a synthetic ras peptide pulsed on antigen presenting cells isolated from peripheral blood (74). This procedure led to generation of cancer cell-specific cellular response, without side effects. However, in all patients tumor progression was observed after the vaccination.

Several strategies for modifying peptides have been attempted to improve their efficiency as cancer vaccines. The clinical use of peptides is limited by their rapid proteolytic digestion. To overcome this limitation Celis et al. designed a peptide construct containing a pan-reactive DR epitope, a CTL epitope and a fatty-acid moiety (75). A lipopeptide-based therapeutic vaccine was able to induce strong CTL responses both in humans and animals (76). Several studies demonstrated a correlation between MHC binding affinity and peptide immunogenicity (77). Peptides derived from gp100, whose anchor residues were modified to fit the optimal HLA-A2 binding motif, stimulated tumor-reactive CTL more efficiently than the natural epitopes (78). An unmodified, gp100-derived peptide, failed to elicit peptide-specific CTL in melanoma patients after subcutaneous administration with incomplete Freund's adjuvant (IFA). In contrast, vaccination with the modified peptide induced CTL responses in 91% of cases (10). None of the 11 patients immunized with the modified peptide in IFA alone experienced an objective tumor response. Interestingly, administration of the modified peptide along with high dose interleukin-2 led to a clinical response rate of 42% in a group of 31 patients. More recently, two modified gp100 peptides were combined with an antibody that abrogated cytotoxic T lymphocyte antigen-4 (CTLA-4) signaling to augment T-cell reactivity (79). In that trial there were two complete responses and one partial response in 14 patients with stage IV melanoma that were maintained beyond 12 months. Another group also utilized the same anti-CTLA-4 antibody in combination with three melanoma peptides (80). Nineteen patients with stage III and IV melanoma were immunized. Nine of 11 patients without autoimmune symptoms have experienced disease relapse, and 3 of 8 patients with autoimmune symptoms experienced relapse. These findings suggest possible correlation between development of autoimmunity and lack of relapse. Several groups reported clinical trials with melanoma patients immunized with the immunogenic peptide MART-1$_{27-35}$ (AAGIGILTV) (81-83). Wang et al. immunized patients with high-risk resected melanoma with MART-1$_{27-35}$ complexed with incomplete Freund's adjuvants, or with Freund's adjuvants mixed with CRL1005, a blocked co-polymer adjuvant. Ten of 22 patients demonstrated an immune response to peptide-pulsed targets or tumor cells by ELISA assay after vaccination, as did 12 of 20 patients by ELISPOT. Immune response by ELISA correlated with prolonged relapse-free survival (81). This data suggests that a significant proportion of patients with resected melanoma mount an antigen-specific immune response against MART-1$_{27-35}$. Another study analyzed antigen-specific T-cell responses induced in the skin and in peripheral blood lymphocytes in a HLA-A2+ melanoma patient. The patient showed major regression of metastatic melanoma under continued immunization with peptides derived from the antigens MART-1, tyrosinase and gp100 (82). The authors demonstrated that intradermal (i.d.) immunization with peptides alone leads to oligoclonal expansion of MART-1-specific CTL. These findings provide strong evidence for the effective induction of specific T-cell responses to MART-1 by i.d. immunization with peptide alone, which accounts for specific cytotoxicity against MART-1-expressing melanoma cells and clinical tumor regression. Brinckerhoff et al. evaluated the stability of the same peptide - MART-1$_{27-35}$ in fresh normal human plasma and possible peptide modifications that convey protection against enzymatic destruction without loss of immunogenicity (83). When this peptide was incubated in plasma prior to pulsing on target cells, CTL reactivity was lost within 3 hours. The stability of MART-1$_{27-35}$ was markedly prolonged by C-terminal amidation and/or N-terminal acetylation, or by polyethylene-glycol modification of the C-terminus. These modified peptides were recognized by CTL. This study suggests that the immunogenicity of the peptide vaccines might be enhanced by creating modifications that increase their stability.

We investigated the effectiveness of several synthetic insertion signal sequences in enhancing the presentation of the HLA-A2.1 restricted melanoma epitope MART-1$_{27-35}$ (84). An important step in presentation of the class I-restricted antigens is the translocation of processed proteins from the cytosol across the endoplasmic reticulum membrane mediated by transporter associated with antigen processing proteins (TAP), or as an alternative, by endoplasmic reticulum-insertion signal sequences located at the NH$_2$-terminus of the precursor molecules (85). Using a technique known as osmotic lysis of pinocytic vesicles (86), we loaded several synthetic peptide constructs into the cytosol of antigen processing deficient T2 cells, TAP-expressing human melanoma cells, and dendritic cells. We examined whether the natural signal sequences ES (derived from the adenovirus E3/19K glycoprotein) (87), and IS (derived from IFN-β(88) could enhance and prolong presentation of MART-1$_{27-35}$. We found that the addition of signal sequence at the N-terminus, but not at the C-terminus, of MART-1$_{27-35}$ greatly enhanced its presentation in both TAP-deficient and TAP-expressing cells. A newly designed peptide construct, composed of the epitope replacing the hydrophobic part of a natural signal sequence, was also effective. Interestingly, an artificial signal sequence containing the epitope was the most efficient construct for enhancing its presentation. These peptide constructs facilitated epitope presentation in a TAP-independent manner when loaded into the cytosol of TAP-deficient T2 cells. In addition, loading of these constructs into TAP-expressing melanoma cells also led to a more efficient presentation than the loading of the minimal peptide. Most importantly, loading of human dendritic cells with the same constructs resulted in a prolonged presentation of this melanoma epitope (84). The efficient presentation of MART-1$_{27-35}$, loaded into TAP-expressing tumor cells and DC, may be explained by the availability of intact TAP transporters in these cells. In this case, some of the loaded MART-1$_{27-35}$ may have been translocated by TAP from the cytosol even 8 days after loading. The size of MART-1$_{27-35}$ (9 amino acids) is appropriate for optimal translocation by TAP (3). Still, fusion peptides were more effective than MART-1$_{27-35}$, probably because of their translocation by both TAP-dependent and TAP-independent pathway. The later mechanism of peptide translocation may be important for antigen presentation especially in cancers that fail to utilize the classical MHC class I pathway (89).

These findings may be of practical significance for the development of synthetic anticancer vaccines and *in vitro* immunization of CTL for adoptive immunotherapy.

Various methods have been exploited to improve the peptide vaccine antigenicity. The most common are a combination of the peptide administered with cytokines and/or with an adjuvant. Slingluff et al. implemented a phase II trial to test whether low-dose IL-2 is capable of enhancing T-cell immune responses to a multipeptide melanoma vaccine (90). Forty melanoma patients were randomly vaccinated with four gp100- and tyrosinase-derived peptides that were restricted by HLA-A1, -A2, and –A3. After either one week or 28 days a tetanus helper peptide as well as IL-2 were administered daily. A higher response was found in the second group (tetanus helper peptide and IL-2 administered after 28 days). This study also found that the tyrosinase peptides DAEKSDICTDEY and YMDGTMSQV were more immunogenic than the gp100 peptides YLEPGPVTA and ALLAVGATK. The disease-free survival estimates were 39% for the first group and 50% for the second group at two years. In another trial, the effect of IL-12 on the immune response to a resected metastatic melanoma multipeptide vaccine was studied in 48 patients with melanoma (91). The patients were immunized with two peptides derived from gp100 (209-217)(210M) and tyrosinase (368-376)(370D) emulsified with IFA. The peptide/adjuvant was either administered with or without IL-12. Out of forty patients, thirty-four developed a positive skin test response to only the gp100 peptide and not the tyrosinase peptide. Out of 38 patients, 33 showed an immune response as determined by ELISA, and 37 of 42 patients showed a response by a tetramer assay. These findings indicate that IL-12 may augment the immune response to certain peptides. These findings were confirmed by Peterson et al. who found in a phase II study that recombinant IL-12 when administered with Mart-1/Melan-A, is effective as an adjuvant in melanoma patients (92). Another recent trial determined that the melanoma peptides MAGE-A1 (96-104), MAGE-A10 (254-262), and gp 100(614-622) are immunogenic when combined with granulocyte-macrophage colony-stimulating factor (GM-CSF) and montanide ISA-51 adjuvant and administered as part of a multipeptide vaccine (93). Hersey et al. undertook a phase I/II trial with 36 patients with melanoma half of which were given peptides derived from gp100, MART-1, tyrosinase, and MAGE-3 in the Montanide-ISA-720 adjuvant, and half the patients were given GM-CSF s.c. for 4 days following each injection (94). The authors concluded that the peptides were more effective when given with the adjuvant Montanide-ISA-720. In another trial the peptides MART-1(26-35 (27L)), gp100(209-217 (210M)),and tyrosinase (368-376 (370D)) were emulsified with incomplete Freund's adjuvant and administered with SD-9427 (progenipoietin) – an agonist of granulocyte colony-stimulating factor and the FLT-3 receptor (95). This study found that the SD-9427 combined with a multipeptide vaccine was generally well tolerated, and that the majority of patients with resected melanoma mounted an antigen-specific immune response against the multipeptide vaccine. Butterfield et al. studied the induction of T-cell responses to HLA-A*0201 immunodominant peptides derived from alpha-fetoprotein (AFP) in patients with hepatocellular cancer (96). In this study the authors tested the immunological paradigm that high concentrations of soluble protein contribute to the maintenance of peripheral tolerance/ignorance to self-protein. They confirmed that the patients' T-cell repertoire was capable of recognizing AFP in the context of MHC class I even in an environment of high circulating levels of this oncofetal protein. Our group identified two HLA-A2-restricted peptides derived from human telomerase reverse transcriptase (hTRT), and induced hTRT-specific CTL *in vitro* (22). Importantly, we also demonstrated that the hTRT-specific CTL lysed a variety of HLA-A2-positive cancer cell lines, but not HLA-A2-negative cancer cell lines. All of these cancer cell lines were hTRT positive as determined by the TRAPeze assay (Intergen). A Phase I clinical trial was performed by Vonderheide et al. to evaluate the clinical and immunological impact of vaccinating advanced cancer patients with the HLA-A2-restricted hTRT I540 peptide presented with keyhole limpet hemocyanin by ex vivo generated autologous dendritic cells (97). It was found that hTRT-specific T lymphocytes were induced in 4 of 7 patients with advanced breast or prostate carcinoma after vaccination with dendritic cells pulsed with hTRT peptide. It is important to note that no significant toxicity was observed despite concerns of telomerase activity in rare normal cells. These results demonstrated the immunological feasibility of vaccinating patients against telomerase and provided rationale for targeting self-antigens with critical roles in oncogenesis. An interesting study utilized the flt3 ligand as a systemic vaccine adjuvant with the E75 HLA-A2 epitope from HER-2/neu (98). Twenty patients with advanced stage prostate cancer were enrolled in this study. Dendritic cells were markedly increased in the peripheral blood of subjects receiving flt3 ligand with each repetitive cycle, but augmentation of antigen-presenting cells within the dermis was not observed. No significant peptide-specific T-cell responses were detected. The authors concluded that the inability of flt3 ligand to augment the number of peripheral skin antigen-presenting cells may have contributed to the absence of robust peptide-specific immunity detectable in the peripheral blood of immunized subjects treated with flt3 ligand.

A difficulty with the use of peptide vaccines is the fact that the T cell responses usually do not last long enough to have a significant effect on the tumor. To address this issue Davila et al. examined the role of synthetic oligodeoxynucleotide (ODN) adjuvants containing unmethylated cytosine-guanine motifs (CpG-ODN) and CTLA-4 blockade in enhancing the antitumor effectiveness of peptide vaccines intended to elicit CTL responses (99). This study found that combination immunotherapy consisting of vaccination with a synthetic peptide corresponding to an immunodominant CTL epitope derived from tyrosinase-related protein-2 administered with CpG-ODN adjuvant and followed by systemic injection of anti-CTLA-4 antibodies increased the survival of mice against the poorly immunogenic B16 melanoma. These findings suggest that peptide vaccination applied in combination with a strong adjuvant and CTLA-4 blockade, is capable of eliciting durable antitumor T cell responses that provide survival benefit.These findings bear clinical significance for the design of peptide-based therapeutic vaccines for human cancer patients.

From a clinical perspective, immunization with peptides may be preferable to immunization with recombinant vaccinia viruses because of its safety and because it is not associated with diminished immune responses in patients immunized against smallpox. Immunizing with minimal determinant constructs may avoid the possible oncogenic effect of full-length proteins containing ras, p53 or other potential oncogenes. In addition to their safety, peptide vaccines can be designed to induce well-defined immune responses, and synthesized in large quantities with very high purity and reproducibility. Another potential advantage of peptide vaccines over whole proteins or DNA vaccines is the ability to identify the specific epitopes of the tumor antigens to which an individual is able to mount an immune response, but not a state of immune tolerance (100). In addition, *in vivo* or *in vitro* immunization with peptide antigens "packaged" in dendritic cells or other antigen-presenting cells (discussed below) opens an exciting opportunity for eliciting powerful CTL-responses.

A disadvantage of peptide vaccines is their poor immunogenicity and monospecificity of the induced immune response. Another limiting factor for the use of peptide vaccines in outbred populations is that T cells from individuals expressing different MHC molecules recognize different peptides from tumor or viral antigens in the context of self-MHC. However, the use of synthetic peptides from tumor-associated antigens that are presented by common MHC molecules may overcome this problem. Poor immunogenicity caused by rapid degradation of the peptides by serum peptidases may be corrected by modifications or incorporation of the peptides into controlled release formulations.

3.2 Recombinant Viruses As Vaccines

Many different viruses have been used to construct recombinant vaccines. These vaccines have the advantage of inducing both humoral and cell-mediated immune responses, in some cases even after a single application. However, possible disadvantages of recombinant viruses include recombinantion with wild type viruses, conversion to virulence, oncogenic potential, or immunosuppression. We will briefly discuss current strategies to overcome some of these obstacles in order to develop efficient recombinant viral vaccines.

Vaccinia virus (VV) was demonstrated to be a safe and very effective immunogen in the smallpox eradication campaign, where it was administered to over one billion people. Large amounts of foreign DNA can be stably inserted into the VV genome by homologous recombination (101). Another advantage of this vector is a very efficient post-translational processing of the inserted genes within host cell cytoplasm. However, due to the induction of high titers of anti-vaccinia antibodies, recombinant vaccinia viruses may be given only once or twice (102). It was demonstrated that intratumoral inoculation of vaccinia virus induced very high levels of antivaccinia antibodies in serum. Surprisingly however, it was possible to sustain viral gene function by repeatedly injecting vaccinia in the tumor site (103). A promising strategy to increase the efficiency of recombinant viral vaccines is to use two different vectors for priming and boosting vaccinations (104). This approach was much more effective in generating antigen-specific CTL responses than the use of one vector for both priming and boosting. In a recent study, a recombinant vaccinia virus (rVV) expressing CD40 ligand or CD154 (CD154rVV) was constructed and the effects of CD154rVV infection on antigen presenting cells (APC) activation and its consequences on T cell stimulation were evaluated. In the presence of CD154rVV-activated APC, significantly higher numbers of specific cytotoxic CD8+ T cells were detected, as compared with cultures performed in the presence of wild type vaccinia virus or in the absence of virus. The authors concluded that functional CD154 expression from rVV-infected cells could promote APC activation, thereby enhancing antigen-specific T cell generation. Therefore, this vector might help bypass the requirement for activated helper cells during CTL priming, thus qualifying as a potentially relevant vector in the generation of CD8+ T cell responses in cancer immunotherapy (105).

Since vaccinia is a replication competent virus, it may cause disseminated viremia especially in immunosuppressed individuals (106).Therefore, several research groups attempted to develop recombinant vaccines based on non-replicating viruses (107). Utilizing recombinant fowlpox virus, which does not replicate in mammalian cells, Wang et al. were able to treat established tumors in mice (108). An important aspect of this work was the finding that prior immunization with vaccinia virus did not abrogate the immune responses elicited by the recombinant fowlpox virus. A different non-replicating virus, canarypox virus (ALVAC), was used to generate recombinant viruses, able to elicit immune responses against a variety of antigens (109). A clinical trial with vaccinia-CEA in patients with colorectal cancer resulted in eliciting of cell-mediated immune responses against CEA-derived peptide (110). In this study rejection of the vaccinia virus itself was not observed. More recently, the same group performed the first clinical trial with a nonreplicating ALVAC-CEA vector in patients with advanced carcinoma (111). Although no objective antitumor responses were observed, the vaccine was very well tolerated and no significant toxicity was reported. In 7 of 9 patients evaluated, statistically significant increases in CTL precursors specific for CEA were observed in PBMC after vaccination. T cell responses elicited by patients before and after vaccination with the ALVAC-CEA recombinants were further characterized in another study (112). This study demonstrated the ability to vaccinate cancer patients with an avipox recombinant as well as to derive T cells that are capable of lysing allogenic and autologous tumor cells in a MHC-restricted manner. Phase I trial of a recombinant vaccinia virus encoding CEA in 20 patients with metastatic adenocarcinoma showed that the toxicity was limited to local inflamation as well as low grade fever, each affecting fewer than 20% of the patients (113). No objective clinical responses to the vaccine were observed among this population of patients with widely metastatic andenocarcinoma. The antibody response to CEA in patients was studied by Conry et al. (114). This group used recombinant vaccinia viruses encoding full-length of internally deleted cDNAs for human CEA to vaccinate 32 patients with CEA-expressing adenocarcinomas of colorectal origin. The detected CEA autoantibodies were predominantly IgG1, with a minority of patients also demonstrating IgM autoantibodies. A non-replicating vaccinia virus, known as modified vaccinia virus Ankara (MVA), is avirulent in normal and immunosuppressed animals and was shown to have no significant side effects after inoculation of 120,000 humans (115). Since replication of MVA is blocked at a step of virion assembly (116), rather than at an early stage, MVA vectors produce recombinant proteins in amounts similar to those of wild type viruses. In addition, the immunogenicity of MVA recombinants in mice is similar to that of virulent strains (117). Therefore, MVA is a very promising vector for the development of recombinant vaccines for cancer. This vector was recently used for expression of human tyrosinase, a melanoma specific differentiation antigen (118). Stable recombinant viruses (MVA-hTyr) were constructed that have deleted selection marker lacZ and efficiently expressed human tyrosinase in primary human cells and cell lines. An efficient tyrosinase- and melanoma-specific CTL response was induced in vitro using MVA-hTyr-infected autologous dendritic cells as activators for PBMCs derived from HLA-A2.1-positive melanoma patients, despite prior vaccination against smallpox. A new recombinant poxvirus vaccine that codes for 10 HLA-A2-restricted epitopes derived from 5 melanoma antigens conjoined in an artificial polyepitope or polytope construct was recently designed (119). Multiple epitopes within the polytope construct were shown to be individually immunogenic, which illustrated the feasibility of the polytope approach for melanoma immunotherapy. Tumor escape from CTL surveillance, through down regulation of individual tumor antigens and MHC alleles, might be overcome by polytope vaccines, which simultaneously target multiple cancer antigens. Fifty-four patients with metastatic melanoma were immunized with recombinant adenoviruses encoding MART-1 and gp100 melanoma antigens alone, or followed by the administration of IL2 (120). One of 16 patients receiving the recombinant adenovirus MART-1 alone, experienced a complete clinical response. However, immunologic assays showed no consistent immunization to the MART-1 or gp100 transgenes expressed by the recombinant adenoviruses. This study found that high doses of recombinant adenoviruses could be safely administered to cancer patients. Another study tested a recombinant adeno-associated virus expressing human papillomavirus type 16 E7 peptide DNA fused with heat shock protein DNA as a potential vaccine for cervical cancer (121). It was demonstrated that this vaccine can eliminate tumor cells in syngeneic animals and induce CD4- and CD8-dependant CTL activity *in vitro*. This study indicates that this chimeric gene delivered by adeno-associated virus has potential as a cervical cancer vaccine. Prostate cancer recurrence, evidenced by rising PSA levels after radical prostatectomy, is an increasingly prevalent clinical problem. A clinical study was undertaken to evaluate the safety and biologic effects of vaccinia-PSA (PROSTVAC) administered to 6 patients with post-prostatectomy recurrence of prostate cancer (122). Toxicity was minimal, and primary anti-PSA IgG antibody activity was induced after vaccinia-PSA immunization in one subject, although such antibodies were detectable in several subjects at baseline. More recently, a phase I/II clinical trial in metastatic melanoma patients was performed using a UV-inactivated nonreplicating recombinant vaccinia virus expressing three endoplasmic reticulum-targeted HLA-A0201-restricted epitopes (Melan-A/MART-1(27-35), gp100(280-288), and tyrosinase(1-9)), together with CD80 and CD86 costimulatory molecules. No major clinical toxicity was reported. Of the 17 patients, three demonstrated regression of individual metastases, seven had stable disease, and progressive disease was observed in seven patients. These results, in terms of safety and immunogenicity, support the use of this reagent in active specific immunotherapy (123).

In recent years, the use of recombinant virus vaccines has tremendously influenced advances in the fight against prostate cancer. A clinical trial was performed that sought to analyze toxicity, immunogenicity and time to treatment failure using vaccine, anti-androgen therapy or their sequential use (124). The vaccine consisted of recombinant vaccinia viruses containing the PSA and B7.1 costimulatory genes as prime vaccinations, and avipox-PSA as boosters. Although the results did not definitively support the use of one method over another, they served to warrant further investigations on the role of combining vaccine with anti-androgen therapy or vaccine followed by vaccine plus anti-androgen therapy in this patient population. Another trial involving patients with intermediate to high risk prostate cancer was performed to determine the safety of intra-prostatic administration of a replication-competent, oncolytic adenovirus containing a cytosine deaminase (CD)/herpes simplex virus thymidine kinase (HSV-1 TK) fusion gene concomitant with increasing durations of 5-fluorocytosine and valganciclovir prodrug therapy and conventional-dose three-dimensional conformal radiation therapy (3D-CRT). Results demonstrated that replication-competent adenovirus-mediated double-suicide gene therapy can be combined safely with conventional-dose 3D-CRT" to augment the antitumor effects as seen by the decrease in the PSA half-life (125). A phase I trial of antigen-specific gene therapy using a recombinant vaccinia virus encoding MUC-1 and IL-2 in MUC-1-positive patients with advanced prostate cancer showed increased immune responses (126). The results of these and other ongoing clinical trials will help to direct the future use of the recombinant virus-based vaccines.

These early clinical studies with recombinant viruses as vaccine vectors are very encouraging. In contrast to other vaccine vectors, viruses elicit strong and long-lasting immune response, and are able to infect nearly all host cells, as well as to ensure intracellular translation, degradation and efficient trafficking of peptide antigens to the cell surface. The potential drawbacks of the viral vectors are related to their safety and pre-existing immunity, particularly to vaccinia virus and adenoviruses. However, the safety of the viral vaccines can be ensured by using non-replicating, highly attenuated or genetically modified viruses, while the problem of pre-existing immunity may be circumvented by the use of non-mammalian viruses, such as the avian poxviruses. It is now established that recombinant viruses can be useful to break immune tolerance against tumor-associated antigens specifically expressed by human cancers (127). Therefore, the use of recombinant viruses as cancer vaccines is very promising.

3.3 DNA-Based Vaccines

This novel approach involves direct inoculation of expression plasmids, which results in the induction of long-lasting immune responses against the expressed antigens. Fynan et al. compared six routes of inoculation of naked DNA for their relative efficacies (128). In this study, intramuscular injection of DNA generated the best response, whereas inoculation of DNA-coated gold particles using "gene gun" required significantly lower doses of DNA. It was found that the uptake of the injected DNA is an active energy-dependent process (129). Once inside the cell, plasmid DNA can get through the nuclear membrane and persists as a non-replicating episomal molecule, which explains the long-lived foreign gene expression (130). The low, but long-lasting expression of the encoded antigens is an important feature of this approach (131). The duration of expression seems to be more important than the dose of the antigen for induction of CTL responses, although DNA immunization has been shown to result in both cellular and humoral immune responses, and in generation of antigen-specific CD8+ and CD4+ T cells (132, 133). Irvine et al. reported effective treatment of established pulmonary metastases, using a "gene gun" for DNA immunization (134). In this study, recombinant cytokines enhanced the therapeutic effects of this approach. Enhancement of the immune response against a model tumor antigen was also observed after cotransfection of the genes coding for the cytokine GM-CSF and the costimulatory molecule B7-1 (135). Several elegantly designed studies addressed the important question of the mechanism of DNA immunization (136-138). Results demonstrate that the antigen presenting cells can be transfected directly or they can acquire the antigens expressed by other transfected cells. However, only professional APCs are able to initiate primary immune responses as a result of DNA immunization. These findings are extremely important in the development of DNA-based vaccines for clinical application. A promising DNA vaccine has been developed against a B-cell lymphoma (139). Another plasmid for clinical application encodes human CEA and the HBV surface antigen (HbsAg), each of them under a separate CMV promoter (135).

Recent clinical trials have supported the continued research of DNA vaccines for cancer treatment. In a Phase I/II trial of patients with follicular lymphoma, 7 of 12 patients mounted either humoral or T-cell-proliferative responses after vaccination with plasmids encoding tumor-specific idiotypes (140). In a safety study of human CEA DNA vaccine, patients had no objective clinical response with mild toxicity. However, 4 of 17 patients did have induction of lymphoproliferative response (141).

DNA vaccines may be particularly useful in combination with conventional chemotherapy treatment. In animal studies, the injection of recombinant DNA and modified vaccinia virus, in combination with metronomic dosing of alkylating agent cyclophosphamide

(CTX), initiated a specific CTL response in mice, leading to increased resistance to challenge with the murine melanoma B16 compared to CTX alone (142). Similar findings occurred with the combination of 5-Aza and DNA vaccine treatment. Intradermal injection of plasmids encoding hsp70 and a suicide gene transcriptionally targeted to melanocytes led to CD8+ T cell response eradicating systemically established melanoma B16 tumors. When combined with 5-Aza this immunotherapy led to a significant decrease in tumors compared to the use of the demethylating agent alone (143).

Interesting work has recently been completed utilizing DNA vaccines as anti-angiogenic agents to target cancer metastases and primary tumors. One specific study looked at attenuated Salmonella typhimurium directed against vascular endothelial growth factor receptor-2, or fetal liver kinase-1 (FLK-1), and transcription factor Fos-related antigen-1 (Fra-1) (144). It was found that the FLK-1 and Fra-1 vaccines circumvented T-cell tolerance in order to suppress the tumor angiogenesis and stimulate cell-mediated immunity. Another study, combining suppression of angiogenesis with apoptosis found that CTL induced by a DNA vaccine encoding secretory chemokine CCL21 and survivin specifically targeted proliferating endothelial cells in the tumor vasculature and tumor cells. Surprisingly, this anti-tumor effect in the treated mice did not inhibit wound healing or fertility (145).

While DNA vaccines elicit sustained cellular and humoral immune responses, their overall immune stimulation remains weak. To boost the immune response Bronte et al. utilized CD40 agonist as an adjuvant to sustain tumor-specific T lymphocyte survival, leading to a dramatic increase in the number of specific CD8+ T lymphocytes, in a phase dependent manner (146). Others have attempted to enhance the immune response with DNA fusion vaccines and electroporation, leading to a "homologous prime/boost approach" (147). Electroporation (EP) appears to effectively increase expression without introducing additional competing antigens (148). Specifically, Zhang et al injected micron-size gold particles and DNA intramuscularly into mice, followed by EP of the vaccine, leading to protection against tumor challenge with HbsAg+ cancer cells (149). Yet another option are the polytope DNA vaccines, which elicit powerful immune responses. For example, Doan et al. demonstrated significant increases of CTL responses against HPV 16 oncoprotein E7 following vaccination with murine (H-2b) and human (HLA-A*0201)-restricted epitopes (150). Likewise, blocking CTLA-4 interaction with APC's B7 augments T-cell responses and tumor immunity elicited by DNA vaccines (151). Finally, increases in the suppressive effects of DNA vaccines has been described through the use of Pan-IA DNA vaccines (152).

Occasionally, tolerance may lead to decreased efficacy of plasmid DNA vaccines. Jia et al overcame this difficulty through neutralization of TGF-beta, enhancing the response to DNA vaccine and successfully inducing anti-tumor immunity against melanoma-associated antigens (153). DNA vaccination alone led to partial breaking of tolerance in ErbB-2 tolerant mice (154). This result was confirmed when Pupa et al reported that xenogeneic DNA immunization could brake tolerance to the mouse (m) neu proto-oncogene product m-p185(neu). This led to significant inhibition of mammary carcinoma development in HER-2/neu transgenic mice" (155).

Tumor immunogenicity may also be increased through the use of specific cytokines. The combination of antibodies and T cells releasing specific cytokines (such as IFN-gamma) is essential for tumor clearance (156). Also, over expression of intratumoral CCL5, a chemokine involved in the recruitment of a wide spectrum of immunocompetent cells, lead to increased recruitment of immunocompetent cells and effector function, hinting at the usefulness of chimeric CCL5-Ig DNA in cancer treatment (157). Yet, the effects of dual cytokine use have proven unpredictable. For example, genetic engineering of tumor cells expressing both granulocyte-macrophage colony-stimulating factor (GM-CSF) and interleukin (IL)-2 may enhance or inhibit immune response (158). Interestingly, the fusion of GM-CSF and IL-2 led to a significant antitumor effect, greater than the GM-CSF/IL-2 combination (158). A recent study showed that the targeting of transcription factor Fos-related antigen 1 (Fra-1) by co-expressing secretory cytokines led to the induction of specific CD8+ T cell-mediated immunity. This immune response led to the elimination of pulmonary and breast cancer metastases (159).

While research into DNA vaccines for melanoma, cervical cancer, colon cancer, and lymphomas has been well established, encouraging studies have been recently completed on the use of DNA vaccines for treatment of brain tumors. Immunogene therapy with the improved Sindbis virus vector expressing xenogeneic gp100 and syngenic IL-18 may be an excellent approach for developing a new treatment protocol. Thus, the Sindbis DNA system may represent a novel approach for the treatment of malignant brain tumors (160). Likewise, a DNA vaccine expressing tyrosinase-related protein-2 (a melanoma-associated antigen) induced T-cell-mediated partial protection against subcutaneous, intravenous, or intracerebral challenge with mouse glioblastoma cells. This effect was augmented by the addition of IL-12 (161).

DNA vaccines have several potential advantages over peptide and recombinant viral vaccines. DNA vaccines are simpler and cheaper to produce. DNA immunization is not associated with an anamnestic immune response, which is responsible for the rapid clearance of viral constructs. Another major advantage is that DNA vaccination induces very long-lasting immune responses. Addressing a major concern for the clinical use of DNA-based vaccines – their safety – Kurth et al. calculated that the probability of tumor-promoting events by plasmid DNA integration was below the statistical events leading to a mutation within the lifetime of an individual (162). In all, DNA-based vaccines seem to be a promising approach for the treatment of cancer.

3.4 Dendritic Cell-Based Vaccines

Dendritic cells play multiple roles in the immune system. They capture, process and present antigens, stimulate lymphocytes, migrate from the periphery to lymphoid organs, and secrete cytokines. In fact, dendritic cells have already been proven to be the most potent antigen presenting cells for T cell priming (163). In many cases the patients with cancer are profoundly immunosuppressed, making it essential to activate both innate and acquired immunity for optimal tumor immunotherapy (164). DC-based vaccines effectively accomplish this end.

In addition to their ability to efficiently acquire and process antigens (165, 166), DC express high levels of MHC Class I and Class II molecules as well as costimulatory molecules (167, 168) essential in antigen presentation. Therefore, many investigators attempted to immunize with peptide-pulsed DC. It was found that immunization with peptide-pulsed DC is superior to injection of peptide in adjuvant in inducing potent cytotoxic T-cell responses (169). A similar strategy was also reported by others to be successful in eliciting T lymphocyte-mediated protective anti-tumor immunity (170) (171, 172). A possible disadvantage of peptide pulsing is the short half-life (2-10 hours) of most MHC-restricted epitopes (173), which creates the requirement for several injections of peptide-pulsed DC to achieve effective immune responses (172, 174, 175). Therefore, development of different methods for loading of antigens allowing DC to utilize their own intracellular pathways is highly desirable. The antigens of interest must be present in the cytosol of the DC in order to enter the intracellular pathway leading to their loading onto MHC class I molecules and the subsequent activation of CD8+ T cells. Surprisingly, Paglia et al. were able to prime murine CTL against tumor antigen by incubating DC with whole protein *in vitro* (176). Another group reported the generation of specific CTL in mice vaccinated with DC pulsed with RNA from an ovalbumin-expressing tumor (177). In this approach however, rapid degradation of RNA limits the duration of antigen expression. Another study showed that treatment of pulmonary metastases in mice with bone marrow-derived DC, transduced with retroviral vector encoding a model antigen was very effective (178). The reduction of the metastatic nodules was associated with induction of antigen-specific CTL. Adenovirus vectors were also used to transduce DC with genes coding for tumor antigens. It was demonstrated in a murine breast cancer model that a single injection with transduced DC provided complete protection against tumor cell challenge (179). This approach was not limited by hepatic toxicity and the development of neutralizing antibodies associated with the direct administration of the adenoviral vectors (180, 181). It was also demonstrated that adenovirus vectors are a promising vehicle for genetically engineering of human DC (182). A comparison of various gene transfer methods in human DC showed that adenovirus vectors were the most efficient in transducing human DC, with transduction efficiencies exceeding 95% at higher multiplicity of infection. Bronte et al. studied the antigen expression by DC infected with a panel of recombinant vaccinia viruses in which a murine model tumor antigen was expressed under different promoters (183). Interestingly, DC were found to express the model antigen only under the control of early promoters, even though late promoters were more active in other cell types. This study suggests that the use of promoters capable of driving the expression of tumor-associated antigens in DC is essential in development of recombinant anti-cancer vaccines. Another group described the effective generation of DC expressing tumor-associated antigens by particle-mediated gene transfer (184). These DC were able to induce antigen-specific CTL *in vivo* and to reduce the growth of murine tumors expressing tumor-associated viral or "self" antigens. With our signal sequence method, we showed that human DC could be loaded successfully with fusion peptides incorporating the melanoma epitope MART-1$_{27-35}$ (84). We found that the addition of signal sequence at the NH$_2$-terminus, but not at the COOH-terminus, of this epitope greatly prolonged its presentation in DC. A newly designed peptide construct, composed of the MART-1$_{27-35}$ epitope replacing the hydrophobic part of a natural signal sequence, was also effective. Interestingly, as with our earlier work with T2 cells, an artificial signal sequence containing the epitope was the most efficient construct for enhancing its presentation. These findings may be of practical significance for the development of synthetic anticancer vaccines and in vitro immunization of CTL for adoptive immunotherapy. Although viral vectors are efficient vehicles for gene transfer into DC, non-viral delivery of antigens has its advantages too. Fusion peptides can be readily produced in large quantities, and are very stable. In addition their application is not associated with immune responsiveness to vector-derived immunogens, or with risk of recombination.

Recent methods have been devised to improve the immunogenicity of DC vaccines. RNA-transfected DC could induce immune reactions against a variety of epitopes (185). For example, tumor cells from patients with acute myeloid leukemia as well as other malignant hemopoietic cell lines were effectively targeted by CTL stimulated with autologous dendritic cells transfected with survivin-RNA (186). Exosomes have recently received attention for their activity on DC and tumor cells alike. The tumor cell exosomes coated in tumor antigens, and released by DC were found to be very immunogenic (187). In DC, exosomes present molecules required for antigen presentation, such as MHC class I, MHC class II, and costimulatory molecules. These MHC molecules contained in the DC exosomes were immunogenic when loaded either directly or indirectly with antigenic peptides (188).

One key step in the process of cancer vaccine development is ensuring the maturation of DC. This process potentiates T cell activation and leads to increased migration of DC. For example, a recent prospective randomized phase II trial of patients with metastatic melanoma showed that, when comparing peptide-loaded immature and mature DC, only the mature cells were effective in stimulating antigen-specific cytolytic effector responses (189). This lack of maturation may explain the non-immunogenic nature of apoptotic tumor cells (ATC). To avoid the restriction of working only with identified antigens, DC loading could occur instead with ATC, exposing the DC to a plethora of yet undescribed tumor antigens. To overcome the non-immunogenic nature of ATC and allow DC to efficiently stimulate the immune system with a variety of unknown tumor-associated antigens, Akiyama et al. took advantage of ATC that have been opsonized with IgG (ATC-immune complexes, ATC-ICs) so as to target them to FcR for IgG (FcgammaReceptors) on DC. The result was a prominent internalization of ATC-ICs by DC via the Fcgamma receptors. This process effectively induced maturation of DC (190). Importantly, ATC-IC loading was shown to be more efficient than ATC alone in its capacity for inducing antitumor immunity *in vivo*, in terms of cytotoxic T cell induction and tumor rejection. These results show that using ATC-ICs may overcome the limitations and may enhance the immune response of current ATC-based DC vaccination therapy.

Cytokines play an essential role in the maturation and efficacy of DC vaccines. DC expressing TNF-alpha genes have improved cellular maturation and consequent robust T-cell activation (191). Likewise, IFN-beta and IL-3 appear to enhance mature dendritic cells priming of CTL (192). IL-12 continues to play an essential role in DC vaccines, enhancing *in vivo* antitumor immunity (193). Positive results were also demonstrated using a gene construct simultaneously expressing tumor-associated antigens and IL-12 (194). Exogenous soluble CD40 ligand (sCD40L) augmented DC IL-12 secretion and melanoma specific CTL induction in RNA-transfected DC preparations (195).

The encouraging pre-clinical results as well as improved techniques for in vitro immunization and expansion of DC support the initial attempts to immunize patients with DC expressing tumor antigens. Development of an efficient method for isolation and partial purification of DC (196, 197) led to the infusion of antigen-pulsed DC into four patients with follicular low-grade B cell lymphoma (198). Complete remission was observed in two patients, one patient had a partial response, and one patient had stable disease. In contrast, immunization with the antigen (monoclonal surface immunoglobulin) alone or emulsified in adjuvants did not induce regression of lymphoma (199). Another clinical study showed that DC pulsed with idiotypic protein derived from serum in patients with multiple myeloma induced a specific CTL response in one patient (200). DC infected with poxviruses encoding MART-1 were able to sensitize T lymphocytes from melanoma patients in vitro (201). This study suggests that the prolonged endogenous expression of tumor-associated antigens by the DC might be utilized for induction of CTL responses in patients.

The source of the DC for vaccination and the frequency of the CTL precursors in cancer patients should be carefully evaluated. In patients with a low frequency of peptide-specific precursors, the efficient activation of antigen-specific CTL required the use of peptide-loaded CD34+-derived, but not monocyte-derived, DC (202). This suggested that DC derived from CD34+ cells and monocytes were not functionally equivalent for the activation of CTL in patients with a low CTL precursor frequency. Antimelanoma CTL were generated *in vitro* from healthy donors (203) and melanoma patients (204) with DC pulsed with melanoma-derived peptides. It was also shown that vaccination of patients with melanoma with DC pulsed with MAGE-1-derived peptide elicited melanoma-specific CTL *in vivo* (71). In another clinical study sixteen melanoma patients were immunized with peptide-pulsed or tumor lysate-pulsed DC (205). Vaccination was well tolerated in all patients. Objective clinical responses were observed in 5 out of 16 patients with regression of metastases in various organs. These encouraging clinical trials suggest that a variety of tumor types may be responsive to DC-based immunotherapy.

Mixed but encouraging clinical trial results have been achieved with minimal toxicity. The kinetics of DC vaccine's induction of the tumor specific CTL is rapid. In a study of 18 HLA A*0201 patients with stage IV melanoma, even a single injection of CD34+ progenitor-derived dendritic cell vaccine could lead to induction of T-cell immunity in patients with stage IV melanoma (206). This reaction may have been brief, but could be observed in 7 of 11 patients, and the induced memory response lasted for over a six-month period (207). Thirty-five renal cell carcinoma (RCC) and metastatic melanoma patients were vaccinated with autologous tumor and allogeneic dendritic hybrid cells. Almost 75% of the patients had stable disease for over one and a half years following immunization. Fourteen percent of the patients suffering from RCC had objective responses (208). Immunization with autologous dendritic cells pulsed with human recombinant prostate-specific antigen (PSA) (Dendritophage-rPSA) was attempted in a phase I trial of complementary vaccine treatment for twenty-four prostate cancer patients. This study found that six patients initially with circulating prostate cancer cells, had undetectable levels at 6 and 12 months. Likewise, the PSA decreased anywhere from 6% to 39% (209). Another still ongoing study involves the use of human telomerase reverse transcriptase (hTRT) transfected DC vaccines for the treatment of patients with metastatic prostate cancer (210). DCs pulsed with necrotic pulmonary tumor cells were injected intranodally to lung cancer patients. Modest increases in T-cell response occurred in six of eight patients. Of these six patients, the two patients with superior T-cell responses also had more sustained disease control (211). In a study for the treatment of non-small cell lung cancer, patients received surgery, chemoradiation or multimodality treatment including DC-based vaccines. Independent of clinical outcome five of the sixteen patients immunized with DC vaccines showed a tumor-antigen independent response and six of sixteen showed an antigen specific response (212). In a phase I/II trial, breast cancer patients with metastatic disease received ex vivo expanded DCs from CD34+ progenitor cells. Toxicity was mild, with two patients showing a partial response to therapy, and two others producing tumor specific CTLs (213). A newly developed fusion cell vaccine was given to patients with metastatic breast cancer or metastatic renal cancer. Disease regression occurred in two of ten patients with breast cancer and five of thirteen patients with renal cancer (214). In another study, patients with colorectal cancer were immunized intranodally with DCs pulsed with HLA-A*0201- or HLA-A*2402-restricted carcinoembryonic antigen (CEA) -derived peptides. CEA-specific T cells were found in 70% of patients, and 20% of patients had three months of stable disease (215). Immunotherapy of cancer has also been proven to be safe for children. In a Phase I study of 11 pediatric neuroblastoma patients, dendritic cells pulsed with tumor RNA were found to be both safe and feasible (216).

Immune therapy has recently been used to treat one of the most aggressive and devastating cancers, malignant glioma. The DC immunizations for brain tumors have began to address the questions of central nervous system immune privilege and suppression of the immune system by the glioma itself (217). Gliomas and malignant melanomas share common antigens at the RNA level. In a study by Prins et al, two murine glioma cell lines expressing melanoma antigens gp100 and tyrosinase-related protein 2 were effectively targeted to immune therapy (218). DC pulsed with tumour lysate appeared to considerably benefit survival of mice with glioblastomas (219). Most of the immunized rats with the glioblastoma 9L showed substantial immune response to a DC vaccine injected with processed GM-CSF secreting 9L cells. Not surprisingly, the curative responses corresponded to CTL activity and IFN-gamma production. All of the rats with remission efficiently withstood a re-challenge with the parental cells (220). Fifteen patients with malignant glioma were immunized with fusions of dendritic and glioma cells augmented with recombinant human interleukin 12. After treatment, four patients had decreased tumor size by more than a half, determined by MRI (221). Another Phase I study of ten patients with glioblastoma multiforme and anaplastic astrocytoma looked at tumor lysate-pulsed DC immunization. Six of these patients manifested aggressive cytotoxicity, and of six that underwent tumor resection after treatment, three had intratumoral T-cell infiltrate (222). Phase 1 trials found that MART-1$_{27-35}$-peptide-pulsed immature dendritic cells had both immunologic and clinical results. An interesting phase II study found that sequential CTLA4 blockade was beneficial for DC vaccination (223).

As with other vaccine approached, the attack of tumor angiogenesis remains crucial to the tumor's defeat. One specific study monitored vascular endothelial growth factor, platelet-derived endothelial cell growth factor, and thrombospondin-1, to determine the effect of DC immunization. In fact, the detectable amount of circulating angiogenic factors was sufficiently sensitive to DC immunotherapy, and was increased in patients with more advanced disease (224).

Some of the early clinical trials may have been suboptimal secondary to the fact that tumor cells secrete various immunosuppressive factors. These include TGF-beta, which significantly reduces the potency of DC vaccines. It is suggested that the vaccine effectiveness may be increased by neutralizing TGF-beta (225). It also appears that allogeneic DC vaccines help to recover cancer patient immune function (226).

While DC vaccines have made great advances over the last decade, multiple hurdles still remain. Significant research is still required in the areas of DC loading, maturation, and migration. This treatment approach is time and resource expensive, not to mention the difficulty in constructing a universal vaccine rather than one for an individual tumor/patient. Difficulties such as T cell "exhaustion" and tumor antigen regulatory T cells have yet to be surmounted (227). There is still a great deal of discussion regarding the optimal antigen loading protocols. In summary, the completed clinical trials have shown that this form of vaccination is feasible and safe. In some cases, clinical responses were observed, but the future trials should address the technical difficulties of manipulating human DC, as well as the development of standardized clinical protocols.

4. Prospects

The growing number of TAA identified in many tumor types becomes a solid basis for vaccine development. However, the antigenic profile of human tumors is very complex, and consists of many peptides originating from various classes of protein. This fact should be considered carefully in designing anti-cancer vaccines. An important question is which tumor antigens are the most important in tumor regression *in vivo*. Differentiation antigens may play an important role in tumor regression, which is suggested by the positive correlation between the development of vitiligo and a good clinical response to immunotherapy in melanoma patients (228). Promising candidates are also MAGE, BAGE, and GAGE antigens since they are expressed in a variety of cancer cells, but not in normal cells except testis. Mutated epitopes such as CDK-4 and β-Catenin are tumor specific, but immunotherapy using these antigens is likely to be applicable only to individual patients. Most recent vaccine studies focused on class I-restricted antigens as targets for cancer-specific CTL. The characterization of class II-restricted antigens as targets for CD4+ T cell responses will allow concurrent immunization with class I and class II epitopes in order to generate more potent immune responses. In any case, the ideal vaccine most likely will consists of a cocktail of tumor antigens or proteins. However, the number of epitopes in the vaccine cocktail should be evaluated carefully since CTL responses in AIDS patients directed to fewer epitopes are associated with better clinical outcome (229). In this case it appears that the stimulation of multiple simultaneous CTL responses is clinically inefficient. Very important is also the dose of antigen and the speed of antigen release in the vaccine formulations. High doses of antigen released faster may induce T-cell tolerance (230). Immune tolerance may be due to fast expansion and subsequent elimination of specific T-cell clones, or to apoptosis induced by repeated stimulation of already stimulated T-cells in cell cycle (231, 232). Therefore, it is essential to select as immunogens those epitopes against which tolerance has not been induced (233, 234).

Future cancer vaccine strategies will most likely focus on more potent approaches for immunization. The use of the entire antigenic proteins might well be superior to peptide vaccines. A whole protein may provide several T-cell epitopes presented by different MHC molecules. An additional advantage of the whole protein vaccines may be the induction of humoral immune responses (235). Alone, or in conjunction with surgery, radiotherapy and/or chemotherapy, immunotherapy of prostate cancer and breast cancer can be effective in eliminating micro-metastases, in decreasing the immunosuppressive effects of the chemotherapy or radiotherapy, and in increasing the resistance to viral or bacterial infections frequently occurring in cancer patients.

Many challenges exist in the development of safe and effective vaccines for cancer. Cancer cells can undergo genetic alterations that result in loss of antigen expression or loss of the ability to present the tumor antigens. Recent advances in the design of polyvalent vaccines targeting several antigens may solve this problem. In addition, the possibility to treat patients with vaccines earlier in the course of the disease and to combine vaccines with other treatment modalities may also improve the vaccine efficacy. Further understanding of the mechanisms of the antitumor immune responses will provide a basis for improvement of the cancer vaccine approaches in the future. As a result, immunotherapy may become a major treatment modality of cancer.

REFERENCES

[1] Rammensee, H. G. Antigen presentation--recent developments. Int.Arch.Allergy Immunol., *110:* 299-307, 1996.

[2] Yewdell, J. W. and Bennink, J. R. Cell biology of antigen processing and presentation to major histocompatibility complex class I molecule-restricted T lymphocytes. Advances in Immunology, *52:* 1-123, 1992.

[3] Heemels, M. T. and Ploegh, H. Generation, translocation, and presentation of MHC class I- restricted peptides. Annu.Rev.Biochem., *64:* 463-491, 1995.

[4] Liu, C. C., Young, L. H., and Young, J. D. Lymphocyte-mediated cytolysis and disease. N.Engl.J.Med., *335:* 1651-1659, 1996.

[5] Van Pel, A., van der Bruggen, P., Coulie, P. G., Brichard, V. G., Lethe, B., van den Eynde, B., Uyttenhove, C., Renauld, J. C., and Boon, T. Genes coding for tumor antigens recognized by cytolytic T lymphocytes. Immunological Reviews, *145:* 229-250, 1995.

[6] De Plaen, E., Lurquin, C., Lethe, B., van der Bruggen, P., Brichard, V., Renauld, J. C., Coulie, P., Van Pel, A., and Boon, T. Identification of genes coding for tumor antigens recognized by cytolytic T lymphocytes. Methods, *12:* 125-142, 1997.

[7] Rosenberg, S. A. Cancer vaccines based on the identification of genes encoding cancer regression antigens. Immunol.Today, *18:* 175-182, 1997.

[8] Wang, R. F. Human tumor antigens: implications for cancer vaccine development. Journal of Molecular Medicine, *77:* 640-655, 1999.

[9] Nestle, F. O., Alijagic, S., Gilliet, M., Sun, M., Grabbe, S., Dummer, R., Burg, G., and Schadendorf, D. Vaccination of melanoma patients with peptide- or tumor lysate-pulsed dendritic cells. Nature Medicine, *4:* 328-332, 1998.

[10] Rosenberg, S. A., Yang, J. C., Schwartzentruber, D. J., Hwu, P., Marincola, F. M., Topalian, S. L., Restifo, N. P., Dudley, M. E., Schwarz, S. L., Spiess, P. J., Wunderlich, J. R., Parkhurst, M. R., Kawakami, Y., Seipp, C. A., Einhorn, J. H., and White, D. E. Immunologic and therapeutic evaluation of a synthetic peptide vaccine for the treatment of patients with metastatic melanoma. . Nature Medicine, *4:* 321-327, 1998.

[11] Thurner, B., Haendle, I., Reoder, C., Dieckmann, D., Keikavoussi, P., Jonuleit, H., Bender, A., Maczek, C., Schreiner, D., von den Driesch, P., Breocker, E. B., Steinman, R. M., Enk, A., Keampgen, E., and Schuler, G. Vaccination with mage-3A1 peptide-pulsed mature, monocyte-derived dendritic cells expands specific cytotoxic T cells and induces regression of some metastases in advanced stage IV melanoma. Journal of Experimental Medicine, *190:* 1669-1678, 1999.

[12] Kawakami, Y., Nishimura, M. I., Restifo, N. P., Topalian, S. L., O'Neil, B. H., Shilyansky, J., Yannelli, J. R., and Rosenberg, S. A. T-cell recognition of human melanoma antigens. J.Immunother., *14:* 88-93, 1993.

[13] Kawakami, Y., Eliyahu, S., Delgado, C. H., Robbins, P. F., Sakaguchi, K., Appella, E., Yannelli, J. R., Adema, G. J., Miki, T., and Rosenberg, S. A. Identification of a human melanoma antigen recognized by tumor- infiltrating lymphocytes associated with in vivo tumor rejection. Proc.Natl.Acad.Sci.U.S.A., *91:* 6458-6462, 1994.

[14] Brichard, V., Van Pel, A., Wölfel, T., Wölfel, C., De Plaen, E., Lethé, B., Coulie, P., and Boon, T. The tyrosinase gene codes for an antigen recognized by autologous

cytolytic T lymphocytes on HLA-A2 melanomas. Journal of Experimental Medicine, *178:* 489-495, 1993.

[15] Storkus, W. J., Zeh, H. J. d., Maeurer, M. J., Salter, R. D., and Lotze, M. T. Identification of human melanoma peptides recognized by class I restricted tumor infiltrating T lymphocytes. J.Immunol., *151:* 3719-3727, 1993.

[16] Cox, A. L., Skipper, J., Chen, Y., Henderson, R. A., Darrow, T. L., Shabanowitz, J., Engelhard, V. H., Hunt, D. F., and Slingluff, C. L. J. Identification of a peptide recognized by five melanoma-specific human cytotoxic T cell lines. Science, *264:* 716-719, 1994.

[17] Christinck, E. R., Luscher, M. A., Barber, B. H., and Williams, D. B. Peptide binding to class I MHC on living cells and quantitation of complexes required for CTL lysis. Nature, *352:* 67-70, 1991.

[18] Rammensee, H. G., Friede, T., and Stevanoviic, S. MHC ligands and peptide motifs: first listing. Immunogenetics, *41:* 178-228, 1995.

[19] Nakamura, T. M., Morin, G. B., Chapman, K. B., Weinrich, S. L., Andrews, W. H., Lingner, J., Harley, C. B., and Cech, T. R. Telomerase catalytic subunit homologs from fission yeast and human [see comments]. Science, *277:* 955-959, 1997.

[20] Ruppert, J., Sidney, J., Celis, E., Kubo, R. T., Grey, H. M., and Sette, A. Prominent role of secondary anchor residues in peptide binding to HLA-A2.1 molecules. Cell, *74:* 929-937, 1993.

[21] Parker, K. C., Bednarek, M. A., and Coligan, J. E. Scheme for ranking potential HLA-A2 binding peptides based on independent binding of individual peptide side-chains. Journal of Immunology, *152:* 163-175, 1994.

[22] Minev, B., Hipp, J., Firat, H., Schmidt, J. D., Langlade-Demoyen, P., and Zanetti, M. Cytotoxic T cell immunity against telomerase reverse transcriptase in humans. Proceedings of the National Academy of Sciences of the United States of America, *97:* 4796-4801, 2000.

[23] Mitchell, M. S., Kan-Mitchell, J., Minev, B. R., Edman, C., and Deans, R. J. A novel melanoma gene (MG50) encoding the interleukin 1 receptor antagonist and six epitopes recognized by human cytolytic T lymphocytes. Cancer Research, *60:* 6448-6456, 2000.

[24] Sahin, U., Teureci, O., and Pfreundschuh, M. Serological identification of human tumor antigens. Current Opinion in Immunology, *9:* 709-716, 1997.

[25] Bystryn, J. C., Rigel, D., Friedman, R. J., and Kopf, A. Prognostic significance of hypopigmentation in malignant melanoma. Arch.Dermatol., *123:* 1053-1055, 1987.

[26] Rosenberg, S. A. and White, D. E. Vitiligo in patients with melanoma: normal tissue antigens can be targets for cancer immunotherapy. J.Immunother.Emphasis.Tumor Immunol., *19:* 81-84, 1996.

[27] van der Bruggen, P., Traversari, C., Chomez, P., Lurquin, C., De Plaen, E., Van den Eynde, B., Knuth, A., and Boon, T. A gene encoding an antigen recognized by cytolytic T lymphocytes on a human melanoma. Science, *254:* 1643-1647, 1991.

[28] Chaux, P., Luiten, R., Demotte, N., Vantomme, V., Stroobant, V., Traversari, C., Russo, V., Schultz, E., Cornelis, G. R., Boon, T., and van der Bruggen, P. Identification of five MAGE-A1 epitopes recognized by cytolytic T lymphocytes obtained by in vitro stimulation with dendritic cells transduced with MAGE-A1. Journal of Immunology, *163:* 2928-2936, 1999.

[29] Boel, P., Wildmann, C., Sensi, M. L., Brasseur, R., Renauld, J. C., Coulie, P., Boon, T., and van der Bruggen, P. BAGE: a new gene encoding an antigen recognized on human melanomas by cytolytic T lymphocytes. Immunity., *2:* 167-175, 1995.

[30] Van den Eynde, B., Peeters, O., De Backer, O., Gaugler, B., Lucas, S., and Boon, T. A new family of genes coding for an antigen recognized by autologous cytolytic T lymphocytes on a human melanoma. J.Exp.Med., *182:* 689-698, 1995.

[31] Gaugler, B., Brouwenstijn, N., Vantomme, V., Szikora, J. P., Van der Spek, C. W., Patard, J. J., Boon, T., Schrier, P., and Van den Eynde, B. J. A new gene coding for an antigen recognized by autologous cytolytic T lymphocytes on a human renal carcinoma. Immunogenetics, *44:* 323-330, 1996.

[32] Lee, L., Wang, R. F., Wang, X., Mixon, A., Johnson, B. E., Rosenberg, S. A., and Schrump, D. S. NY-ESO-1 may be a potential target for lung cancer immunotherapy [see comments]. Cancer Journal from Scientific American, *5:* 20-25, 1999.

[33] Jeager, E., Chen, Y. T., Drijfhout, J. W., Karbach, J., Ringhoffer, M., Jeager, D., Arand, M., Wada, H., Noguchi, Y., Stockert, E., Old, L. J., and Knuth, A. Simultaneous humoral and cellular immune response against cancer-testis antigen NY-ESO-1: definition of human histocompatibility leukocyte antigen (HLA)-A2-binding peptide epitopes. Journal of Experimental Medicine, *187:* 265-270, 1998.

[34] Jeager, E., Jeager, D., Karbach, J., Chen, Y. T., Ritter, G., Nagata, Y., Gnjatic, S., Stockert, E., Arand, M., Old, L. J., and Knuth, A. Identification of NY-ESO-1 epitopes presented by human histocompatibility antigen (HLA)-DRB4*0101-0103 and recognized by CD4(+) T lymphocytes of patients with NY-ESO-1-expressing melanoma. Journal of Experimental Medicine, *191:* 625-630, 2000.

[35] De Plaen, E., Lurquin, C., Van Pel, A., Mariame', B., Szikora, J.-P., Wölfel, T., Sibille, C., Chomez, P., and Boon, T. Immunogenic (tum⁻) variants of mouse tumor P815: cloning of the gene of tum⁻ antigen P91A and identification of the tum⁻ mutation. Proc.Natl.Acad.Sci.USA, *85:* 2274-2278, 1988.

[36] Wolfel, T., Hauer, M., Schneider, J., Serrano, M., Wolfel, C., Klehmann-Hieb, E., De Plaen, E., Hankeln, T., Meyer zum Buschenfelde, K. H., and Beach, D. A p16INK4a-insensitive CDK4 mutant targeted by cytolytic T lymphocytes in a human melanoma. Science, *269:* 1281-1284, 1995.

[37] Coulie, P. G., Lehmann, F., Lethe, B., Herman, J., Lurquin, C., Andrawiss, M., and Boon, T. A mutated intron sequence codes for an antigenic peptide recognized by cytolytic T lymphocytes on a human melanoma. Proc.Natl.Acad.Sci.U.S.A., *92:* 7976-7980, 1995.

[38] Robbins, P. F., el-Gamil, M., Li, Y. F., Kawakami, Y., Loftus, D., Appella, E., and Rosenberg, S. A. A mutated beta-catenin gene encodes a melanoma-specific antigen recognized by tumor infiltrating lymphocytes. J.Exp.Med., *183:* 1185-1192, 1996.

[39] Gendler, S., Taylor-Papadimitriou, J., Duhig, T., Rothbard, J., and Burchell, J. A highly immunogenic region of a human polymorphic epithelial mucin expressed by carcinomas is made up of tandem repeats. J.Biol.Chem., *263:* 12820-12823, 1988.

[40] Magarian-Blander, J., Domenech, N., and Finn, O. J. Specific and effective T-cell recognition of cells transfected with a truncated human mucin cDNA. Ann.N.Y.Acad.Sci., *690:* 231-243, 1993.

[41] Takahashi, T., Makiguchi, Y., Hinoda, Y., Kakiuchi, H., Nakagawa, N., Imai, K., and Yachi, A. Expression of MUC1 on myeloma cells and induction of HLA- unrestricted

CTL against MUC1 from a multiple myeloma patient. J.Immunol., *153:* 2102-2109, 1994.

[42] Jerome, K. R., Barnd, D. L., Bendt, K. M., Boyer, C. M., Taylor-Papadimitriou, J., McKenzie, I. F., Bast, R. C., Jr., and Finn, O. J. Cytotoxic T-lymphocytes derived from patients with breast adenocarcinoma recognize an epitope present on the protein core of a mucin molecule preferentially expressed by malignant cells. Cancer.Res., *51:* 2908-2916, 1991.

[43] Pietersz, G. A., Li, W., Osinski, C., Apostolopoulos, V., and McKenzie, I. F. Definition of MHC-restricted CTL epitopes from non-variable number of tandem repeat sequence of MUC1. Vaccine, *18:* 2059-2071, 2000.

[44] Coussens, L., Yang-Feng, T. L., Liao, Y. C., Chen, E., Gray, A., McGrath, J., Seeburg, P. H., Libermann, T. A., Schlessinger, J., and Francke, U. Tyrosine kinase receptor with extensive homology to EGF receptor shares chromosomal location with neu oncogene. Science, *230:* 1132-1139, 1985.

[45] Toikkanen, S., Helin, H., Isola, J., and Joensuu, H. Prognostic significance of HER-2 oncoprotein expression in breast cancer: a 30-year follow-up. J.Clin.Oncol., *10:* 1044-1048, 1992.

[46] Disis, M. L., Smith, J. W., Murphy, A. E., Chen, W., and Cheever, M. A. In vitro generation of human cytolytic T-cells specific for peptides derived from the HER-2/neu protooncogene protein. Cancer Res., *54:* 1071-1076, 1994.

[47] Fisk, B., Blevins, T. L., Wharton, J. T., and Ioannides, C. G. Identification of an immunodominant peptide of HER-2/neu protooncogene recognized by ovarian tumor-specific cytotoxic T lymphocyte lines. J.Exp.Med., *181:* 2109-2117, 1995.

[48] Lustgarten, J., Theobald, M., Labadie, C., LaFace, D., Peterson, P., Disis, M. L., Cheever, M. A., and Sherman, L. A. Identification of Her-2/Neu CTL epitopes using double transgenic mice expressing HLA-A2.1 and human CD.8. Hum.Immunol., *52:* 109-118, 1997.

[49] Toes, R. E. M., Ossendorp, F., Offringa, R., and Melief, C. J. M. CD4 T cells and their role in antitumor immune responses. Journal of Experimental Medicine, *189:* 753-756, 1999.

[50] Topalian, S. L., Rivoltini, L., Mancini, M., Markus, N. R., Robbins, P. F., Kawakami, Y., and Rosenberg, S. A. Human CD4+ T cells specifically recognize a shared melanoma- associated antigen encoded by the tyrosinase gene. Proc.Natl.Acad.Sci.U.S.A., *91:* 9461-9465, 1994.

[51] Chaux, P., Vantomme, V., Stroobant, V., Thielemans, K., Corthals, J., Luiten, R., Eggermont, A. M., Boon, T., and van der Bruggen, P. Identification of MAGE-3 epitopes presented by HLA-DR molecules to CD4(+) T lymphocytes [see comments]. Journal of Experimental Medicine, *189:* 767-778, 1999.

[52] Wang, R. F., Wang, X., Atwood, A. C., Topalian, S. L., and Rosenberg, S. A. Cloning genes encoding MHC class II-restricted antigens: mutated CDC27 as a tumor antigen. Science, *284:* 1351-1354, 1999.

[53] Zarour, H. M., Kirkwood, J. M., Kierstead, L. S., Herr, W., Brusic, V., Slingluff, C. L., Jr., Sidney, J., Sette, A., and Storkus, W. J. Melan-A/MART-1(51-73) represents an immunogenic HLA-DR4-restricted epitope recognized by melanoma-reactive CD4(+) T cells. Proceedings of the National Academy of Sciences of the United States of America, *97:* 400-405, 2000.

[54] Baxevanis, C. N., Voutsas, I. F., Tsitsilonis, O. E., Gritzapis, A. D., Sotiriadou, R., and Papamichail, M. Tumor-specific CD4+ T lymphocytes from cancer patients are required for optimal induction of cytotoxic T cells against the autologous tumor. Journal of Immunology, *164:* 3902-3912, 2000.

[55] Schulz, M., Zinkernagel, R. M., and Hengartner, H. Peptide-induced antiviral protection by cytotoxic T cells. Proc.Natl.Acad.Sci.U.S.A., *88:* 991-993, 1991.

[56] Cormier, J. N., Salgaller, M. L., Prevette, T., Barracchini, K. C., Rivoltini, L., Restifo, N. P., Rosenberg, S. A., and Marincola, F. M. Enhancement of cellular immunity in melanoma patients immunized with a peptide from MART-1/Melan A [see comments]. Cancer J.Sci.Am., *3:* 37-44, 1997.

[57] Lipford, G. B., Hoffman, M., Wagner, H., and Heeg, K. Primary in vivo responses to ovalbumin. Probing the predictive value of the Kb binding motif. Journal of Immunology, *150:* 1212-1222, 1993.

[58] Zhou, F., Rouse, B. T., and Huang, L. Prolonged survival of thymoma-bearing mice after vaccination with a soluble protein antigen entrapped in liposomes: a model study. Cancer.Res., *52:* 6287-6291, 1992.

[59] Mossman, S. P., Evans, L. S., Fang, H., Staas, J., Tice, T., Raychaudhuri, S., Grabstein, K. H., Cheever, M. A., and Johnson, M. E. Development of a CTL vaccine for Her-2/neu using peptide-microspheres and adjuvants. Vaccine, *23:* 3545-3554, 2005.

[60] Zhou, F., Rouse, B. T., and Huang, L. Induction of cytotoxic T lymphocytes in vivo with protein antigen entrapped in membranous vehicles. Journal of Immunology, *149:* 1599-1604, 1992.

[61] Harty, J. T. and Bevan, M. J. CD8+ T cells specific for a single nonamer epitope of Listeria monocytogenes are protective in vivo. J.Exp.Med., *175:* 1531-1538, 1992.

[62] Noguchi, Y., Chen, Y. T., and Old, L. J. A mouse mutant p53 product recognized by CD4+ and CD8+ T cells. Proc.Natl.Acad.Sci.U.S.A., *91:* 3171-3175, 1994.

[63] Mayordomo, J. I., Zorina, T., Storkus, W. J., Zitvogel, L., Garcia-Prats, M. D., DeLeo, A. B., and Lotze, M. T. Bone marrow-derived dendritic cells serve as potent adjuvants for peptide-based antitumor vaccines. Stem.Cells, *15:* 94-103, 1997.

[64] Minev, B. R., McFarland, B. J., Spiess, P. J., Rosenberg, S. A., and Restifo, N. P. Insertion signal sequence fused to minimal peptides elicits specific CD8+ T-cell responses and prolongs survival of thymoma- bearing mice. Cancer Res., *54:* 4155-4161, 1994.

[65] Jager, E., Ringhoffer, M., Arand, M., Karbach, J., Jager, D., Ilsemann, C., Hagedorn, M., Oesch, F., and Knuth, A. Cytolytic T cell reactivity against melanoma-associated differentiation antigens in peripheral blood of melanoma patients and healthy individuals. Melanoma.Res., *6:* 419-425, 1996.

[66] Rivoltini, L., Kawakami, Y., Sakaguchi, K., Southwood, S., Sette, A., Robbins, P. F., Marincola, F. M., Salgaller, M. L., Yannelli, J. R., Appella, E., and et al. Induction of tumor-reactive CTL from peripheral blood and tumor-infiltrating lymphocytes of melanoma patients by in vitro stimulation with an immunodominant peptide of the human melanoma antigen MART-1. Journal of Immunology, *154:* 2257-2265, 1995.

[67] Visseren, M. J., van Elsas, A., van der Voort, E. I., Ressing, M. E., Kast, W. M., Schrier, P. I., and Melief, C. J. CTL specific for the tyrosinase autoantigen can be induced from healthy donor blood to lyse melanoma cells. Journal of Immunology, *154:* 3991-3998, 1995.

[68] Marchand, M., Weynants, P., Rankin, E., Arienti, F., Belli, F., Parmiani, G., Cascinelli, N., Bourlond, A., Vanwijck, R., and Humblet, Y. Tumor regression responses in melanoma patients treated with a peptide encoded by gene MAGE-3 [letter]. Int.J.Cancer, *63:* 883-885, 1995.

[69] Marchand, M., van Baren, N., Weynants, P., Brichard, V., Dreno, B., Tessier, M. H., Rankin, E., Parmiani, G., Arienti, F., Humblet, Y., Bourlond, A., Vanwijck, R., Lienard, D., Beauduin, M., Dietrich, P. Y., Russo, V., Kerger, J., Masucci, G., Jager, E., De Greve, J., Atzpodien, J., Brasseur, F., Coulie, P. G., van der Bruggen, P., and Boon, T. Tumor regressions observed in patients with metastatic melanoma treated with an antigenic peptide encoded by gene MAGE-3 and presented by HLA-A1. Int J Cancer, *80:* 219-230, 1999.

[70] Salgaller, M. L., Afshar, A., Marincola, F. M., Rivoltini, L., Kawakami, Y., and Rosenberg, S. A. Recognition of multiple epitopes in the human melanoma antigen gp100 by peripheral blood lymphocytes stimulated in vitro with synthetic peptides. Cancer Res., *55:* 4972-4979, 1995.

[71] Mukherji, B., Chakraborty, N. G., Yamasaki, S., Okino, T., Yamase, H., Sporn, J. R., Kurtzman, S. K., Ergin, M. T., Ozols, J., and Meehan, J. Induction of antigen-specific cytolytic T cells in situ in human melanoma by immunization with synthetic peptide-pulsed autologous antigen presenting cells. Proc.Natl.Acad.Sci.U.S.A., *92:* 8078-8082, 1995.

[72] Jaeger, E., Bernhard, H., Romero, P., Ringhoffer, M., Arand, M., Karbach, J., Ilsemann, C., Hagedorn, M., and Knuth, A. Generation of cytotoxic T-cell responses with synthetic melanoma- associated peptides in vivo: implications for tumor vaccines with melanoma-associated antigens. Int.J.Cancer, *66:* 162-169, 1996.

[73] Jager, E., Gnjatic, S., Nagata, Y., Old, L. J., and Knuth, A. Induction of primary NY-ESO-1 immunity: CD8+ T lymphocyte and antibody responses in peptide-vaccinated patients with NY-ESO-1+ cancers. P.N.A.S., *97:* 12198-12202, 2000.

[74] Gjertsen, M. K., Bakka, A., Breivik, J., Saeterdal, I., Gedde-Dahl, T 3rd, Stokke, K. T., Solheim, B. G., Egge, T. S., Soreide, O., Thorsby, E., and Gaudernack, G. Ex vivo ras peptide vaccination in patients with advanced pancreatic cancer: results of a phase I/II study. Int.J.Cancer, *65:* 450-453, 1996.

[75] Celis, E., Tsai, V., Crimi, C., DeMars, R., Wentworth, P. A., Chesnut, R. W., Grey, H. M., Sette, A., and Serra, H. M. Induction of anti-tumor cytotoxic T lymphocytes in normal humans using primary cultures and synthetic peptide epitopes. Proc.Natl.Acad.Sci.U.S.A., *91:* 2105-2109, 1994.

[76] Vitiello, A., Ishioka, G., Grey, H. M., Rose, R., Farness, P., LaFond, R., Yuan, L., Chisari, F. V., Furze, J., and Bartholomeuz, R. Development of a lipopeptide-based therapeutic vaccine to treat chronic HBV infection. I. Induction of a primary cytotoxic T lymphocyte response in humans. J.Clin.Invest., *95:* 341-349, 1995.

[77] Sette, A., Alexander, J., Ruppert, J., Snoke, K., Franco, A., Ishioka, G., and Grey, H. M. Antigen analogs/MHC complexes as specific T cell receptor antagonists. Annu.Rev.Immunol., *12:* 413-431, 1994.

[78] Parkhurst, M. R., Salgaller, M. L., Southwood, S., Robbins, P. F., Sette, A., Rosenberg, S. A., and Kawakami, Y. Improved induction of melanoma-reactive CTL with peptides from the melanoma antigen gp100 modified at HLA-A*0201-binding residues. J.Immunol., *157:* 2539-2548, 1996.

[79] Phan, G. Q., Yang, J. C., Sherry, R. M., Hwu, P., Topalian, S. L., Schwartzentruber, D. J., Restifo, N. P., Haworth, L. R., Seipp, C. A., Freezer, L. J., Morton, K. E., Mavroukakis, S. A., Duray, P. H., Steinberg, S. M., Allison, J. P., Davis, T. A., and Rosenberg, S. A. Cancer regression and autoimmunity induced by cytotoxic T lymphocyte-associated antigen 4 blockade in patients with metastatic melanoma. Proc Natl Acad Sci U S A, *100:* 8372-8377, 2003.

[80] Sanderson, K., Scotland, R., Lee, P., Liu, D., Groshen, S., Snively, J., Sian, S., Nichol, G., Davis, T., Keler, T., Yellin, M., and Weber, J. Autoimmunity in a phase I trial of a fully human anti-cytotoxic T-lymphocyte antigen-4 monoclonal antibody with multiple melanoma peptides and Montanide ISA 51 for patients with resected stages III and IV melanoma. J Clin Oncol, *23:* 741-750, 2005.

[81] Wang, F., Bade, E., Kuniyoshi, C., Spears, L., Jeffery, G., Marty, V., Groshen, S., and Weber, J. Phase I trial of a MART-1 peptide vaccine with incomplete Freund's adjuvant for resected high-risk melanoma. Clinical Cancer Research, *5:* 2756-2765, 1999.

[82] Jeager, E., Maeurer, M., Heohn, H., Karbach, J., Jeager, D., Zidianakis, Z., Bakhshandeh-Bath, A., Orth, J., Neukirch, C., Necker, A., Reichert, T. E., and Knuth, A. Clonal expansion of Melan A-specific cytotoxic T lymphocytes in a melanoma patient responding to continued immunization with melanoma-associated peptides. International Journal of Cancer, *86:* 538-547, 2000.

[83] Brinckerhoff, L. H., Kalashnikov, V. V., Thompson, L. W., Yamshchikov, G. V., Pierce, R. A., Galavotti, H. S., Engelhard, V. H., and Slingluff, C. L., Jr. Terminal modifications inhibit proteolytic degradation of an immunogenic MART-1(27-35) peptide: implications for peptide vaccines. International Journal of Cancer, *83:* 326-334, 1999.

[84] Minev, B. R., Chavez, F. L., Dudouet, B. M., and Mitchell, M. S. Synthetic insertion signal sequences enhance MHC class I presentation of a peptide from the melanoma antigen MART-1. Eur. J. Immunol., *30:* 2115-2124, 2000.

[85] Anderson, K., Cresswell, P., Gammon, M., Hermes, J., Williamson, A., and Zweerink, H. Endogenously synthesized peptide with an endoplasmic reticulum signal sequence sensitizes antigen processing mutant cells to class I-restricted cell-mediated lysis. Journal of Experimental Medicine, *174:* 489-492, 1991.

[86] Okada, C. Y. and Rechsteiner, M. Introduction of macromolecules into cultured mammalian cells by osmotic lysis of pinocytic vesicles. Cell, *29:* 33-41, 1982.

[87] Persson, H., Jornvall, H., and Zabielski, J. Multiple mRNA species for the precursor to an adenovirus-encoded glycoprotein: identification and structure of the signal sequence. Proc.Natl.Acad.Sci.U.S.A., *77:* 6349-6353, 1980.

[88] Houghton, M., Stewart, A. G., Doel, S. M., Emtage, J. S., Eaton, M. A., Smith, J. C., Patel, T. P., Lewis, H. M., Porter, A. G., Birch, J. R., Cartwright, T., and Carey, N. H. The amino-terminal sequence of human fibroblast interferon as deduced from reverse transcripts obtained using synthetic oligonucleotide primers. Nucleic.Acids.Res., *8:* 1913-1931, 1980.

[89] Restifo, N. P., Esquivel, F., Kawakami, Y., Yewdell, J. W., Mule, J. J., Rosenberg, S. A., and Bennink, J. R. Identification of human cancers deficient in antigen processing. J.Exp.Med., *177:* 265-272, 1993.

[90] Slingluff, C. L., Jr., Petroni, G. R., Yamshchikov, G. V., Hibbitts, S., Grosh, W. W., Chianese-Bullock, K. A., Bissonette, E. A., Barnd, D. L., Deacon, D. H., Patterson, J.

W., Parekh, J., Neese, P. Y., Woodson, E. M., Wiernasz, C. J., and Merrill, P. Immunologic and clinical outcomes of vaccination with a multiepitope melanoma peptide vaccine plus low-dose interleukin-2 administered either concurrently or on a delayed schedule. J Clin Oncol, *22:* 4474-4485, 2004.

[91] Lee, P., Wang, F., Kuniyoshi, J., Rubio, V., Stuges, T., Groshen, S., Gee, C., Lau, R., Jeffery, G., Margolin, K., Marty, V., and Weber, J. Effects of interleukin-12 on the immune response to a multipeptide vaccine for resected metastatic melanoma. J Clin Oncol, *19:* 3836-3847., 2001.

[92] Peterson, A. C., Harlin, H., and Gajewski, T. F. Immunization with Melan-A peptide-pulsed peripheral blood mononuclear cells plus recombinant human interleukin-12 induces clinical activity and T-cell responses in advanced melanoma. J Clin Oncol, *21:* 2342-2348, 2003.

[93] Chianese-Bullock, K. A., Pressley, J., Garbee, C., Hibbitts, S., Murphy, C., Yamshchikov, G., Petroni, G. R., Bissonette, E. A., Neese, P. Y., Grosh, W. W., Merrill, P., Fink, R., Woodson, E. M., Wiernasz, C. J., Patterson, J. W., and Slingluff, C. L., Jr. MAGE-A1-, MAGE-A10-, and gp100-derived peptides are immunogenic when combined with granulocyte-macrophage colony-stimulating factor and montanide ISA-51 adjuvant and administered as part of a multipeptide vaccine for melanoma. J Immunol, *174:* 3080-3086, 2005.

[94] Hersey, P., Menzies, S. W., Coventry, B., Nguyen, T., Farrelly, M., Collins, S., Hirst, D., and Johnson, H. Phase I/II study of immunotherapy with T-cell peptide epitopes in patients with stage IV melanoma. Cancer Immunol Immunother, *54:* 208-218, 2005.

[95] Pullarkat, V., Lee, P. P., Scotland, R., Rubio, V., Groshen, S., Gee, C., Lau, R., Snively, J., Sian, S., Woulfe, S. L., Wolfe, R. A., and Weber, J. S. A phase I trial of SD-9427 (progenipoietin) with a multipeptide vaccine for resected metastatic melanoma. Clin Cancer Res, *9:* 1301-1312, 2003.

[96] Butterfield, L. H., Ribas, A., Meng, W. S., Dissette, V. B., Amarnani, S., Vu, H. T., Seja, E., Todd, K., Glaspy, J. A., McBride, W. H., and Economou, J. S. T-cell responses to HLA-A*0201 immunodominant peptides derived from alpha-fetoprotein in patients with hepatocellular cancer. Clin Cancer Res, *9:* 5902-5908, 2003.

[97] Vonderheide, R. H., Domchek, S. M., Schultze, J. L., George, D. J., Hoar, K. M., Chen, D. Y., Stephans, K. F., Masutomi, K., Loda, M., Xia, Z., Anderson, K. S., Hahn, W. C., and Nadler, L. M. Vaccination of cancer patients against telomerase induces functional antitumor CD8+ T lymphocytes. Clin Cancer Res, *10:* 828-839, 2004.

[98] McNeel, D. G., Knutson, K. L., Schiffman, K., Davis, D. R., Caron, D., and Disis, M. L. Pilot study of an HLA-A2 peptide vaccine using flt3 ligand as a systemic vaccine adjuvant. J Clin Immunol, *23:* 62-72, 2003.

[99] Davila, E., Kennedy, R., and Celis, E. Generation of antitumor immunity by cytotoxic T lymphocyte epitope peptide vaccination, CpG-oligodeoxynucleotide adjuvant, and CTLA-4 blockade. Cancer Res, *63:* 3281-3288, 2003.

[100] Celis, E., Sette, A., and Grey, H. M. Epitope selection and development of peptide based vaccines to treat cancer. Semin.Cancer Biol., *6:* 329-336, 1995.

[101] Moss, B. Vaccinia virus: a tool for research and vaccine development. Science, *252:* 1662-1667, 1991.

[102] Etlinger, H. M. and Altenburger, W. Overcoming inhibition of antibody responses to a malaria recombinant vaccinia virus caused by prior exposure to wild type virus. Vaccine, *9:* 470-472, 1991.

[103] Mastrangelo, M. J., Maguire, H. C., and McCue, P. A pilot study demonstrating the feasibility of using intratumoral vaccinia injections as a vector for gene transfer. Vaccine Research, *4:* 55-69, 1995.

[104] Irvine, K. R., Chamberlain, R. S., Shulman, E. P., Surman, D. R., Rosenberg, S. A., and Restifo, N. P. Enhancing efficacy of recombinant anticancer vaccines with prime/boost regimens that use two different vectors. J.Natl.Cancer Inst., *89:* 1595-1601, 1997.

[105] Feder-Mengus, C., Schultz-Thater, E., Oertli, D., Marti, W. R., Heberer, M., Spagnoli, G. C., and Zajac, P. Nonreplicating recombinant vaccinia virus expressing CD40 ligand enhances APC capacity to stimulate specific CD4+ and CD8+ T cell responses. Hum Gene Ther, *16:* 348-360, 2005.

[106] McElrath, M. J. Selection of potent immunological adjuvants for vaccine construction. Semin.Cancer Biol., *6:* 375-385, 1995.

[107] Baxby, D. and Paoletti, E. Potential use of non-replicating vectors as recombinant vaccines. Vaccine, *10:* 8-9, 1992.

[108] Wang, M., Bronte, V., Chen, P. W., Gritz, L., Panicali, D., Rosenberg, S. A., and Restifo, N. P. Active immunotherapy of cancer with a nonreplicating recombinant fowlpox virus encoding a model tumor-associated antigen. J.Immunol., *154:* 4685-4692, 1995.

[109] Cox, W. I., Tartaglia, J., and Paoletti, E. Induction of cytotoxic T lymphocytes by recombinant canarypox (ALVAC) and attenuated vaccinia (NYVAC) viruses expressing the HIV-1 envelope glycoprotein. Virology, *195:* 845-850, 1993.

[110] Tsang, K. Y., Zaremba, S., Nieroda, C. A., Zhu, M. Z., Hamilton, J. M., and Schlom, J. Generation of human cytotoxic T cells specific for human carcinoembryonic antigen epitopes from patients immunized with recombinant vaccinia-CEA vaccine. J.Natl.Cancer Inst., *87:* 982-990, 1995.

[111] Marshall, J. L., Hawkins, M. J., Tsang, K. Y., Richmond, E., Pedicano, J. E., Zhu, M. Z., and Schlom, J. Phase I study in cancer patients of a replication-defective avipox recombinant vaccine that expresses human carcinoembryonic antigen. Journal of Clinical Oncology, *17:* 332-337, 1999.

[112] Zhu, M. Z., Marshall, J., Cole, D., Schlom, J., and Tsang, K. Y. Specific cytolytic T-cell responses to human CEA from patients immunized with recombinant avipox-CEA vaccine. Clinical Cancer Research, *6:* 24-33, 2000.

[113] Conry, R. M., Khazaeli, M. B., Saleh, M. N., Allen, K. O., Barlow, D. L., Moore, S. E., Craig, D., Arani, R. B., Schlom, J., and LoBuglio, A. F. Phase I trial of a recombinant vaccinia virus encoding carcinoembryonic antigen in metastatic adenocarcinoma: comparison of intradermal versus subcutaneous administration. Clinical Cancer Research, *5:* 2330-2337, 1999.

[114] Conry, R. M., Allen, K. O., Lee, S., Moore, S. E., Shaw, D. R., and LoBuglio, A. F. Human autoantibodies to carcinoembryonic antigen (CEA) induced by a vaccinia-CEA vaccine. Clinical Cancer Research, *6:* 34-41, 2000.

[115] Meyer, H., Sutter, G., and Mayr, A. Mapping of deletions in the genome of the highly attenuated vaccinia virus MVA and their influence on virulence. J.gen.Virol., *72:* 1031-1038, 1991.

[116] Sutter, G. and Moss, B. Nonreplicating vaccinia vector efficiently expresses recombinant genes. Proc.Natl.Acad.Sci.U.S.A., *89:* 10847-10851, 1992.

[117] Sutter, G., Wyatt, L. S., Foley, P. L., Bennink, J. R., and Moss, B. A recombinant vector derived from the host range-restricted and highly attenuated MVA strain of vaccinia virus stimulates protective immunity in mice to influenza virus. Vaccine, *12:* 1032-1040, 1994.

[118] Drexler, I., Antunes, E., Schmitz, M., Weolfel, T., Huber, C., Erfle, V., Rieber, P., Theobald, M., and Sutter, G. Modified vaccinia virus Ankara for delivery of human tyrosinase as melanoma-associated antigen: induction of tyrosinase- and melanoma-specific human leukocyte antigen A*0201-restricted cytotoxic T cells in vitro and in vivo. Cancer Research, *59:* 4955-4963, 1999.

[119] Mateo, L., Gardner, J., Chen, Q., Schmidt, C., Down, M., Elliott, S. L., Pye, S. J., Firat, H., Lemonnier, F. A., Cebon, J., and Suhrbier, A. An HLA-A2 polyepitope vaccine for melanoma immunotherapy. Journal of Immunology, *163:* 4058-4063, 1999.

[120] Rosenberg, S. A., Zhai, Y., Yang, J. C., Schwartzentruber, D. J., Hwu, P., Marincola, F. M., Topalian, S. L., Restifo, N. P., Seipp, C. A., Einhorn, J. H., Roberts, B., and White, D. E. Immunizing patients with metastatic melanoma using recombinant adenoviruses encoding MART-1 or gp100 melanoma antigens. Journal of the National Cancer Institute, *90:* 1894-1900, 1998.

[121] Liu, D. W., Tsao, Y. P., Kung, J. T., Ding, Y. A., Sytwu, H. K., Xiao, X., and Chen, S. L. Recombinant adeno-associated virus expressing human papillomavirus type 16 E7 peptide DNA fused with heat shock protein DNA as a potential vaccine for cervical cancer. Journal of Virology, *74:* 2888-2894, 2000.

[122] Sanda, M. G., Smith, D. C., Charles, L. G., Hwang, C., Pienta, K. J., Schlom, J., Milenic, D., Panicali, D., and Montie, J. E. Recombinant vaccinia-PSA (PROSTVAC) can induce a prostate-specific immune response in androgen-modulated human prostate cancer. Urology, *53:* 260-266, 1999.

[123] Zajac, P., Oertli, D., Marti, W., Adamina, M., Bolli, M., Guller, U., Noppen, C., Padovan, E., Schultz-Thater, E., Heberer, M., and Spagnoli, G. Phase I/II clinical trial of a nonreplicative vaccinia virus expressing multiple HLA-A0201-restricted tumor-associated epitopes and costimulatory molecules in metastatic melanoma patients. Hum Gene Ther, *14:* 1497-1510, 2003.

[124] Arlen, P. M., Gulley, J. L., Todd, N., Lieberman, R., Steinberg, S. M., Morin, S., Bastian, A., Marte, J., Tsang, K. Y., Beetham, P., Grosenbach, D. W., Schlom, J., and Dahut, W. Antiandrogen, vaccine and combination therapy in patients with nonmetastatic hormone refractory prostate cancer. J Urol, *174:* 539-546, 2005.

[125] Freytag, S. O., Stricker, H., Pegg, J., Paielli, D., Pradhan, D. G., Peabody, J., DePeralta-Venturina, M., Xia, X., Brown, S., Lu, M., and Kim, J. H. Phase I study of replication-competent adenovirus-mediated double-suicide gene therapy in combination with conventional-dose three-dimensional conformal radiation therapy for the treatment of newly diagnosed, intermediate- to high-risk prostate cancer. Cancer Res, *63:* 7497-7506, 2003.

[126] Pantuck, A. J., van Ophoven, A., Gitlitz, B. J., Tso, C. L., Acres, B., Squiban, P., Ross, M. E., Belldegrun, A. S., and Figlin, R. A. Phase I trial of antigen-specific gene therapy using a recombinant vaccinia virus encoding MUC-1 and IL-2 in MUC-1-positive patients with advanced prostate cancer. J Immunother, *27:* 240-253, 2004.

[127] Bonnet, M. C., Tartaglia, J., Verdier, F., Kourilsky, P., Lindberg, A., Klein, M., and Moingeon, P. Recombinant viruses as a tool for therapeutic vaccination against human cancers. Immunology Letters, *74:* 11-25, 2000.

[128] Fynan, E. F., Webster, R. G., Fuller, D. H., Haynes, J. R., Santoro, J. C., and Robinson, H. L. DNA vaccines: protective immunizations by parenteral, mucosal, and gene-gun inoculations. Proc.Natl.Acad.Sci.U.S.A., *90:* 11478-11482, 1993.

[129] Wolff, J. A., Dowty, M. E., Jiao, S., Repetto, G., Berg, R. K., Ludtke, J. J., Williams, P., and Slautterback, D. B. Expression of naked plasmids by cultured myotubes and entry of plasmids into T tubules and caveolae of mammalian skeletal muscle. J.Cell Sci., *103:* 1249-1259, 1992.

[130] Wolff, J. A., Ludtke, J. J., Acsadi, G., Williams, P., and Jani, A. Long-term persistence of plasmid DNA and foreign gene expression in mouse muscle. Hum.Mol.Genet., *1:* 363-369, 1992.

[131] Yankauckas, M. A., Morrow, J. E., Parker, S. E., Abai, A., Rhodes, G. H., Dwarki, V. J., and Gromkowski, S. H. Long-term anti-nucleoprotein cellular and humoral immunity is induced by intramuscular injection of plasmid DNA containing NP gene. DNA Cell Biol., *12:* 771-776, 1993.

[132] Fuller, D. H. and Haynes, J. R. A qualitative progression in HIV type 1 glycoprotein 120- specific cytotoxic cellular and humoral immune responses in mice receiving a DNA-based glycoprotein 120 vaccine. AIDS Res.Hum.Retroviruses, *10:* 1433-1441, 1994.

[133] Pertmer, T. M., Eisenbraun, M. D., McCabe, D., Prayaga, S. K., Fuller, D. H., and Haynes, J. R. Gene gun-based nucleic acid immunization: elicitation of humoral and cytotoxic T lymphocyte responses following epidermal delivery of nanogram quantities of DNA. Vaccine, *13:* 1427-1430, 1995.

[134] Irvine, K. R., Rao, J. B., Rosenberg, S. A., and Restifo, N. P. Cytokine enhancement of DNA immunization leads to effective treatment of established pulmonary metastases. J.Immunol., *156:* 238-245, 1996.

[135] Conry, R. M., Widera, G., LoBuglio, A. F., Fuller, J. T., Moore, S. E., Barlow, D. L., Turner, J., Yang, N. S., and Curiel, D. T. Selected strategies to augment polynucleotide immunization. Gene Ther., *3:* 67-74, 1996.

[136] Corr, M., Lee, D. J., Carson, D. A., and Tighe, H. Gene vaccination with naked plasmid DNA: mechanism of CTL priming. J.Exp.Med., *184:* 1555-1560, 1996.

[137] Ulmer, J. B., Deck, R. R., Dewitt, C. M., Donnhly, J. I., and Liu, M. A. Generation of MHC class I-restricted cytotoxic T lymphocytes by expression of a viral protein in muscle cells: antigen presentation by non-muscle cells. Immunology, *89:* 59-67, 1996.

[138] Condon, C., Watkins, S. C., Celluzzi, C. M., Thompson, K., and Falo, L. D. J. DNA-based immunization by in vivo transfection of dendritic cells. Nat.Med., *2:* 1122-1128, 1996.

[139] Syrengelas, A. D., Chen, T. T., and Levy, R. DNA immunization induces protective immunity against B-cell lymphoma. Nat.Med., *2:* 1038-1041, 1996.

[140] Timmerman, J. M., Singh, G., Hermanson, G., Hobart, P., Czerwinski, D. K., Taidi, B., Rajapaksa, R., Caspar, C. B., Van Beckhoven, A., and Levy, R. Immunogenicity of a plasmid DNA vaccine encoding chimeric idiotype in patients with B-cell lymphoma. Cancer Res, *62:* 5845-5852, 2002.

[141] Conry, R. M., Curiel, D. T., Strong, T. V., Moore, S. E., Allen, K. O., Barlow, D. L., Shaw, D. R., and LoBuglio, A. F. Safety and immunogenicity of a DNA vaccine encoding carcinoembryonic antigen and hepatitis B surface antigen in colorectal carcinoma patients. Clin Cancer Res, 8: 2782-2787, 2002.

[142] Hermans, I. F., Chong, T. W., Palmowski, M. J., Harris, A. L., and Cerundolo, V. Synergistic effect of metronomic dosing of cyclophosphamide combined with specific antitumor immunotherapy in a murine melanoma model. Cancer Res, 63: 8408-8413, 2003.

[143] Sanchez-Perez, L., Kottke, T., Diaz, R. M., Ahmed, A., Thompson, J., Chong, H., Melcher, A., Holmen, S., Daniels, G., and Vile, R. G. Potent selection of antigen loss variants of B16 melanoma following inflammatory killing of melanocytes in vivo. Cancer Res, 65: 2009-2017, 2005.

[144] Reisfeld, R. A., Niethammer, A. G., Luo, Y., and Xiang, R. DNA vaccines suppress tumor growth and metastases by the induction of anti-angiogenesis. Immunol Rev, 199: 181-190, 2004.

[145] Xiang, R., Mizutani, N., Luo, Y., Chiodoni, C., Zhou, H., Mizutani, M., Ba, Y., Becker, J. C., and Reisfeld, R. A. A DNA vaccine targeting survivin combines apoptosis with suppression of angiogenesis in lung tumor eradication. Cancer Res, 65: 553-561, 2005.

[146] Bronte, V., Cingarlini, S., Apolloni, E., Serafini, P., Marigo, I., De Santo, C., Macino, B., Marin, O., and Zanovello, P. Effective genetic vaccination with a widely shared endogenous retroviral tumor antigen requires CD40 stimulation during tumor rejection phase. J Immunol, 171: 6396-6405, 2003.

[147] Buchan, S., Gronevik, E., Mathiesen, I., King, C. A., Stevenson, F. K., and Rice, J. Electroporation as a "prime/boost" strategy for naked DNA vaccination against a tumor antigen. J Immunol, 174: 6292-6298, 2005.

[148] Stevenson, F. K., Ottensmeier, C. H., Johnson, P., Zhu, D., Buchan, S. L., McCann, K. J., Roddick, J. S., King, A. T., McNicholl, F., Savelyeva, N., and Rice, J. DNA vaccines to attack cancer. Proc Natl Acad Sci U S A, 101 Suppl 2: 14646-14652, 2004.

[149] Zhang, L., Widera, G., Bleecher, S., Zaharoff, D. A., Mossop, B., and Rabussay, D. Accelerated immune response to DNA vaccines. DNA Cell Biol, 22: 815-822, 2003.

[150] Doan, T., Herd, K., Ramshaw, I., Thomson, S., and Tindle, R. W. A polytope DNA vaccine elicits multiple effector and memory CTL responses and protects against human papillomavirus 16 E7-expressing tumour. Cancer Immunol Immunother, 54: 157-171, 2005.

[151] Gregor, P. D., Wolchok, J. D., Ferrone, C. R., Buchinshky, H., Guevara-Patino, J. A., Perales, M. A., Mortazavi, F., Bacich, D., Heston, W., Latouche, J. B., Sadelain, M., Allison, J. P., Scher, H. I., and Houghton, A. N. CTLA-4 blockade in combination with xenogeneic DNA vaccines enhances T-cell responses, tumor immunity and autoimmunity to self antigens in animal and cellular model systems. Vaccine, 22: 1700-1708, 2004.

[152] Teramoto, K., Kontani, K., Ozaki, Y., Sawai, S., Tezuka, N., Nagata, T., Fujino, S., Itoh, Y., Taguchi, O., Koide, Y., Asai, T., Ohkubo, I., and Ogasawara, K. Deoxyribonucleic acid (DNA) encoding a pan-major histocompatibility complex class II peptide analogue augmented antigen-specific cellular immunity and suppressive effects on tumor growth elicited by DNA vaccine immunotherapy. Cancer Res, 63: 7920-7925, 2003.

[153] Jia, Z. C., Zou, L. Y., Ni, B., Wan, Y., Zhou, W., Lv, Y. B., Geng, M., and Wu, Y. Z. Effective induction of antitumor immunity by immunization with plasmid DNA encoding TRP-2 plus neutralization of TGF-beta. Cancer Immunol Immunother, *54:* 446-452, 2005.

[154] Piechocki, M. P., Ho, Y. S., Pilon, S., and Wei, W. Z. Human ErbB-2 (Her-2) transgenic mice: a model system for testing Her-2 based vaccines. J Immunol, *171:* 5787-5794, 2003.

[155] Pupa, S. M., Iezzi, M., Di Carlo, E., Invernizzi, A., Cavallo, F., Meazza, R., Comes, A., Ferrini, S., Musiani, P., and Menard, S. Inhibition of mammary carcinoma development in HER-2/neu transgenic mice through induction of autoimmunity by xenogeneic DNA vaccination. Cancer Res, *65:* 1071-1078, 2005.

[156] Quaglino, E., Iezzi, M., Mastini, C., Amici, A., Pericle, F., Di Carlo, E., Pupa, S. M., De Giovanni, C., Spadaro, M., Curcio, C., Lollini, P. L., Musiani, P., Forni, G., and Cavallo, F. Electroporated DNA vaccine clears away multifocal mammary carcinomas in her-2/neu transgenic mice. Cancer Res, *64:* 2858-2864, 2004.

[157] Lavergne, E., Combadiere, C., Iga, M., Boissonnas, A., Bonduelle, O., Maho, M., Debre, P., and Combadiere, B. Intratumoral CC chemokine ligand 5 overexpression delays tumor growth and increases tumor cell infiltration. J Immunol, *173:* 3755-3762, 2004.

[158] Stagg, J., Wu, J. H., Bouganim, N., and Galipeau, J. Granulocyte-macrophage colony-stimulating factor and interleukin-2 fusion cDNA for cancer gene immunotherapy. Cancer Res, *64:* 8795-8799, 2004.

[159] Luo, Y., Zhou, H., Mizutani, M., Mizutani, N., Liu, C., Xiang, R., and Reisfeld, R. A. A DNA vaccine targeting Fos-related antigen 1 enhanced by IL-18 induces long-lived T-cell memory against tumor recurrence. Cancer Res, *65:* 3419-3427, 2005.

[160] Yamanaka, R. and Xanthopoulos, K. G. Induction of antigen-specific immune responses against malignant brain tumors by intramuscular injection of sindbis DNA encoding gp100 and IL-18. DNA Cell Biol, *24:* 317-324, 2005.

[161] O, I., Blaszczyk-Thurin, M., Shen, C. T., and Ertl, H. C. A DNA vaccine expressing tyrosinase-related protein-2 induces T-cell-mediated protection against mouse glioblastoma. Cancer Gene Ther, *10:* 678-688, 2003.

[162] Kurth, R. Risk potential of the chromosomal insertion of foreign DNA. Ann.N.Y.Acad.Sci., *772:* 140-151, 1995.

[163] Figdor, C. G., de Vries, I. J., Lesterhuis, W. J., and Melief, C. J. Dendritic cell immunotherapy: mapping the way. Nat Med, *10:* 475-480, 2004.

[164] Ikeda, H., Chamoto, K., Tsuji, T., Suzuki, Y., Wakita, D., Takeshima, T., and Nishimura, T. The critical role of type-1 innate and acquired immunity in tumor immunotherapy. Cancer Sci, *95:* 697-703, 2004.

[165] Nijman, H. W., Kleijmeer, M. J., Ossevoort, M. A., Oorschot, V. M., Vierboom, M. P., van de Keur, M., Kenemans, P., Kast, W. M., Geuze, H. J., and Melief, C. J. Antigen capture and major histocompatibility class II compartments of freshly isolated and cultured human blood dendritic cells. J.Exp.Med., *182:* 163-174, 1995.

[166] Sallusto, F., Cella, M., Danieli, C., and Lanzavecchia, A. Dendritic cells use macropinocytosis and the mannose receptor to concentrate macromolecules in the major histocompatibility complex class II compartment: downregulation by cytokines and bacterial products [see comments]. J.Exp.Med., *182:* 389-400, 1995.

[167] Kiertscher, S. M. and Roth, M. D. Human CD14+ leukocytes acquire the phenotype and function of antigen-presenting dendritic cells when cultured in GM-CSF and IL-4. J.Leukoc.Biol., *59:* 208-218, 1996.

[168] Zhou, F. and Huang, L. Delivery of protein antigen to the major histocompatibility complex class I-restricted antigen presentation pathway. J.Drug Target., *3:* 91-109, 1995.

[169] Porgador, A. and Gilboa, E. Bone marrow-generated dendritic cells pulsed with a class I- restricted peptide are potent inducers of cytotoxic T lymphocytes. J.Exp.Med., *182:* 255-260, 1995.

[170] Ossevoort, M. A., Feltkamp, M. C., van Veen, K. J., Melief, C. J., and Kast, W. M. Dendritic cells as carriers for a cytotoxic T-lymphocyte epitope- based peptide vaccine in protection against a human papillomavirus type 16-induced tumor. J.Immunother.Emphasis.Tumor Immunol., *18:* 86-94, 1995.

[171] Mayordomo, J. I., Zorina, T., Storkus, W. J., Zitvogel, L., Celluzzi, C., Falo, L. D., Melief, C. J., Ildstad, S. T., Kast, W. M., Deleo, A. B., and et al. Bone marrow-derived dendritic cells pulsed with synthetic tumour peptides elicit protective and therapeutic antitumour immunity. Nature Medicine, *1:* 1297-1302, 1995.

[172] Celluzzi, C. M., Mayordomo, J. I., Storkus, W. J., Lotze, M. T., and Falo, L. D. J. Peptide-pulsed dendritic cells induce antigen-specific CTL- mediated protective tumor immunity [see comments]. J.Exp.Med., *183:* 283-287, 1996.

[173] Eberl, G., Widmann, C., and Corradin, G. The functional half-life of H-2Kd-restricted T cell epitopes on living cells. Eur.J.Immunol., *26:* 1993-1999, 1996.

[174] Zitvogel, L., Mayordomo, J. I., Tjandrawan, T., DeLeo, A. B., Clarke, M. R., Lotze, M. T., and Storkus, W. J. Therapy of murine tumors with tumor peptide-pulsed dendritic cells: dependence on T cells, B7 costimulation, and T helper cell 1-associated cytokines [see comments]. J.Exp.Med., *183:* 87-97, 1996.

[175] Mayordomo, J. I., Zorina, T., Storkus, W. J., Zitvogel, L., Celluzzi, C., Falo, L. D., Melief, C. J., Ildstad, S. T., Kast, W. M., and DeLeo, A. B. Bone marrow-derived dendritic cells pulsed with synthetic tumour peptides elicit protective and therapeutic antitumour immunity. Nat.Med., *1:* 1297-1302, 1995.

[176] Paglia, P., Chiodoni, C., Rodolfo, M., and Colombo, M. P. Murine dendritic cells loaded in vitro with soluble protein prime cytotoxic T lymphocytes against tumor antigen in vivo [see comments]. J.Exp.Med., *183:* 317-322, 1996.

[177] Boczkowski, D., Nair, S. K., Snyder, D., and Gilboa, E. Dendritic cells pulsed with RNA are potent antigen-presenting cells in vitro and in vivo. J.Exp.Med., *184:* 465-472, 1996.

[178] Specht, J. M., Wang, G., Do, M. T., Lam, J. S., Royal, R. E., Reeves, M. E., Rosenberg, S. A., and Hwu, P. Dendritic cells retrovirally transduced with a model antigen gene are therapeutically effective against established pulmonary metastases. J.Exp.Med., *186:* 1213-1221, 1997.

[179] Wan, Y., Bramson, J., Carter, R., Graham, F., and Gauldie, J. Dendritic cells transduced with an adenoviral vector encoding a model tumor-associated antigen for tumor vaccination. Hum.Gene Ther., *8:* 1355-1363, 1997.

[180] Fisher, K. J., Jooss, K., Alston, J., Yang, Y., Haecker, S. E., High, K., Pathak, R., Raper, S. E., and Wilson, J. M. Recombinant adeno-associated virus for muscle directed gene therapy. Nat.Med., *3:* 306-312, 1997.

[181] Yang, Y., Li, Q., Ertl, H. C., and Wilson, J. M. Cellular and humoral immune responses to viral antigens create barriers to lung-directed gene therapy with recombinant adenoviruses. J.Virol., *69:* 2004-2015, 1995.

[182] Arthur, J. F., Butterfield, L. H., Roth, M. D., Bui, L. A., Kiertscher, S. M., Lau, R., Dubinett, S., Glaspy, J., McBride, W. H., and Economou, J. S. A comparison of gene transfer methods in human dendritic cells. Cancer Gene Ther., *4:* 17-25, 1997.

[183] Bronte, V., Carroll, M. W., Goletz, T. J., Wang, M., Overwijk, W. W., Marincola, F., Rosenberg, S. A., Moss, B., and Restifo, N. P. Antigen expression by dendritic cells correlates with the therapeutic effectiveness of a model recombinant poxvirus tumor vaccine. Proc.Natl.Acad.Sci.U.S.A., *94:* 3183-3188, 1997.

[184] Tuting, T., Zorina, T., Ma, D. I., Wilson, C. C., De Cesare, C. M., De Leo, A. B., Lotze, M. T., and Storkus, W. J. Development of dendritic cell-based genetic vaccines for cancer. Adv.Exp.Med.Biol., *417:* 511-518, 1997.

[185] Grunebach, F., Muller, M. R., and Brossart, P. New developments in dendritic cell-based vaccinations: RNA translated into clinics. Cancer Immunol Immunother, *54:* 517-525, 2005.

[186] Zeis, M., Siegel, S., Wagner, A., Schmitz, M., Marget, M., Kuhl-Burmeister, R., Adamzik, I., Kabelitz, D., Dreger, P., Schmitz, N., and Heiser, A. Generation of cytotoxic responses in mice and human individuals against hematological malignancies using survivin-RNA-transfected dendritic cells. J Immunol, *170:* 5391-5397, 2003.

[187] Andre, F., Escudier, B., Angevin, E., Tursz, T., and Zitvogel, L. Exosomes for cancer immunotherapy. Ann Oncol, *15 Suppl 4:* iv141-144, 2004.

[188] Hsu, D. H., Paz, P., Villaflor, G., Rivas, A., Mehta-Damani, A., Angevin, E., Zitvogel, L., and Le Pecq, J. B. Exosomes as a tumor vaccine: enhancing potency through direct loading of antigenic peptides. J Immunother, *26:* 440-450, 2003.

[189] Adams, S., O'Neill, D., and Bhardwaj, N. Maturation matters: importance of maturation for antitumor immunity of dendritic cell vaccines. J Clin Oncol, *22:* 3834-3835; author reply 3835, 2004.

[190] Akiyama, K., Ebihara, S., Yada, A., Matsumura, K., Aiba, S., Nukiwa, T., and Takai, T. Targeting apoptotic tumor cells to Fc gamma R provides efficient and versatile vaccination against tumors by dendritic cells. J Immunol, *170:* 1641-1648, 2003.

[191] Zhang, W., Chen, Z., Li, F., Kamencic, H., Juurlink, B., Gordon, J. R., and Xiang, J. Tumour necrosis factor-alpha (TNF-alpha) transgene-expressing dendritic cells (DCs) undergo augmented cellular maturation and induce more robust T-cell activation and anti-tumour immunity than DCs generated in recombinant TNF-alpha. Immunology, *108:* 177-188, 2003.

[192] Renneson, J., Salio, M., Mazouz, N., Goldman, M., Marchant, A., and Cerundolo, V. Mature dendritic cells differentiated in the presence of interferon-beta and interleukin-3 prime functional antigen-specific CD8 T cells. Clin Exp Immunol, *139:* 468-475, 2005.

[193] Suzuki, T., Fukuhara, T., Tanaka, M., Nakamura, A., Akiyama, K., Sakakibara, T., Koinuma, D., Kikuchi, T., Tazawa, R., Maemondo, M., Hagiwara, K., Saijo, Y., and Nukiwa, T. Vaccination of dendritic cells loaded with interleukin-12-secreting cancer cells augments in vivo antitumor immunity: characteristics of syngeneic and allogeneic antigen-presenting cell cancer hybrid cells. Clin Cancer Res, *11:* 58-66, 2005.

[194] Okada, N., Iiyama, S., Okada, Y., Mizuguchi, H., Hayakawa, T., Nakagawa, S., Mayumi, T., Fujita, T., and Yamamoto, A. Immunological properties and vaccine

efficacy of murine dendritic cells simultaneously expressing melanoma-associated antigen and interleukin-12. Cancer Gene Ther, *12:* 72-83, 2005.

[195] Onaitis, M. W., Kalady, M. F., Emani, S., Abdel-Wahab, Z., Tyler, D. S., and Pruitt, S. K. CD40 ligand is essential for generation of specific cytotoxic T cell responses in RNA-pulsed dendritic cell immunotherapy. Surgery, *134:* 300-305, 2003.

[196] Takamizawa, M., Fagnoni, F., Mehta-Damani, A., Rivas, A., and Engleman, E. G. Cellular and molecular basis of human gamma delta T cell activation. Role of accessory molecules in alloactivation. J.Clin.Invest., *95:* 296-303, 1995.

[197] Mehta-Damani, A., Markowicz, S., and Engleman, E. G. Generation of antigen-specific CD8+ CTLs from naive precursors. J.Immunol., *153:* 996-1003, 1994.

[198] Hsu, F. J., Benike, C., Fagnoni, F., Liles, T. M., Czerwinski, D., Taidi, B., Engleman, E. G., and Levy, R. Vaccination of patients with B-cell lymphoma using autologous antigen-pulsed dendritic cells. Nat.Med., *2:* 52-58, 1996.

[199] Kwak, L. W., Campbell, M. J., Czerwinski, D. K., Hart, S., Miller, R. A., and Levy, R. Induction of immune responses in patients with B-cell lymphoma against the surface-immunoglobulin idiotype expressed by their tumors [see comments]. N.Engl.J.Med., *327:* 1209-1215, 1992.

[200] Reichardt, V., Okada, C., Benike, C., Long, G., Engleman, E., Blume, K., and Levy, R. Idiotypic vaccination using dendritic cells for multiple myeloma patients after autologous peripheral blood stem cell transplantation. Blood *88:* 481, 1996.

[201] Kim, C. J., Prevette, T., Cormier, J., Overwijk, W., Roden, M., Restifo, N. P., Rosenberg, S. A., and Marincola, F. M. Dendritic cells infected with poxviruses encoding MART-1/Melan A sensitize T lymphocytes in vitro. J.Immunother., *20:* 276-286, 1997.

[202] Mortarini, R., Anichini, A., Di Nicola, M., Siena, S., Bregni, M., Belli, F., Molla, A., Gianni, A. M., and Parmiani, G. Autologous dendritic cells derived from CD34+ progenitors and from monocytes are not functionally equivalent antigen-presenting cells in the induction of melan-A/Mart-1(27-35)-specific CTLs from peripheral blood lymphocytes of melanoma patients with low frequency of CTL precursors. Cancer Res., *57:* 5534-5541, 1997.

[203] Bakker, A. B., Marland, G., de Boer, A. J., Huijbens, R. J., Danen, E. H., Adema, G. J., and Figdor, C. G. Generation of antimelanoma cytotoxic T lymphocytes from healthy donors after presentation of melanoma-associated antigen-derived epitopes by dendritic cells in vitro. Cancer Res., *55:* 5330-5334, 1995.

[204] Storkus, W. J., Mayordomo, J. I., Deleo, A., Zitvogel, L., Tjandrawan, T., and Lotze, M. T. Dendritic cells pulsed with tumor epitopes elicit potent anti-tumor CTL in vitro and in vivo. *In:* The 9th International Congress of Immunology; Meeting Sponsored by the American Association of Immunologists and the International Union of Immunological Societies, San Francisco, California, USA, July 23-29, 1995, pp. 589. 1995.

[205] Nestle, F. O., Alijagic, S., Gilliet, M., Sun, Y., Grabbe, S., Dummer, R., Burg, G., and Schadendorf, D. Vaccination of melanoma patients with peptide- or tumor lysate-pulsed dendritic cells. Nat Med, *4:* 328-332, 1998.

[206] Palucka, A. K., Dhodapkar, M. V., Paczesny, S., Burkeholder, S., Wittkowski, K. M., Steinman, R. M., Fay, J., and Banchereau, J. Single injection of CD34+ progenitor-

derived dendritic cell vaccine can lead to induction of T-cell immunity in patients with stage IV melanoma. J Immunother, *26:* 432-439, 2003.

[207] Palucka, A. K., Dhodapkar, M. V., Paczesny, S., Ueno, H., Fay, J., and Banchereau, J. Boosting vaccinations with peptide-pulsed CD34+ progenitor-derived dendritic cells can expand long-lived melanoma peptide-specific CD8+ T cells in patients with metastatic melanoma. J Immunother, *28:* 158-168, 2005.

[208] Barbuto, J. A., Ensina, L. F., Neves, A. R., Bergami-Santos, P., Leite, K. R., Marques, R., Costa, F., Martins, S. C., Camara-Lopes, L. H., and Buzaid, A. C. Dendritic cell-tumor cell hybrid vaccination for metastatic cancer. Cancer Immunol Immunother, *53:* 1111-1118, 2004.

[209] Barrou, B., Benoit, G., Ouldkaci, M., Cussenot, O., Salcedo, M., Agrawal, S., Massicard, S., Bercovici, N., Ericson, M. L., and Thiounn, N. Vaccination of prostatectomized prostate cancer patients in biochemical relapse, with autologous dendritic cells pulsed with recombinant human PSA. Cancer Immunol Immunother, *53:* 453-460, 2004.

[210] Su, Z., Dannull, J., Yang, B. K., Dahm, P., Coleman, D., Yancey, D., Sichi, S., Niedzwiecki, D., Boczkowski, D., Gilboa, E., and Vieweg, J. Telomerase mRNA-transfected dendritic cells stimulate antigen-specific CD8+ and CD4+ T cell responses in patients with metastatic prostate cancer. J Immunol, *174:* 3798-3807, 2005.

[211] Chang, G. C., Lan, H. C., Juang, S. H., Wu, Y. C., Lee, H. C., Hung, Y. M., Yang, H. Y., Whang-Peng, J., and Liu, K. J. A pilot clinical trial of vaccination with dendritic cells pulsed with autologous tumor cells derived from malignant pleural effusion in patients with late-stage lung carcinoma. Cancer, *103:* 763-771, 2005.

[212] Hirschowitz, E. A., Foody, T., Kryscio, R., Dickson, L., Sturgill, J., and Yannelli, J. Autologous dendritic cell vaccines for non-small-cell lung cancer. J Clin Oncol, *22:* 2808-2815, 2004.

[213] Dees, E. C., McKinnon, K. P., Kuhns, J. J., Chwastiak, K. A., Sparks, S., Myers, M., Collins, E. J., Frelinger, J. A., Van Deventer, H., Collichio, F., Carey, L. A., Brecher, M. E., Graham, M., Earp, H. S., and Serody, J. S. Dendritic cells can be rapidly expanded ex vivo and safely administered in patients with metastatic breast cancer. Cancer Immunol Immunother, *53:* 777-785, 2004.

[214] Vanchieri, C. Excitement tempered by long road ahead for dendritic cell vaccines. J Natl Cancer Inst, *96:* 1350-1351, 2004.

[215] Liu, K. J., Wang, C. C., Chen, L. T., Cheng, A. L., Lin, D. T., Wu, Y. C., Yu, W. L., Hung, Y. M., Yang, H. Y., Juang, S. H., and Whang-Peng, J. Generation of carcinoembryonic antigen (CEA)-specific T-cell responses in HLA-A*0201 and HLA-A*2402 late-stage colorectal cancer patients after vaccination with dendritic cells loaded with CEA peptides. Clin Cancer Res, *10:* 2645-2651, 2004.

[216] Caruso, D. A., Orme, L. M., Amor, G. M., Neale, A. M., Radcliff, F. J., Downie, P., Tang, M. L., and Ashley, D. M. Results of a Phase I study utilizing monocyte-derived dendritic cells pulsed with tumor RNA in children with Stage 4 neuroblastoma. Cancer, *103:* 1280-1291, 2005.

[217] Fecci, P. E., Mitchell, D. A., Archer, G. E., Morse, M. A., Lyerly, H. K., Bigner, D. D., and Sampson, J. H. The history, evolution, and clinical use of dendritic cell-based immunization strategies in the therapy of brain tumors. J Neurooncol, *64:* 161-176, 2003.

[218] Prins, R. M., Odesa, S. K., and Liau, L. M. Immunotherapeutic targeting of shared melanoma-associated antigens in a murine glioma model. Cancer Res, *63:* 8487-8491, 2003.

[219] Pellegatta, S. and Finocchiaro, G. Cell therapies in neuro-oncology. Neurol Sci, *26 Suppl 1:* S43-45, 2005.

[220] Driessens, G., Hamdane, M., Cool, V., Velu, T., and Bruyns, C. Highly successful therapeutic vaccinations combining dendritic cells and tumor cells secreting granulocyte macrophage colony-stimulating factor. Cancer Res, *64:* 8435-8442, 2004.

[221] Kikuchi, T., Akasaki, Y., Abe, T., Fukuda, T., Saotome, H., Ryan, J. L., Kufe, D. W., and Ohno, T. Vaccination of glioma patients with fusions of dendritic and glioma cells and recombinant human interleukin 12. J Immunother, *27:* 452-459, 2004.

[222] Yu, J. S., Liu, G., Ying, H., Yong, W. H., Black, K. L., and Wheeler, C. J. Vaccination with tumor lysate-pulsed dendritic cells elicits antigen-specific, cytotoxic T-cells in patients with malignant glioma. Cancer Res, *64:* 4973-4979, 2004.

[223] 223.   Ribas, A., Glaspy, J. A., Lee, Y., Dissette, V. B., Seja, E., Vu, H. T., Tchekmedyian, N. S., Oseguera, D., Comin-Anduix, B., Wargo, J. A., Amarnani, S. N., McBride, W. H., Economou, J. S., and Butterfield, L. H. Role of dendritic cell phenotype, determinant spreading, and negative costimulatory blockade in dendritic cell-based melanoma immunotherapy. J Immunother, *27:* 354-367, 2004.

[224] Brostjan, C., Bayer, A., Zommer, A., Gornikiewicz, A., Roka, S., Benko, T., Yaghubian, R., Jakesz, R., Steger, G., Gnant, M., Friedl, J., and Stift, A. Monitoring of circulating angiogenic factors in dendritic cell-based cancer immunotherapy. Cancer, *98:* 2291-2301, 2003.

[225] Kao, J. Y., Gong, Y., Chen, C. M., Zheng, Q. D., and Chen, J. J. Tumor-derived TGF-beta reduces the efficacy of dendritic cell/tumor fusion vaccine. J Immunol, *170:* 3806-3811, 2003.

[226] Neves, A. R., Ensina, L. F., Anselmo, L. B., Leite, K. R., Buzaid, A. C., Camara-Lopes, L. H., and Barbuto, J. A. Dendritic cells derived from metastatic cancer patients vaccinated with allogeneic dendritic cell-autologous tumor cell hybrids express more CD86 and induce higher levels of interferon-gamma in mixed lymphocyte reactions. Cancer Immunol Immunother, *54:* 61-66, 2005.

[227] Banchereau, J. and Palucka, A. K. Dendritic cells as therapeutic vaccines against cancer. Nat Rev Immunol, *5:* 296-306, 2005.

[228] Nordlund, J. J., Kirkwood, J. M., Forget, B. M., Milton, G., Albert, D. M., and Lerner, A. B. Vitiligo in patients with metastatic melanoma: a good prognostic sign. J.Am.Acad.Dermatol., *9:* 689-696, 1983.

[229] Nowak, M. A., May, R. M., Phillips, R. E., Rowland-Jones, S., Lalloo, D. G., McAdam, S., Klenerman, P., Koppe, B., Sigmund, K., and Bangham, C. R. Antigenic oscillations and shifting immunodominance in HIV-1 infections [see comments]. Nature, *375:* 606-611, 1995.

[230] Toes, R. E., Offringa, R., Blom, R. J., Melief, C. J., and Kast, W. M. Peptide vaccination can lead to enhanced tumor growth through specific T-cell tolerance induction. Proc.Natl.Acad.Sci.U.S.A., *93:* 7855-7860, 1996.

[231] Webb, S., Morris, C., and Sprent, J. Extrathymic tolerance of mature T cells: clonal elimination as a consequence of immunity. Cell, *63:* 1249-1256, 1990.

[232] Aichele, P., Brduscha-Riem, K., Zinkernagel, R. M., Hengartner, H., and Pircher, H. T cell priming versus T cell tolerance induced by synthetic peptides. J.Exp.Med., *182:* 261-266, 1995.

[233] Benichou, G., Fedoseyeva, E., Olson, C. A., Geysen, H. M., McMillan, M., and Sercarz, E. E. Disruption of the determinant hierarchy on a self-MHC peptide: concomitant tolerance induction to the dominant determinant and priming to the cryptic self-determinant. Int.Immunol., *6:* 131-138, 1994.

[234] Sercarz, E. E., Lehmann, P. V., Ametani, A., Benichou, G., Miller, A., and Moudgil, K. Dominance and crypticity of T cell antigenic determinants. Annu.Rev.Immunol., *11:* 729-766, 1993.

[235] Hoon, D. S., Yuzuki, D., Hayashida, M., and Morton, D. L. Melanoma patients immunized with melanoma cell vaccine induce antibody responses to recombinant MAGE-1 antigen. J.Immunol., *154:* 730-737, 1995.

In: Leading Topics in Cancer Research
Editor: Lee P. Jeffries, pp. 293-310

ISBN 1-60021-332-4
© 2007 Nova Science Publishers, Inc.

Chapter 11

CANCER VACCINES FOR HORMONE IMMUNE-DEPRIVATION: THE EGF VACCINE APPROACH

Gisela González and Agustín Lage

Center of Molecular Immunology, Havana, Cuba;
Hermanos Ameijeiras Hospital, Havana, Cuba.

ABSTRACT

Experimental and clinical evidences strongly indicate that the immune system can naturally prevent tumour development and provide new support to the old idea of treating tumours with therapeutic vaccines.

Several cancer vaccines are currently under clinical testing, using a wide diversity of tumour antigens and platforms for delivering them to the immune system. Most of them intend to elicit citotoxic-T-lymphocyte responses or antibody responses against antigens expressed by tumour cells.

However, in parallel to this mainstream, a different cancer vaccine approach has been developed, focusing the activation of an immune response against some self extra cellular proteins (mainly hormones and growth factors) which participate in the control of cell proliferation.

These vaccines are composed by the self hormone linked to a carrier and administered in an adjuvant. Immunization provokes specific anti-hormone antibodies that block the binding to the receptor, avoiding the "start up" of signal transduction mechanisms derived from this binding. These vaccines are not intended to mobilize the effector's branch of the immune system for a direct cytolysis but to inhibit hormonal mechanisms which in turn, influence tumour development.

The field of anticancer drugs has experienced recently a paradigm shift, beyond unspecific anti-proliferative drugs, to specific targets related to growth factors and signal transduction. Cancer vaccines aiming to interfere with hormone and growth factor mediated cell proliferation represent an equivalent idea, in the field of active immunotherapy.

The rationale of hormone immunosuppresion can be found in autoimmune diseases against hormones and their receptors. Nature has created mechanisms of interaction between hormone systems and immune systems, that, when deregulated, provoke autoimmune diseases. An adequate manipulation of these interactions can be used to fight diseases where hormonal mechanisms are deregulated, i.e. cancer.

In the present chapter we review the current development of several hormone-suppressive active immunotherapies and we provide a wider description of the approach of active immunotherapy for Epidermal Growth Factor (EGF) deprivation developed at our own laboratory.

Insegia™ (G17DT) is an immunogen containing gastrin which provokes an antibody response blocking gastrin-stimulated cell growth. It is actually in clinical trials for pancreatic, colorectal and gastric carcinomas.

Gonadimmune™ (D17DT) is a vaccine containing the gonadotrophin releasing hormone (GnRH) which is being tested in the clinical setting for prostate cancer.

AVICINE^R is a vaccine targeting the human chorionic gonadotrophin (hCG) currently in clinical trials for colorectal and pancreatic cancer.

The EGF vaccine, finally, is a composition of Epidermal Growth Factor linked to a carrier protein, which induces anti-EGF antibodies which in turn block the binding of EGF to the EGF-Receptor (EGFR). It is currently in Phase 2 clinical trials for the treatment of non-small cell lung carcinoma (NSCLC). Additionally, a similar vaccine is being developed to target Transforming Growth Factor (TGF), an alternative ligand of the EGFR. This last vaccine is currently under pre-clinical investigation.

Specific antibody responses have been obtained after vaccination with all these self molecules, and for those tested in the clinical setting this antibody response is related with decrease in the targeted hormone levels and with improved survival of vaccinated patients.

Once the initial proof of the concept is becoming a reality, current challenges are how to find the best therapeutic doses and vaccination schedules to expand the immune response and how to maintain it long enough to sustain a chronic treatment.

INTRODUCTION

The frequency of tumour development is relatively low in immunocompetent hosts. This fact has been explained based on the assumption that the immune system might be able to control or eliminate the majority of tumours early in their development. The old theory of Thomas and Burnet in the 60´s about tumour immunosurveillance postulated that the immune system was permanently controlling the appearance of malignant cells [1, 2]. This theory had been challenged, or even abandoned, based on the lack of clear evidence on increased incidence of spontaneous tumours (except those related to viruses) in immunosuppressed animals or in patients under immunosuppressive treatments. However, the immunosurveillance theory has recently received new support from new experimental and clinical data:

- The incidence of spontaneous or chemically induced tumours is much higher in knock-out mice lacking critical molecules of the immune system than in wild type mice strains (for review see [3]). These animal models did not exist at the times of initial polemics about immunosurveillance.

- Lymphocyte infiltration in tumours correlate with improved survival in patients with different malignancies [4,5,6,7,8];
- Patients receiving chronic immunosuppressive treatment after organ transplantation have high incidence in malignancies, a finding that has recently become more evident as larges series of transplanted patients with long survival accumulate [9, 10].

But it is also a fact that tumours evade the natural immune response and produce clinically significant illness and death. Two main hypotheses have been postulated to explain tumour escape: tumour immunoediting [11] and tumour-induced immunosuppresion [12].

In this current scientific knowledge environment, the ancient idea of activating the body's immune system to recognize and destroy tumours has re-emerged and encouraged the development of therapeutic cancer vaccines aiming to activate both cellular and humoral effectors mechanisms against target molecules in the tumour cells [13, 14, 15].

But, in parallel with this main approach, some few vaccines have been designed with a different purpose i.e. to activate an immune response against hormones and / or growth factors that participate in the stimulation of tumour growth.

This parallel approach is mainly based in two previous pieces of knowledge:

1. The results of hormone deprivation in cancer treatment.
2. The evidence that natural tolerance to self is partial and that vaccination can induce an immune response against some self antigens.

HORMONES, GROWTH FACTORS AND CANCER THERAPY

Some tumours, such as breast and prostate cancer, require hormonal stimulation for growth. Hormone – receptor binding regulates the expression of some particular genes that encode proteins related with cell cycle regulation and cell proliferation.

In hormone-dependent cancer, deprivation of hormonal stimulus can induce growth arrest and apoptosis. Endocrine therapy is an old and validated approach in the treatment of hormone dependent tumours [16]. Compared with chemotherapy, hormone therapy has the advantages of less toxicity and feasibility of long term treatments achieving long term responses.

There is currently a wide and growing armamentarium of hormone-therapy procedures, including: surgical castration, radiotherapy castration, androgen therapy for oestrogen-dependent tumours, oestrogen therapy for androgen-dependent tumours, antagonists of LHRH analogist; oestrogen receptor antagonists, androgen receptor antagonists, and aromatase inhibitors blocking the synthesis of estrogens [16].

In addition to hormones, tumour growth can be regulated by growth factors, such as Epidermal Growth Factor, which also bind to specific cell membrane receptors. However, growth factors are secreted systemically (including the tumour environment itself) and a deprivation by surgical ablation of the glands is not feasible.

In fact, many tumours have growth dependence on the EGF or other growth factors. This fact enlarges the hormone-dependence concept and its therapeutic implications to growth factors [17].

Research on new anticancer drugs is increasingly focused in growth factors, their receptors and their signal transduction mechanisms.

Several decades ago a first generation of anti-cancer drugs targeted one of the most obvious capabilities of cancer cells: their continuous and uncontrolled proliferation, and introduced in the therapeutic arsenal alkylating agents, such as cyclophosphamide; intercalating drugs, such as adriamycin and platinum compounds; drugs interfering purine and pyrimidine metabolism, such as methotrexare and 6-mercaptopurine and drugs targeting the mitotic apparatus proteins, such as vinca alkaloids. These drugs improved the efficacy of cancer treatment, but at the price of high toxicity.

Since the last decade, efforts have been directed to a second generation of drugs focusing the cell proliferation machinery. Therapies targeting molecules related with signal transduction cascades are in the top attention of new approaches for cancer treatment [18].

Active immunotherapy, targeting growth factors and its receptors represent an equivalent concept, which looks for more specific therapeutic targets [19, 20, 21, 22, 23, 24, 25, 26]. The practical implementation of this concept requires being able to elicit immune responses against hormones, growth factors and receptors which are essentially self-molecules. As will be explained below, this is considered feasible, according to the current views about immune tolerance.

IMMUNE RESPONSE AGAINST SELF ANTIGENS

Discrimination between what is "self" and what is "non self" has been during years the central problem of Immunology. However, it is currently accepted that the tolerance to self is partial and that, under certain conditions, the immune system can react against self antigens.

The detection of natural autoantibodies [27] and self reactive T cells in healthy subjects [28], the discovery of the role of positive selection of the T cell repertoire by self peptides in the thymus [29], and the existence of a functional immune system in antigen-free animals [30], supported that there naturally exists a background of immune reactivity towards self molecules.

Moreover, it has been noticed that autoimmunity is not random, but directed towards a particular subset of self-antigens. The immunological homunculus is the term that has been coined to describe the natural autoimmune repertoire directed towards self-antigens [31, 32]. Autoimmune disease does not exist against any self-antigen, but against such antigens that the immune system "see" better.

Some hormones and hormone-receptors belong to this family of proteins able to provoke autoimmune responses. In fact, some well known autoimmune diseases are related with hormonal deregulations [33].

In Diabetes mellitus (type 1) , auto-reactive T lymphocytes recognize antigens from the pancreatic islet cells, and there are frequently antibodies to insulin. As the disease progresses, the pancreatic islets are destroyed by lymphocytes infiltrating them, causing the production of insulin to stop.

Myasthenia gravis (MG) is an autoimmune disease of the intramuscular junction. The basic abnormality of MG is a decrease of acetylcholine receptors (AChR) at the neuromuscular junctions due to an antibody-mediated autoimmune response. The specific anti AChR autoantibodies reduce the number of available AChR, provoking impaired neuromuscular transmission.

Graves' disease is caused by abnormal immune system activation against the TSH receptor which in turn causes overproduction of thyroid hormones.

Even when it has not been associated with an auto-immune disease, there are also reports of the existence of natural autoimmune responses against some growth factors, i.e the EGF [34]. It has been found that more than 70% of normal subjects have measurable serum anti-EGF antibodies.

LINKAGE BETWEEN ACTIVE IMMUNOTHERAPY AND HORMONE / GROWTH FACTOR DEPRIVATION FOR CANCER TREATMENT

Tumour sensitivity to hormone deprivation, the dependence of some tumours on growth factors for cell proliferation, and the fact that some hormones and growth factors are frequently involved in autoimmune disorders, provide a rationale for the development of vaccines aiming to provoke an immune-deprivation of hormones and growth factors.

Because diseases involving hormones are not pathogen-driven, they have not viewed traditionally as being susceptible to treatment using the body's immune system. Instead, the traditional pharmaceutical industry approach to these diseases has been to treat them with synthetic drugs. These drugs typically must be administered in relatively large quantities and on a daily or more frequent basis, with accumulating side effects and frequent problems with patient compliance with the treatment.

Classic vaccinology has been successful in immunize people against pathogen-related antigens that, naturally, after pathogen infection, provoke an immune response. No such good results have been observed when trying to vaccinate against pathogens that do not provoke natural immunity. In some way, such therapeutic interventions can not do anything better than nature can do.

Reversing the same argument it should be expected that, antigens able to provoke some natural auto-immune responses, are better targets for therapeutic active immunotherapy. As previously said, this is the case of some hormones and growth factors.

Being hormone-therapy a validated intervention in cancer treatment, it could be expected that other approaches of hormone deprivation, i.e., by using active immunotherapy, can be also a novel and useful therapeutically tool.

In the same direction, as the EGFR system has also become an important target for cancer treatment, growth factor deprivation by active immunotherapy can also be evaluated as an alternative way to interfere with the signal transduction cascade related to cell proliferation.

It is surprising that this field has not been explored too much, mainly because cancer vaccines are being designed to provoke anti-tumor CTL or antibody responses.

Nevertheless some few hormone and growth factor based cancer vaccines are currently under pre-clinical and clinical evaluation, such as:

- A cancer vaccine targeting the hormone Gastrin
- Cancer vaccines targeting the hormone LHRH / GnRH
- Cancer vaccines targeting the human Chorionic Gonadotrophin itself (hCG)
- A cancer vaccine targeting the Epidermal Growth Factor (EGF)
- A cancer vaccine targeting the Transforming Growth Factor alpha (TGFα).

We will now update the results emerging in the literature about the development of these novel cancer vaccine approaches.

VACCINES DESIGNED TO PROVOKE HORMONE OR GROWTH FACTORS DEPRIVATION

1. Cancer Vaccine Targeting the Hormone Gastrin

Gastrin 17 is a growth factor for pancreatic, stomach and colorectal cancers. An anti-gastrin vaccine (Insegia^{TM}) has been developed by Aphton Corporation, in alliance with Aventis Pasteur, and is composed by the immunogen G17DT. This anti-gastrin immunogen, consist of a synthetic peptide, which is similar to a portion of the gastrin 17 hormone linked to Diphtheria Toxoid (DT) as carrier protein.

When administered to patients, G17DT induces an immune response, eliciting antibodies that neutralize the target hormone and prevent its interaction with cancer cells.

Since 1996, Watson and cols reported that immunization with G17 provokes a specific antibody response and has anti-tumour effect in pre-clinical models [35].

The vaccine was further moved into clinical trials and, in 2000, results from a Phase I-II trial in advanced colorectal cancer were published by Smith et al [36]. The main objectives of this trial were to asses the safety and efficacy of immunization with G17DT; and the results demonstrated that 80% of vaccinated patients produced measurable anti-G17 antibody titers with an affinity high enough to compete with the cholecystokinin B/ gastrin receptor for binding to G17. The treatment was well tolerated with no systemic side effects seen.

In 2002, results from a Phase II study in advanced pancreatic cancer were reported [37]. This trial included two different doses of the immunogen and the 82% of patients treated with the higher dose developed antibody responses with a significantly greater response rate than the group of patients treated with the lower dose (46% of antibody responders). It was also reported that antibody responders survived significantly more than non-responders.

Gilliam AD et al published in 2004 the results from a Phase II study in gastric carcinoma [38]. It was also a dose scale up trial, where 3 different doses cohorts were tested. Higher rates of antibody responders correlated with increased doses in stages I-III patients, but not in stages IV patients. Antibodies displaced iodinated gastrin from its receptor, with the level of displacement correlating with antibody titers.

In the American Society of Clinical Oncology (ASCO) meeting (June 2004) positive results from a Phase III trial testing GD17 as monotherapy were presented, including patients with advanced pancreatic cancer who were unable to tolerate or unwilling to take chemotherapy [39]. Survival of patients treated with the G17DT immunogen was significantly increased as compared with patients treated with placebo. A significantly longer time to deterioration of Karnofsky Performance Score (KPS) in G17DT treated patients was also described.

In this same ASCO meeting, results of a study determining the immune response to GD17 as a predictor for survival in Colorectal, Gastric and Pancreatic Cancers were presented [40]. Data from three clinical trials in three different gastrointestinal cancers were analyzed, to asses the predictive ability of typical baseline parameters with regards to anti-G17DT immune response and to demonstrate that anti-GD17DT response is a significant predictor for survival that is independent of the covariates identified. Results indicated that subjects, with advanced colorectal, gastric or pancreatic cancers, that generate antibodies to G17 following administration of G17DT, had significantly prolonged survival compared to those who did not. This effect was independent of other covariates analyzed.

More recently, in the 2005 ASCO meeting, the final results from a Phase III trial of Insegia™ in combination with Gemzar (gemcitabine; Lilly) in advanced pancreatic cancer were presented [41]. The primary objective of this trial was to asses the impact of vaccination in overall survival; the secondary objectives were the impact of vaccination in overall tumour response, time to progression and evaluation of survival related to antibody response levels.

No significant difference in survival was detected between vaccinated and controls and the trial failed for its primary objective. However, there was a 75% of responder patient's and the evaluation of survival by antibody response showed that patients who achieved the highest antibody levels survived significantly more than controls.

In general, survival data for antibody responders after vaccination with Insegia™ are consistent with the hypothesis that neutralizing gastrin produces a survival benefit.

2. Cancer Vaccines Targeting the Hormone LHRH/GnRH:

The luteinizing hormone–releasing hormone (LHRH), also known as gonadotropin releasing hormone (GnRH), is synthesized in the hypothalamus and transported by the hypothalamic-hypophyseal portal system to the anterior pituitary where it acts to effect secretion of gonadotropins, luteinizing hormones (LH) and follicle stimulating hormone (FSH).

In males, LHRH induces maturation of the testosterone-secreting interstitial cells of the testis. Testosterone is converted to dihydrotestosterone, the form of the hormone that interacts with androgen receptors on prostate epithelial cells to control their proliferation and apoptosis.

Huggins and Hodges first discovered that androgen deprivation is an effective treatment for prostate cancer [42]. Many hormonal therapies have been developed for reducing androgens. LHRH antagonists had shown to bind LHRH receptors in the prostate and to exhibit a direct inhibitory effect on androgen independent cancer cells [43, 44, 45, 46].

By the1990's, LHRH based vaccines had been tested in men to achieve androgen deprivation as a treatment of prostate cancer [47, 48].

The first reports of clinical trials came from Talwar et al [49]. They focused the hormone immune castration approach for both, contraception vaccines and cancer vaccines. They reported that, in Phase I-II trials with an LHRH based cancer vaccine, vaccination elicits anti-LHRH antibody titers, together with a decline in the concentrations of LH, FSH and testosterone, and also accompanied by a reduction in PSA antigen and with many patients showing a clinical improvement.

In their first trials, Talwar et al used a semi synthetic vaccine composed by LHRL coupled with diphtheria or tetanus toxoid as carrier proteins, but this vaccines induced suppression of antibody response after repeated immunizations. To overcome this limitation, they synthesized two recombinant proteins in which the tetanus or diphtheria toxoids were replaced by synthetic T-helper cell epitopes [50]. With these vaccines, immunogenicity, efficacy and safety were demonstrated in rats. All animals generated anti-LHRH antibodies, which caused the decline of testosterone to castration levels and a significant prostate atrophy.

In parallel with this group of authors, Aphton (in alliance with GlaxoSmithKline) developed another GnRH based cancer vaccine (Gonadimmune^{TM} – D17DT). This vaccine consists in a decapeptide from GnRH linked to diphtheria toxoid.

In August 2000, Simms et al [48] reported results from a pilot clinical trial, designed to assess the tolerance and immunogenicity of D17DT in advanced prostate cancer patients amenable to receive hormone therapy. Two different doses of the vaccine were tested (30 or 100ug). Immunogenicity and safety was demonstrated, with a significant reduction in serum testosterone and PSA in 5 from 12 vaccinated patients while castration levels of testosterone were achieved in 4 of them and maintained for up to 9 month. Patients with the highest antibody titers had the best responses in terms of testosterone suppression.

More recently, the same authors reported results from a Phase I study [51] where two lower vaccine doses were tested (3 and 15 ug). No responses were observed in the group treated with 3ug dose, while 2 from 6 subjects in the 15ug dose group showed significant anti-GnRH antibody titers together with suppression of testosterone to castration levels, and with a significant and prolonged reduction in PSA.

In 2005, Triozzi et al reported results from a Pilot Study designed to determine how to best combine GnRH-DT vaccination with potentially immunosuppressive chemotherapy [52]. They demonstrated, in patients with metastatic, hormone refractory prostate cancer, that the administration of docetaxel with high-dose dexamethasone did not inhibit their ability to develop an antibody response when immunized with the GnRH-DT vaccine.

Norelin TM (YMBiosciences) is other vaccine approach targeting the same hormone. In May 2005, the Company announced results from a clinical trial in men with hormone dependent prostate cancer, which was designed to asses for the immunogenicity and safety of vaccination. Vaccinated patients developed anti-GnRH antibody responses. Castration levels of testosterone were observed in long-term immunized patients associated with normalization of PSA [53].

3. Cancer Vaccines Targeting the Hormone hCG

The human chorionic gonadotropin β sub-unit (hCGβ), is normally produced during pregnancy and facilitates foetal development. It is only produced by foetal and placental cells with the only exception of some cancer cells. This onco-foetal antigen is expressed by several carcinomas and it is a prognostic factor in renal, colorectal, bladder and pancreatic cancers.

Curiously, the very first approach of immunization with hormones was conceived by Talwar et al in the 1970´s, for fertility control [54]. At this time, they reported results of immunization with hCGβ conjugated with tetanus toxoid as carrier protein. Different animal species (mice, rabbits, a goat and monkeys) were immunized and anti-hCG and antibody titers were developed. A Phase I trial in humans was initiated in 1974, and all immunized subjects responded positively with the development of anti-hCG antibodies. The antibody immune response was long lasting and boosteable and the anti-hCG antibodies bound (*in vivo*) to the hCG. Almost 20 years latter, the same group of authors, reported that, after successful completion of Phase 1 trials with this vaccine, it had entered in Phase 2 trials [55]. In 1997, they reported the completion of such Phase 2 trial which provided evidences for the prevention of pregnancy in humans [56]. Then, the very first clinical "proof of the concept" of the active immunotherapy for hormone deprivation concept came from this vaccine to prevent pregnancy.

Results from clinical trials with hCG based cancer vaccines were reviewed by Triozzi et al in 1999 [57]. Immunizations with a vaccine targeting the carboxy-terminal peptide of hCG, corroborated that the immune tolerance against this self molecule can be broken. As a consequence of vaccination, humoral responses as well as cellular responses against the hCG were generated.

These authors further published results from a Phase II trial in patients with metastatic colorectal cancer [58]. A synthetic vaccine composed by the carboxy- terminal peptide of βhCG (CTP37) conjugated to diphtheria toxoid (DT) was administered intramuscularly and patients were randomized to two dose levels. This vaccine, from then on developed by Avi BioPharma and named AVICINE[R], provoked an antibody response in the 95% of immunized patients. Differences in antibody responses and survival were not observed between the two dose groups. However, patients who developed anti-hCG antibody titers higher than, or equal to, the median value showed a significant increase in survival as compared with those that did not reached such antibody levels. In contrast, no significant difference was observed when comparing survival based upon the level of anti-DT antibodies. That means that induction of anti-hCG antibodies, but not of anti-DT antibodies was associated with patient's survival.

The clinical development of this vaccine included also a Phase II trial in patients with pancreatic cancer. Results from this trial were presented at the 2002 ASCO meeting [59]. Fifty five patients were randomized to receive AVICINE[R] alone or AVICINE[R] plus gemcitabine. Some anti-hCG antibody titers were found in the 9% of patients previously to vaccination, but such titers did not influence the magnitude of antibody response to vaccination or patient survival. There was not significant difference in anti-hCG antibody titers between patients randomized to receive the vaccine alone and those receiving the vaccine plus gemcitabine, indicating that gemcitabine did not influence the immune response to the self-antigen. However, the group of patients that received gemcitabine, had significantly lower anti-DT antibody titers as compared with patients receiving the vaccine alone, indicating that gemcitabine significantly inhibited the response to the recall carrier antigen. Survival was better in the group of patients receiving the combination AVICINE[R] + gemcitabine, as compared with either patients receiving only AVICINE[R] in the trial or patients treated with chemotherapy alone as reported in the previous literature.

Based on these results, AviBiopharma announced in 2002 plans to initiate a Phase III trial in pancreatic cancer with 3 arms comparing: AVICINE[R] + gemcitabine with gemcitabine alone and with AVICINE[R] alone. Results from this Phase III trial have still not been disclosed.

More recently, other hCG based cancer vaccine has been reported, which elicits cellular immune response to the antigen [60]. In this case, the hCG was coupled genetically to a human anti- Dendritic Cells (DC) antibody. In a human cell in vitro model, the resulting fusion protein functionally promoted the uptake and processing of the antigen by DCs, which led to the generation of tumor specific class I and class II-restricted T cell responses, including CTLs capable of killing human cancer cell lines expressing hCGβ.

4. Cancer Vaccine Targeting the Epidermal Growth Factor (EGF):

The system composed by the EGFR and its ligands, is emerging as a very important target for cancer therapy (for review see [18]). One appealing approach for targeting this system is active immunotherapy with immunogenic preparations of EGF.

Studies in healthy donor's sera samples demonstrated that there exists a natural immune response against the EGF. The 79% of healthy individuals had measurable anti-EGF antibody titers [34]. Based on this natural response and on the tightly regulated antibody response to EGF, it has been claimed that this growth factor belongs to the immunological homunculus [34], and therefore it is a good candidate target for active immunotherapy.

The EGF Vaccine developed at our own laboratory is composed by human recombinant EGF conjugated with a carrier protein and given together with an adequate adjuvant.

Preclinical studies demonstrated that vaccination with EGF is immunogenic and safe in mice, rats and monkeys. Vaccination induces anti-EGF antibody titers and also has an antitumor effect in mice transplanted with EGFR overexpressing tumours. Moreover the increased survival in vaccinated mice correlates with antibody titers [21, 22].

The clinical experience with the EGF Vaccine began in 1995. The first trial had as main goals to test the immunogenicity and safety of immunization with 2 doses of the EGF Vaccine [23]. The secondary goal was to compare two different carrier proteins in the vaccine formulation: tetanic toxoid and the P64k recombinant protein from *Neisseria Meningitides*. The results demonstrated that, vaccination with EGF was immunogenic and safe in humans. The 60% of patients developed anti EGF antibody responses without significant associated toxicity. The P64k was selected as carrier protein for further product development [23].

A Phase I-II trial was then initiated, where, 20 Non Small Cell Lung Cancer (NSCLC) patients (stages IIIB and IV) were randomized to receive the EGF-P64k vaccine in alum or in Montanide ISA51 (Seppic, France) as adjuvants. The main goals were to test for immunogenicity and safety.

In parallel, another Phase I-II trial was performed with the same design, but including a low dose cyclophosphamide treatment three days before the 1rst vaccination.

Pooled results from both trials [24] demonstrated that, the best immunogenicity results were obtained when patients received a low dose cyclophosphamide pre-treatment and then were vaccinated with the EGF-P64K vaccine using Montanide ISA 51 as adjuvant. The vaccine was well tolerated in all treatment groups.

Patients were defined as Good Antibody Responders (GAR) when, after vaccination, developed anti-EGF antibody titers at least up to 1:4000 sera dilution, and at least 4X their original antibody levels; and as Poor Antibody Responders (PAR) otherwise. GAR patients survived significantly more than PAR, indicating an association (not necessarily causation) between vaccinations-induced antibody titers and patient's survival.

In a subsequent dose-scaling trial, forty NSCLC patients (stage IIIB and IV), were randomized, after finishing 1rst line chemotherapy, to receive a single dose (71 ug EGF) or a double dose (142ug EGF) of the EGF-P64k vaccine in Alum. In this trial EGF sera concentration were measured in addition to anti-EGF antibody titers [25]. The geometric mean of anti-EGF antibody titers was higher in the double dose group. There was a significant inverse correlation between antibody titers and sera EGF concentration indicating that vaccination with EGF provoked a deprivation of circulating EGF.

Again, GAR patients survived significantly more than PAR. Moreover, patients whose EGF sera concentration decreased below 168 pcg/ml, (half of the median value), survived significantly more than patients in which EGF levels were not such considerably reduced.

A randomized Phase II trial was then performed, where 80 NSCLC patients (stages IIIb and IV), were randomized, after finishing 1rst line chemotherapy, to receive the EGF vaccine + Best Supportive Care (BSC) or BSC alone. Results from this trial were presented in the 2005 ASCO meeting [61] and in the 2006 TAT conference (Amsterdam, April 2006). The 53% of vaccinated patients were classified as GAR and 59% decreased their sera EGF concentration below 168pcg/ml.

A significant inverse correlation between anti-EGF antibody titers and sera EGF concentration was observed in vaccinated patients but not in the control group.

GAR patients had a significant increase in survival as compared with PAR. Patients whose sera EGF concentration decreased to levels below 168pcg/ml, survived significantly more than patients that did not reached such reduction. There was a trend, not yet reaching statistical significance, to increase in survival of all vaccinated patients as compared with controls (log rank test: $p=0, 07$).

In the group of patients with ages equal or below 60 years old (n=44), there was a significant increase in survival of all vaccinated patients as compared with non vaccinated controls (log rank test: $p=0,022$).

When stratified by performance status (KPS) and by response to chemotherapy, important trends to better survival were observed, but still not significant, in vaccinated patients with better performance status and previous response to chemotherapy.

Other stratification variables did not influence survival.

A "schedule optimization" trial with the EGF Vaccine is currently ongoing, and partial results were presented in 2004 ASCO meeting [62]. This trial has been conducted as a preliminary investigation to evaluate new vaccination schedules and the feasibility of combinations between vaccination and chemotherapy.

The rationales for the modifications were mainly:

- To create memory cells prior to patient exposure to potentially immunosuppressive chemotherapies: Two doses of the vaccine were given to chemo naïve patients and then, vaccination continue following four to six cycles of the 1rst line chemotherapy
- To increase anti-EGF immune response and reduce the time to induction of the immune response: vaccine dose was increased fourfold compared with previous studies and given in four injection sites.

Updated results showed that, when using this vaccination schedule, anti-EGF antibody titers increased up to 10 times the levels previously obtained, with up to 80% of GAR. The

EGF sera concentration decreased below detectable levels, and continues undetectable during an up to two years follow up.

These results provide a proof of concept for the idea of immune-deprivation of a growth factor.

A definitive proof of the therapeutic value should be obtained in a Phase III trial, already ongoing. The design of this Phase III trial includes stratification of patients by age (60 years cut off) before randomization; fourfold increased doses of the vaccine as compared with the Phase II trial and multiple immunization sites.

5. Cancer Vaccine Targeting the Transforming Growth Factor alpha (TGFα)

Transforming Growth Factor alpha (TGFα) is another ligand of the EGF-Receptor whose blockade could inhibit the initiation of cell signalling proliferation cascade. A TGFα based cancer vaccine is currently in pre-clinical testing in our laboratories [26].

The vaccine is composed by a recombinant fusion protein linking human TGFα (hTGFα) and the P64K protein, and is given together with an adequate adjuvant. Early results show that vaccination with the hTGFα-P64K vaccine in both, alum or Montanide ISA51 as adjuvants, is immunogenic. Specific anti-hTGFα antibodies were obtained after mice vaccination with the fusion protein. The hTGFα immunodominant epitope for this response involved the C-loop/C-terminal region. This region includes key residues for TGFα binding to EGFR.

Mice immune sera recognized natural hTGFα precursor in A421 cells and in hTGFα-transfected 3T3 fibroblasts, as revealed by flow citometry analysis.

Additionally, mice immune sera inhibited the binding of ^{125}I-TGFα to the EGFR; EGFR autophosphorilation and downstream activation of Erk2. Antibody-containing sera also inhibited cell proliferation of two EGFR expressing human carcinoma cell lines. Taken together, all these results strongly suggest the feasibility of TGF-vaccination to inhibit tumour growth.

THE PROOF OF THE CONCEPT

The proof of the concept of hormone or growth factor immune-deprivation for cancer therapy means the demonstration that vaccination with hormones or growth factors could provoke an immune response and that antibodies block the said hormone /growth factor, avoiding their interaction with its receptor with a consequent impact in malignant cell proliferation.

From our review on current approaches, there are several common observations pointing in that direction:

- Vaccination with self hormones / growth factors provokes an immune response, with specific antibodies against these targeted molecules.

- In the different antigenic systems, such antibodies provoke a deprivation of the targeted antigen, and an inhibition of the hormone or growth factor – receptor binding.
- After vaccination, there exists a significant inverse correlation between antibody titers and circulating hormone / growth factor levels.
- There is a significant correlation, in several diverse vaccines and diverse malignancies, between the antibody levels and survival of vaccinated patients.
- There is a significant inverse correlation between the hormone or growth factor concentration (decreased levels reached after vaccination) and patient survival.
- No severe toxicity associated with vaccinations has been observed.

In currently used endocrine anti-cancer therapies, the hormone levels are subrogated markers of treatment effectiveness. Similarly, hormone or growth factor deprivation provoked by vaccination could be considered as a subrogated marker of vaccine's anti-tumoral effect, but this asseveration should be consolidated in further clinical experiences.

Despite the suggestive value of these correlations, the final proof of the therapeutical concept must be obtained in randomized trials showing better survival for all vaccinated patients as compared with controls.

Up to date, such evidence has only been obtained with two of the vaccines and in two specific therapeutic niches:

1. Insegia^{TM} in advanced pancreatic cancer patients who are unable to tolerate or unwilling to take chemotherapy.
2. The EGF Vaccine in stages IIIb and IV NSCLC patients with ages below 60 years.

This is not a singularity from these vaccines: specific effects in some patient's niches are becoming a general trend for novel registered products, specially targeted anticancer therapies, for review see [63].

FUTURE TRENDS

Evidences of the therapeutic effect of immune deprivation of hormones and growth factors are starting to appear. However, as compared with conventional hormone therapy, the critical issues is how deep is the hormone deprivation achieved, and how long it can be maintained.

Profound and long-lasting hormone/growth factor deprivations should be achievable through a smart optimization of vaccine preparations and vaccination schedules.

Some of the variables that should be explored are: doses, treatment timing, vaccine and antibody combinations, and vaccine-chemotherapy (or immune-suppression) combinations (for review see [64]).

At our own experience with the EGF Vaccine, more than complete and partial remissions, what is often observed is long-term disease stabilization, which translates into survival advantage with good quality of life for vaccinated patients.

If these vaccine effects could be optimized , then we could conceive a different way of thinking leading to the management of advanced cancer as any other chronic non communicable disease which, although not-curable, can be controlled for as long as possible with good quality of life.

The main challenges to overcome, when thinking in prolonged vaccination treatments, are the risks of clonal exhaustion in aged patients with a senescent immune system, and un-controlled autoimmunity [64]. Currently ongoing and future clinical trials will insight on these issues.

CONCLUSION

The concept of deprivation of hormones and growth factor through therapeutic vaccination has currently stronger theoretical grounds and emerging clinical evidences. The shift from this scientific evidence grounds to treatments with significant impact in the clinical practice will be dependent upon new research looking for optimization of vaccine preparations and vaccination schedules. If this is achieved, then a fruitful merge between cancer hormone-therapy and cancer immunotherapy will consolidate.

REFERENCES

[1]   Burnet, FM. The concept of immunological surveillance. *Prog.Exp.Tumor Res. 1970, 13, 1-27.*
[2]   Thomas, L. On immunosurveillance in human cancer. *Yale J. Biol. Med. 1982, 55, 329-333.*
[3]   Dunn, GP; Old, LJ.; Schreiber, RD. The three Es of cancer immunoediting. *Ann Rev. Immunol. 2004, 22, 329-360.*
[4]   Zhang, L; Conejo-García, JR; Katsaros, D; Gimotty, PA; Massobrio, M; Regnani, G; Makrigiannakis, A; Gray, H; Schienger, K; Liebam, MN; Rubin, SC; Coukos, G. Intratumoral T cells, recurrence, and survival in ephitelial ovarian cancer. *N. Engl. J. Med. 2003, 204, 203-213.*
[5]   Nakano, O; Sato, M; Naito, Y; Suzuki, K; Orikasa, S; Aizawa, M; Suzuki, Y; Shintaku, I; Nagura, H; Ohtani, H. Proliferative activity of intratumoral CD8+ T-lymphocutes as a prognostic factor in human renal carcinoma: clinicopathologic demonstration of antitumor immunity. *Cancer Res. 2001, 61, 5132-5136*
[6]   Naito, Y; Saito, K; Shiiba, K; Ohuchi, A: Saigenji, K; Nagura, H; Ohtani, H. CD8+ T cells infiltrated within cancer cells nests as a prognostic factor in human colorectal cancer. *Cancer Res, 1998, 58, 3491-3494*
[7]   Marrogi, AJ; Munshi, A; Merogi, AJ; Ohadike, Y; El-Habashi; A; marrogi, OL; Freeman, SM. Study of tumor infiltrating lymphocytes and transforming growth factor-beta as prognostic factors in breast carcinoma. *Int. J. cancer, 1997, 74, 492-501.*
[8]   Schumacher, K; Haensch, W; Roefzaad, C; Schlag, PM. Prognostic significance of activated CD8+ T cell infiltrations within oesophageal carcinomas. *Cancer Res 2001, 61, 3932-3936.*

[9]   Sanchez, EQ; Marubashi, S; Jung, G; Levy, MF; Goldstein, RM; Molmenti, EP; Fasola, CG; Gonwa, TA; Jennings, LW; Brooks, BK; Klintmalm, GB. De novo tumors after liver transplantation: A single institution experience. *Liver Transpl*, 2002, 8, 285-291.

[10] Tenderich, G; Deyerling, W; Schulz, U; Heller, R; Hornik, L; Schulze, B; Jahanyar, J; Koerfer, R. Malignant neoplastic disorders following long-term immunosuppression after orthotopic heart transplantation. *Transplant Proc*. 2001, 33, 3653-3655.

[11] Dunn, GP; Bruce, AT; Ikeda, H; Old, LJ; Schreiber, RD. Cancer immunoediting: from immuosurveillance to tumor escape. *Nat Immunol* 2002, 3, 991-998.

[12] Pardoll, D. Does the immune system see tumors as foreign or self? *Ann Rev Immunol*. 2003, 21, 807-839.

[13] Yu, Z; Restifo, NP. Cancer vaccines: progress reveals new complexities. *J. Clin. Invest*. 2002, 110, 289-294.

[14] Mocellin, S; Mandruzano, S; Bronte, V; Lise, M; Nitti, D. Part I: Vaccines for solid tumors. *Lancet Oncol*. 2004, 5, 681-689.

[15] Berzofsky, JA; Terabe, M; Oh, S; Belyakov, IM; Ahlers, JD; Janik, JE; Morris, JC. Progress on new cancer vaccines strategies for the immunotherapy and prevention of cancer. *J. Clin. Invest*. 2004, 113, 1515-1525.

[16] Cavalli, F; Hansen, HH; Kaye, SB: *Textbook in Medical Oncology. Third edition. Taylor & Francis, London and New York, 2004*.

[17] Rodríguez, RP and Lage, A: Los factores de Crecimiento y sus relaciones con la transformación maligna. *Interferón y Biotecnología, 1986, 3, 179-209*.

[18] Lage, A; Crombet,T; González, G. Targeting epidermal growth factor receptor signalling: early results and future trends in oncology. *Ann Med* 2003, 35, 327-336.

[19] Disis, ML; Gralow, JR; Bernhard, H; Hand, SL; Rubin, WD; Cheever, MA. Peptide-based, but not whole protein, vaccines elicit immunity to HER-2/neu, an oncogenic self protein. *J. Immunol*, 1996, 156, 3151-3158.

[20] Disis, ML; Gooley, TA ; Rinn, K ; Davis, D ; Piepkorn, M ; Cheever, MA ; Knutson, KL; Schiffman, K. Generation of T-cell immunity to the Her-2/neu protein after active immunization with Her-2/neu peptide-based vaccines. *J. Clin. Oncol*. 2002, 20, 2642-2632.

[21] González, G; Sánchez, B; Suarez, E; Beausoleil, I; Perez, O; Lastre, M; Lage, A. Induction of Immune Recognition of Self Epidermal Growth Factor (EGF): Effect on EGF Biodistribution and Tumor Growth. *Vaccine Res*. 1996, 5, 233-244.

[22] González, G; Pardo, OL; Sánchez, B; García, JL; Beausoleil, I; Marinello, P; González, Y; Domarco, A; Guillén, G; Perez, R; Lage, A. Induction of Immune Recognition of Self Epidermal Growth Factor II: Characterization of the Antibody Response and the Use of a Fusion protein. *Vaccine Res*. 1997, 6, 91-100.

[23] González, G; Crombet, T; Catalá, M; Mirabal, V; Hernandez, JC; González; Y; Marinello, P; Guillén, G; Lage, A. A novel cancer vaccine composed of human-recombinant epidermal growth factor linked to a carrier protein: report of a pilot clinical trial. *Ann Onc*, 1998, 9, 431-435.

[24] González, G; Crombet, T; Torres, F; Catalá, M; Alfonso, L; Neninger, E; García, B; Mulet, A; Perez, R; Lage, A. Epidermal growth factor-based cancer vaccine for non-small cell lung cancer therapy. *Ann Onc*. 2003, 14, 461-466.

[25] Crombet, T; Neninger, E; Catala, M; García, B; Leonard,I; Martínez, L; González, G; Pérez, R; Lage, A. Treatment of NSCLC Patients with an EGF- Based cancer Vaccine. *Cancer Biol Ther 2006, 5, 145-149.*

[26] Mulet, A; Garrido, G; Alvarez, A; Menéndez, T; Bohmer, FD; Pérez, R; Fernández, LE. The enlargement of the hormone deprivation concept to the blocking of TGFα-autocrine loop: EGFR signalling inhibition. *Cancer Immunol Immunother. 2006, 55, 628-638.*

[27] Avrameas, S; Guilbert, B; Dighiero, G. Natural antibodies against tubulin, actin, myoglobin, thyroglobulin, fetuin, albumin and transferrin are present in normal human sera, and monoclonal immunoglobulins from multiple myeloma and Waldenstrom´s macroglobulinemia may express similar antibody specificities. *Ann Immunol. 1981, 132C, 231-236*

[28] Cohen, IR. Regulation of autoimmune disease: physiological and therapeutic. *Immunol Rev. 1986, 94, 5-21.*

[29] Nikolic-Zugic, J; Bevan, MJ. Role of self-peptides in positively selecting the T cell repertoire. *Nature 1990, 344, 65-67*

[30] Pereira, P; Forni, L; Larsson, EL; Cooper, M; Heuser, C; Coutinho, A; Autonomous activation of B and T cells in antigen-free mice. *Eur. J. Immunol. 1986, 16, 685-688*

[31] Cohen, IR and Toung, DB. Autoimmunity, microbial immunity and the immunological homunculus. *Immunol Today. 1991, 12, 105-110*

[32] Cohen, IR. The cognitive paradigm and the immunological homunculus. *Immunol Today 1992, 13, 490-494.*

[33] Yehuda Shoenfeld. *The Decade of Autoimmunity, First edition. Elsevier Sciences & Technology Books, 1999.*

[34] González, G; Montero, E; Leon, K; Cohen, LR; Lage. A. Autoimmunization to Epidermal Growth Factor, a component of the immunological homunculus. *Autoimmun Rev 2002, 1, 89-95.*

[35] Watson, SA; Michaeli, D; Grimes, S; Morris, TM; Robinson, G; Varro, A; Justin, TA; Hardcastle, JD. Gastrimune raises antibodies that neutralize amidated and glycine-extended gastrin-17 and inhibit the tumor growth of colon cancer. *Cancer Res. 1996, 15, 880-885.*

[36] Smith, AM; Justin, T; Michaeli, D; Watson, A. Phase I/II study of G17-DT, an anti-gastrin immunogen, in advanced colorectal cancer. *Clin Cancer Res. 2000, 6, 4719-4724.*

[37] Bret, BT; Smith, SC; Bouvier, CV; Michaeli, D; Hochhauserm, D; Davidson, BR; Kurnawinski, TR; Watkinson, AF; Van Someren, N; Pounder, RE; Caplin, ME. Phase II study of anti-gastrin-17 antibodies, raised to G17DT, in advanced pancreatic cancer. *J. Clin. Oncol. 2002, 20, 4225-4231.*

[38] Gillian, AD; Watson, SA; Henwood, M; McKenzie, AJ; Humphreys, JE; Elder, J; Iftikhar, SY; Welch, N; Fielding, J; Broome, P; Michaeli, D. A phase II study of G17DT in gastric carcinoma. *Eur. J. Surg. Oncol. 2004, 30, 536-543.*

[39] Gillian, AD. Randomized, double blind, placebo-controlled, multicenter, group-sequential trial of G17DT in patients with advanced pancreatic cancer. *ASCO meeting, 2004.*

[40] Broome, P; Bruck R, Michaeli D. Immune response to Gastrin-17 as an independent covariate for survival in colorectal, gastric and pancreatic cancers. *ASCO meeting, 2004.*

[41] Shapiro, J; Marshall, H; Karasek, P; Figer, A; Oettle, H; Couture, G; Jeziorski, K; Broome, P; Hawskins R. G17DT + gemcitabine [Gem] versus placebo + Gem in untreated subjects with locally advanced, recurrent or metastatic adenocarcinoma of the pancreas: Results of a rendomized, double-blind, multinational, multicenter study. *J Clin Oncol, Supplement 2005, 23, 1098.*

[42] Huggins,C and Hodges, CV. Studies in prostatic cancer II: The effect of castration on advanced cancer of the prostate gland. *Arch Surg 1941, 43, 209-223.*

[43] Emons, G; Ortmann, O; Schulz, KD; Schally, AV. Growth inhibitory actions of analogues of luteinizing hormone releasing hormone on tumor cells. *Trends Endocrinol. Metab. 1997, 8, 355-361.*

[44] Jungwirth, A; Schally, AV; Pinski, J; Halmos, G; Groot, K; Armantis, P; Vadillo-Buenfil, M. Inhibition of in vivo proliferation of androgen-independent prostate cancers by antagonist of growth hormone-releasing hormone. *J Cancer, 1997, 75, 1585-1592.*

[45] Sakalovic, G; Bokser, L; Radulovic, S; Korkut, E; Schally, AV. Receptors for luteinizing hormone releasing hormone (LHRH) in Dunning R3327 prostate cancers and rat anterior pituitaries after treatment with a sustained delivery system of LHRH antagonist SB-75. *Endocrinology 1990, 127, 3052-2060.*

[46] Halmos, G; Arencibia, JM; Schally, AV; Davis, R; Brostwick, DG. High incidence of receptors for luteinizing hormone releasing hormone (LHRH) and LHRH receptor gene expression in human prostate cancers. *J. Urol. 2000, 163, 623-629.*

[47] Talwar, GP. Vaccine for control of fertility and hormone-dependent cancers. *Immunol Cell Biol. 1997, 75, 184-189*

[48] Simms, MS; Scholfield, DP; Jacobs, E; Michaeli, D; Broome, P; Humphreys, JE; Bishop MC. Anti-GnRH antibodies can induce castrate levels of testosterone in patients with advanced prostate cancer. *Br J Cancer 2000, 83, 443-446.*

[49] Talwar, GP; Singh, O; Pal, R; Chattergie, N. Vaccine for control fertility and hormone dependent cancers. *Int J. Immunopharmacol. 1992, 14, 511-514.*

[50] Talwar, GP; Raina, K; Grupta, JC; Ray, R; Wadhwa, S; Ali, MM. A recombinant luteinizing-hormone-releasing-hormone immunogen bio effective in causing prostatic atrophy. *Vaccine, 2004, 22, 3713-3721.*

[51] Parkinson, RJ; Simms, M; Broome, P; Humphreys, JE; Bishop, MC. A vaccination strategy for a long term suppression of androgens in advanced prostate cancer. *Eur Urol 2004, 45, 171-174.*

[52] Triozzi, PL; Bolger, GB; Neidhart, J; Rinchart, JJ; Saleh, M; Allen, KO; Sellers, S; Waddel, MJ. Effect of doxetacel chemotherapy on the activity of a gonadotropin releasing hormone vaccine in patients with advanced prostate cancer. *Prostate 2005, 65, 316-321.*

[53] www.ymbiosciences.com.

[54] Talwar, GP; Sharma, NC; Dubey, SK; Salahuddin, M; Das, C; Ramakrishnan, S; Kumar, S. Isoimmunization against human chorionic gonadotropin with conjugates of processed β-subunit of the hormone and tetanus toxoid. *Proc Nat Acad Sci USA 1976, 73, 218-222.*

[55] Talwar, GP; Singh, O; Pal, R; Chatterjee, N; Suri, AK; Shaha, C. Vaccines for control fertility. *Indian J Exp Biol. 1992, 30, 947-950.*

[56] Talwar, GP. Vaccines for control fertility and hormone-dependent cancers. *Immunol Cell Biol. 1997, 75, 184-189*

[57] Triozzi, PL and Stevens, VC. Human chorionic gonadotropin as a target for cancer vaccines. *Oncol Rep. 1999, 6, 7-17.*

[58] Moulton, HM; Yoshihara, PH; Mason, DH; Iversen, PL; Triozzi, PL. Active specific immunotherapy with a beta-human chorionic gonadotropin peptide vaccine in patients with metastatic colorectal cancer: antibody response is associated with improved survival. *Clin Cancer Res. 2002, 8, 2044-2051.*

[59] Iversen, PL. Active Beta-hCG-Specific Immunotherapy in Patients with Pancreatic Cancer. *ASCO meeting, 2002.*

[60] He, LZ; Ramakrishna, V; Connolly, JE; Wang, XT; Smith, PA; Jones, CL; Valkova-Valchanova, M; Arunakumari, A; Tremi, JF; Goldstein, J; Wallace, PK; Keler, T; Endres, MJ. A novel human cancer vaccine elicits cellular responses to the tumor-associated antigen, human chorionic gonadotropin beta. *Clin Cancer Res. 2004, 10, 1920-1927*

[61] Neninger, E; Crombet, T; Osorio, M; Catalá, M; Torre, A; Leonard, I; García, B; Marinello, P; González, G; Lage, A. Vaccination with Epidermal Growth Factor specific active immunotherapy improves survival in advanced non small cell lung cancer (NSCLC) patients: interim analysis of a randomized Phase II trial. *ASCO, 2005, Abs N7210.*

[62] Neninger, E; González, G; Crombet, T; Fleites, G; Leonard, I; González, M; badía, T; lage, A. Optimizad phase I-II trial design for vacination with epidermal growth factor (EGF): Effect on immunogenicity and safety. *Proc Am Soc Clin Oncol 2004. 23, Abs 2610.*

[63] Metro, G; Finocchiaro, G; Cappuzo, F. Anti-cancer therapy with EGFR inhibitors; factors of prognostic and predictive significance. *Ann Oncol. 2006, 17 (supplement 2, ii42-ii45*

[64] Lage, A; Pérez, R; Férnandez ; LE. Therapeutic Cancer Vaccines: At Midway between Immunology and Pharmacology. *Current Cancer Drugs Targets, 2005, 5, 611-627.*

INDEX

B

E

F

J

K

L

M

O

P

S

T

W

Y

Z